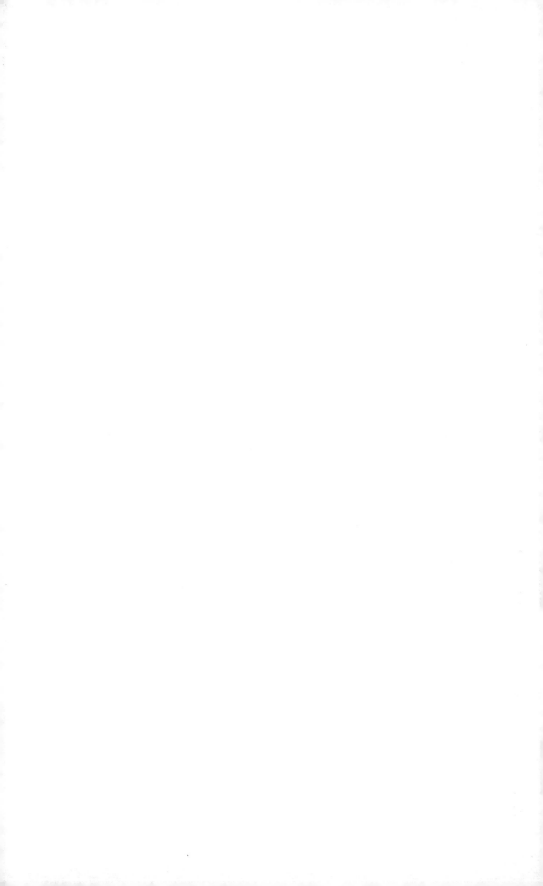

CHAIN DRUG STORES ARE DANGEROUS

How Their Reckless Obsession With the Bottom Line Places You At Risk for Serious Harm or Death

DENNIS MILLER, R.PH.

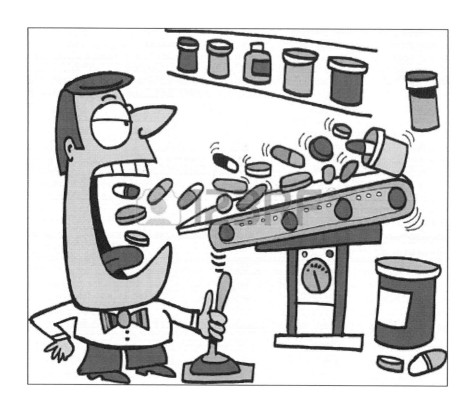

Chain Drug Stores Are Dangerous: How Their
Reckless Obsession With the Bottom Line Places
You At Risk for Serious Harm or Death.
Copyright © 2013 by Dennis B. Miller. All rights reserved.

- The first-ever exposé of pharmacy written by a pharmacist
- This is the book that will change the way America views pharmacy and chain drugstores
- This is the book that the big drugstore chains do not want you to read
- The unreported epidemic of pharmacy mistakes
- Dozens of deaths from pharmacy mistakes and multi-million dollar jury awards
- The disastrous consequences of applying the McDonald's fast food model to pharmacy
- How doctors' illegible handwriting is no laughing matter
- Does your doctor's receptionist have enough knowledge of drug names to phone prescriptions to your drugstore?
- Why electronic prescriptions from doctors are not the panacea they're advertised to be
- How chain drugstores' obsession with speed increases the occurrence of pharmacy mistakes
- How to avoid becoming the victim of a serious pharmacy error
- How poorly trained pharmacy technicians can be a threat to the public safety
- How understaffing increases pharmacy profitability but places the public at risk
- How pharmacists are under tremendous pressure to fill prescriptions at unsafe speeds
- Why it may be safer to have your prescriptions filled at an independent pharmacy rather than at one of the huge drugstore chains
- Why are high school students with after-school jobs routinely allowed to help fill prescriptions in pharmacies across America?
- Why are so many pharmacists not recommending pharmacy as a career for their children?
- What criteria should you look for in deciding whether your pharmacy is thorough in addressing critical details such as potential drug interactions, accurate dosages, drug allergies, proper directions, and therapy duplication?

- How can you determine whether the pills in your bottle are exactly what your doctor prescribed?
- Understaffing sometimes forces pharmacists to take educated guesses when faced with illegible prescriptions or to override potentially significant drug interactions rather than call your doctor
- Due to competitive pressures in the marketplace, pharmacy has been transformed into a high-speed, high-stress, high-stakes enterprise in which powerful prescription drugs are just a blur on a hamburger assembly line
- Drive-thru windows increase mistakes by creating the expectation among customers that prescription drugs should be filled as quickly as McDonald's fills burger orders
- The big drugstore chains run their operations as if pharmacists were dispensing nothing more hazardous than a Big Mac
- Powerful prescription drugs are dispensed across America in a system that is guaranteed to produce errors
- And much, much more
- This book can save your life!

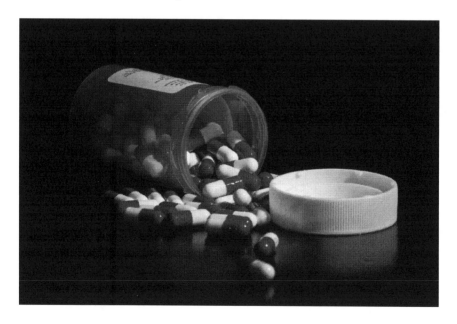

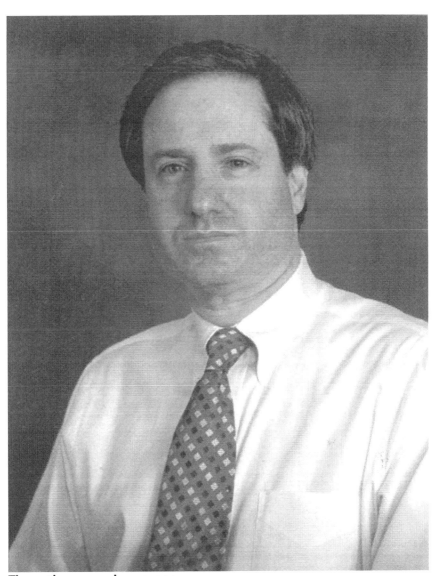

The author several years ago

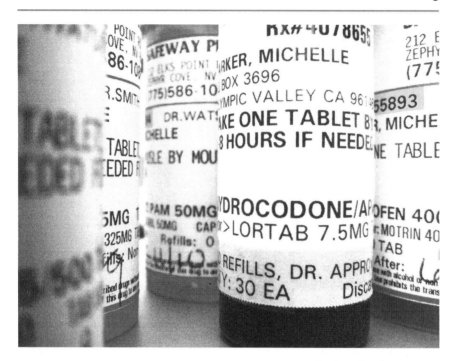

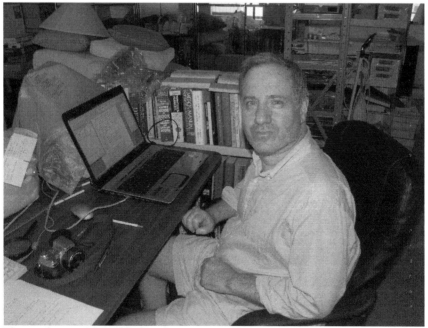

The author writing this book

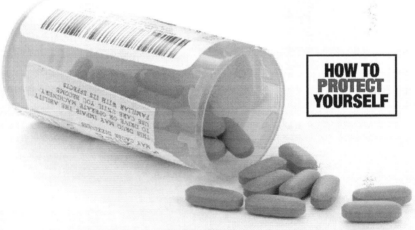

FOREWORD BY JOE GRAEDON
BESTSELLING AUTHOR OF *THE PEOPLE'S PHARMACY*

PHARMACY EXPOSED

DENNIS MILLER, R.PH.

HOW TO PROTECT YOURSELF

1,000 Things That Can Go Deadly Wrong At the Drugstore

The author's first book, a massive 753 pages

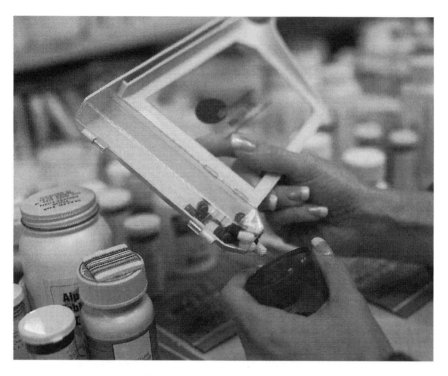

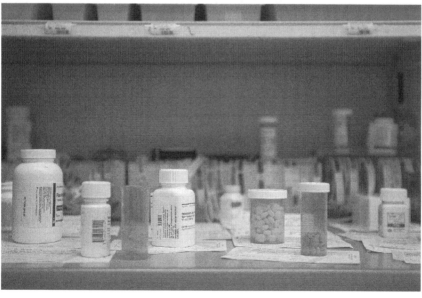

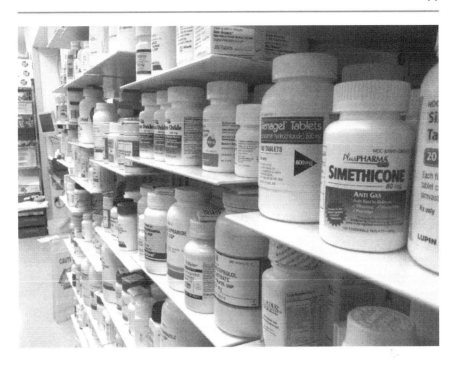

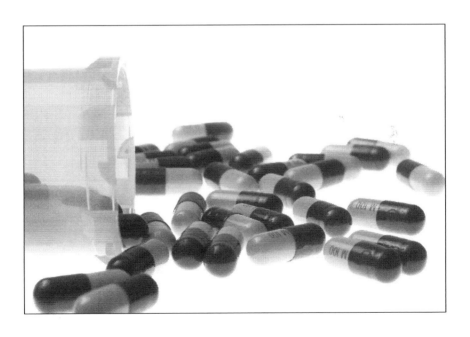

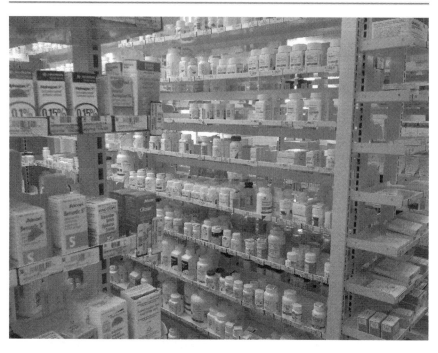

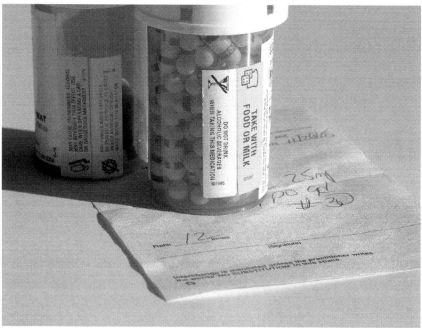

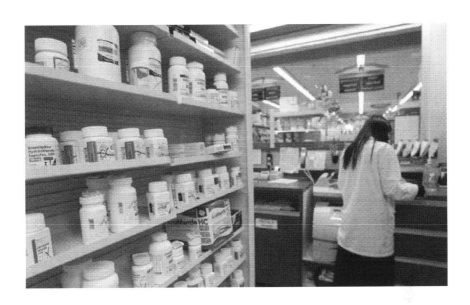

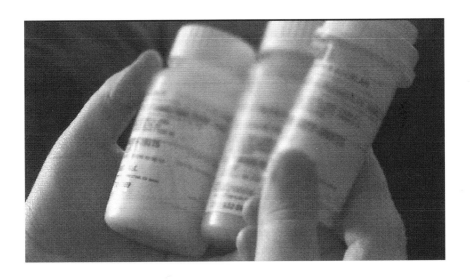

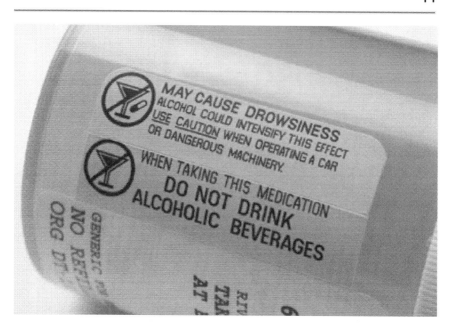

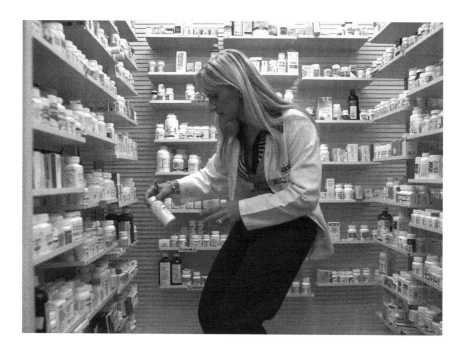

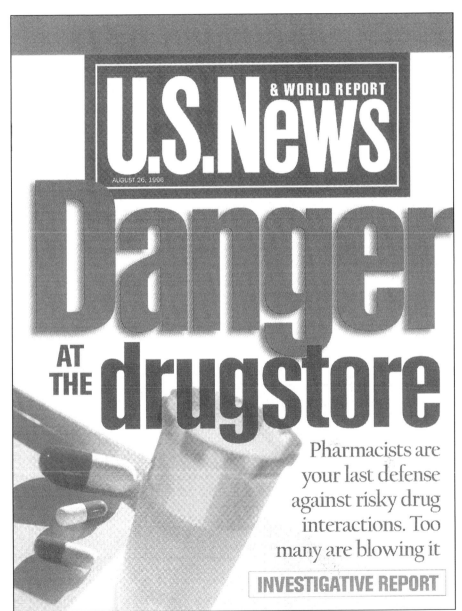

U.S. News & World Report cover story, August 26, 1996

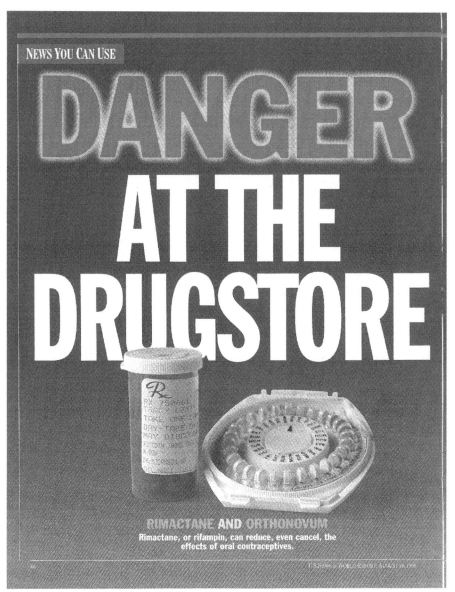

NEWS YOU CAN USE

DANGER

AT THE

DRUGSTORE

RIMACTANE AND ORTHONOVUM

Rimactane, or rifampin, can reduce, even cancel, the effects of oral contraceptives.

U.S. News & World Report, August 26, 1996, page 46

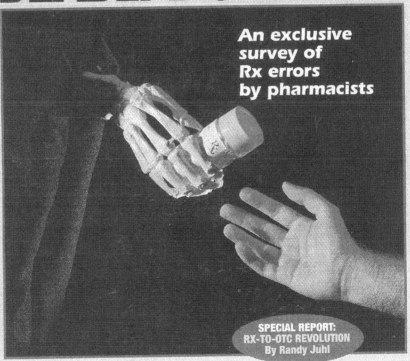

MARCH 3, 1997

DRUG TOPICS®

THE NEWSMAGAZINE FOR PHARMACISTS

Meet the new wave of combo vaccines

What are they: Drugs or cosmetics?

Cognitive pay getting the cold shoulder

R.Ph.s' emerging role in subacute care

FDA launching new cigarette crackdown

New acne Rx drug for women

PLUS For 3 CE credits

NEW DRUG APPROVALS OF 1996–PART 2

DEADLY DISPENSING

An exclusive survey of Rx errors by pharmacists

SPECIAL REPORT: RX-TO-OTC REVOLUTION By Randy Juhl

Drug Topics cover story March 3, 1997 on pharmacy mistakes

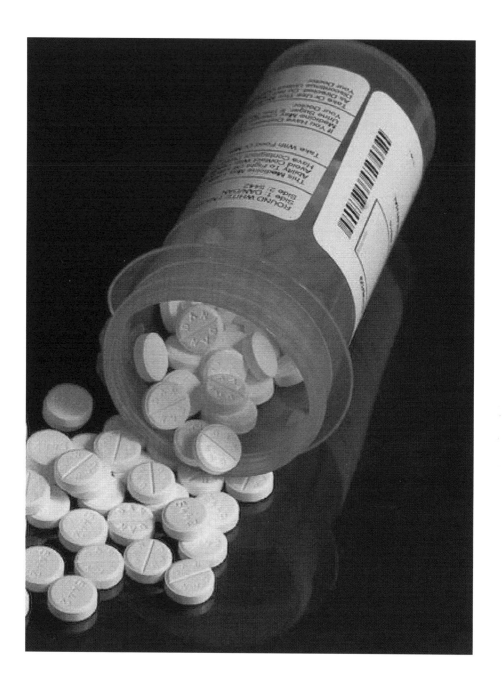

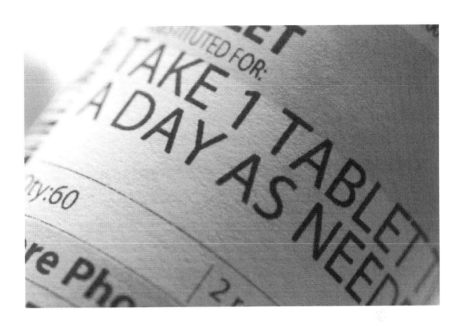

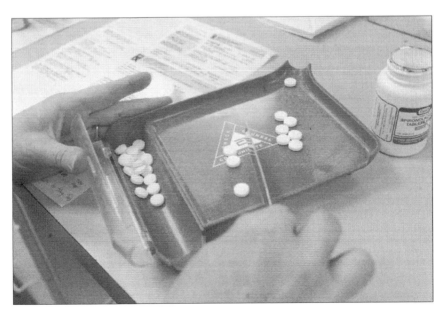

CONTENTS

Contents

PART IX: CHAIN DRUGSTORES

PART X: STATE BOARDS OF PHARMACY

Contents

ACKNOWLEDGEMENTS

For several years, I lived in Oxford, North Carolina which is about thirty miles from Joe Graedon's home in Durham. We used to get together every few months and argue whose perspective on Pharma and modern medicine was more accurate. Occasionally we would meet for lunch at one of the restaurants in Durham. During one phone conversation in which we were discussing where to meet, Joe suggested a particular restaurant and I said, "I'd rather meet at your home so that I can yell at you." He laughed because he knew exactly what I was saying. Our get-togethers usually involved both of us forcefully arguing that our perspective was correct. I want to thank Joe for giving me constant encouragement, criticism, and suggestions as I sought his advice on this book. I first met Joe sometime around 1980. We seldom went more than a few months without speaking on the phone, exchanging e-mails, and yelling at each other.

I would like to thank my brother Jeff for patiently reading most of the chapters in this book and providing criticism. My first drafts of this book way back in the early 1980s were so horrible that Jeff told me he would be embarrassed to let anyone see it. Jeff loves grammar and punctuation and spelling. (He's a math teacher and amateur linguist who maintains several websites, including one titled "Word Oddities and Trivia.") His grammatical suggestions have been invaluable and I am very grateful for his criticisms of the manuscript. All remaining grammar, punctuation, and spelling errors are my fault, not his. I always told Jeff I wanted his "brutally honest" assessment as I e-mailed him each successive chapter. His comments ranged from "terrible," to "not interesting," to "okay" to "very good." Sometimes he said I was including too much detail for a book aimed at a general audience, but I often protested that the pharmacists who read this book may be interested in more detail. So I have included some material that my brother suggested I omit, because I'm hoping it will be of interest to pharmacists.

I want to thank Janice Zoeller who was then editor-in-chief at *American Druggist*. Many years ago, I sent her some of my typewritten pages on the origins of drug brand names and asked whether she was interested in publishing it. When I followed up with a phone call, she said she liked the material and was willing to publish it with a few changes. I was so shocked that I asked her, "Are you serious?" She could plainly see that I was a rookie as a writer. That was back in early 1999 and it became the first article I ever had published. Since she received a lot of favorable mail from pharmacists, she published a second article nearly a year later on an entirely different collection of drug brand names. I was looking forward to writing more articles for *American Druggist* because Janice seemed to be the kind of editor who liked edgy articles written by pharmacists, i.e., just the kind of thing I was interested in. But, unfortunately, *American Druggist* ceased publication shortly after my second article was published in that magazine. I believe I was not to blame.

I looked for another pharmacy magazine that might be willing to publish articles written by a pharmacist with an "attitude." I want to thank Harold Cohen, R.Ph., who was then the editor-in-chief at *Drug Topics*. He subsequently approved several of my "Viewpoint" editorials. When Harold became the editor-in-chief at *U.S. Pharmacist,* Judy Chi moved up to the position of editor-in-chief at *Drug Topics*. I want to thank Judy for continuing to publish more of my Viewpoints over the years. (Judy's mantra: "condense, condense, condense.") When *Drug Topics* moved from New Jersey to Ohio a few years ago, a new editorial staff took over the magazine. I want to thank Julia Talsma (editor-in-chief) and Julianne Stein (managing editor) for publishing two of my Viewpoints from the current editorial offices in Ohio. I have now had a total of eighteen "Viewpoints" published in *Drug Topics*.

I want to thank Carol Ukens who was a senior editor at *Drug Topics* before retiring a few years ago. Carol is an extremely intelligent person who was one of the most perceptive pharmacy writers for many years. I used to call her every few months to run ideas past her. She was always extremely friendly, helpful, and professional. It was rare that there was a pharmacy subject about which she was uninformed. Pharmacy journalism is not the same today without her wisdom and insight.

Each time an article is published, it gives an aspiring author a little more confidence and a little more courage. I gained a little confidence when *Good Housekeeping* magazine used me as a major source for an article on pharmacy mistakes (June 2005). And I gained a little more confidence when James O'Donnell asked me to write a chapter on pharmacy mistakes for the second edition (2005) of his book *Drug Injury: Liability, Analysis, and Prevention.*

I would not have had the courage to continue with this book without the encouragement and criticism I received from these people over the thirty years that I worked on this book. A constant (and, at times, overwhelming) worry during this period was that this book would never see the light of day.

For those pharmacists who feel strongly about pharmacy issues and are yearning to see their words in print, my advice is to keep at it, be persistent, keep improving your writing, and don't be completely discouraged by rejection. I've certainly had my fair share of rejections and discouragements over the last thirty years.

Dennis Miller

INTRODUCTION

It is my hope that *Chain Drug Stores Are Dangerous* becomes a paradigm shifting book. This very controversial book will upset a lot of people in positions of power in the world of pharmacy, particularly those at the highest levels of the big chain drugstores, but also those at the state boards of pharmacy and at this nation's many schools of pharmacy. While readers of this book will not agree with everything I say, I hope to make a very compelling case that the status quo in pharmacy today is completely unacceptable and is, in fact, a prescription for disaster.

I advocate a major overhaul in pharmacy toward one that serves patients' needs rather than corporate interests, and toward one that places the health and well-being of pharmacy customers ahead of corporate profits. I have attempted to say what many pharmacists passionately believe but are afraid to verbalize out of fear of jeopardizing their employment. Too many pharmacists today feel that the chain drugstore model has been disastrous for the public safety and for the profession of pharmacy. So it is not surprising that many pharmacists are not recommending pharmacy as a career for their children.

The pharmacy of today that I describe is one controlled by the bottom line, in which cost-cutting is the core guiding principle. This singular obsession with profits causes the big chains to cut pharmacy staffing to levels that are a threat to the public safety. The chains have embraced the fast food model with disastrous consequences in a system that rewards quantity over quality. This is a system where pharmacists are forced to fill prescriptions as if they were working at McDonald's, Burger King, or Wendy's. It is a system where pharmacists too often don't have enough staffing to adequately answer questions from customers. It is a system that cuts costs by hiring more technicians to do tasks formerly done by pharmacists. It is a system in which insurance companies erect an ever-increasing number of obstacles to dampen utilization while at the same time making policyholders' and pharmacists' lives more complicated. It is a system in which pharmacy mistakes are a horrific yet predictable and inevitable consequence of the chains' obsession with the bottom line.

The pharmacist's daily reality too often consists of arrogant doctors with some or all of the following traits: 1) notoriously illegible handwriting, 2) inadequate knowledge of drug interactions and a rude or dismissive attitude toward pharmacists who call about those potential drugs interactions or questionable doses, and 3) receptionists who too often have a very poor understanding of drug names yet routinely phone prescription orders to the pharmacy. The pharmacist's daily reality also consists of corporate bean counters who only care about numbers, and about how fast pharmacists can fill prescriptions. Pharmacists feel that their speed in filling prescriptions is much more highly valued by the chains than the pharmacist's knowledge of drugs. The pharmacist's daily reality consists of impatient customers who only care about how long they will have to wait for their prescriptions to be filled, and who seem to have no understanding of the potential hazards in the pharmacy and how common pharmacy mistakes are.

A huge number of pharmacists are deeply disgusted with state boards of pharmacy for being too intimidated by the legal and political clout of the chains, and for being too timid to at least try to pass regulations that address the understaffing that is endemic to chain pharmacies. Pharmacists feel that understaffing is at the heart of the epidemic of pharmacy mistakes in America. Pharmacists believe that state boards of pharmacy are doing a breathtakingly poor job in protecting the public safety by failing to mandate staffing levels that are adequate for the safe filling of prescriptions.

Many pharmacists feel that pharmacy schools have grossly misrepresented what conditions are like in the real world. Many pharmacists say they would like to bring a class action lawsuit against the schools of pharmacy for promoting a sugar-coated view of pharmacy, and for promoting a professional model for which the big chains have complete and utter disdain. Pharmacy schools promote a model of the pharmacist as drug expert, but the big chains want nothing to do with that model. The big chains expect pharmacists to fill an ever-increasing number of prescriptions with the same or even decreasing levels of staffing. The big chains seem to have a huge preference for fast pharmacists over knowledgeable or helpful pharmacists.

Ours is a nakedly profit-driven health care system in a culture that demands a quick-fix pill for every ill. It is a culture that prefers pills instead of prevention. It is a culture in which the public has been well-conditioned by pharma advertising to salivate for the latest wonder drug. It is a culture of fast food in which pharmacy drive-thru windows are a threat to the public safety by creating an expectation for service that is as speedy as McDonald's.

It is my hope that *Chain Drug Stores Are Dangerous* serves as an urgently-needed antidote to this madness, showing readers how they can protect themselves and avoid becoming a casualty of a system that is in crisis.

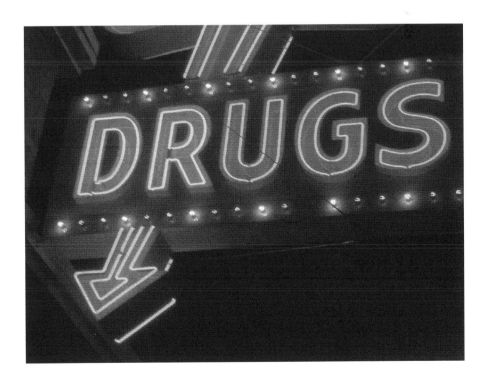

Please note: As is customary, brand name drugs are capitalized and generic names are in lower case.

All pictures are for illustration purposes only—to demonstrate some of the issues discussed in this book. The author is not suggesting or implying in any way that any of the people shown in these pictures do anything less than exemplary work.

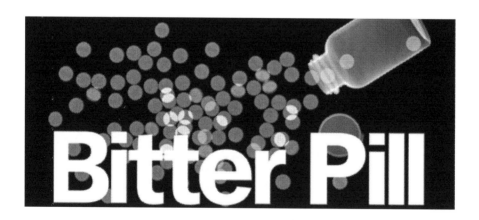

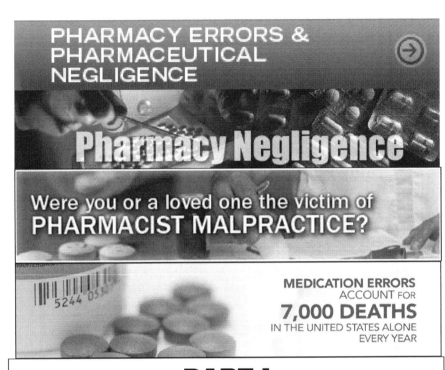

PHARMACY ERRORS &
PHARMACEUTICAL
NEGLIGENCE

Pharmacy Negligence

Were you or a loved one the victim of
PHARMACIST MALPRACTICE?

5244 05

MEDICATION ERRORS
ACCOUNT FOR
7,000 DEATHS
IN THE UNITED STATES ALONE
EVERY YEAR

PART I

DANGER AT THE DRUGSTORE

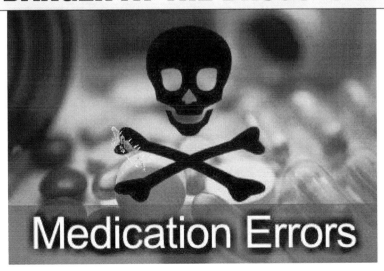

Medication Errors

<table>
<tr><td align="center">**1**</td></tr>
</table>

Memorable misfills during my career in chain drugstores

Every pharmacist has his own horror stories that are seared into his brain. Here are some that stand out in my mind from twenty-five years as a pharmacist.

1. A pharmacist, upon discovering his own error, closed the store and rushed to the customer's house to retrieve the wrong medication.

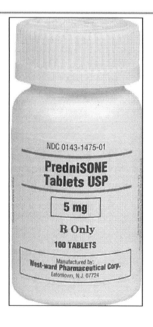 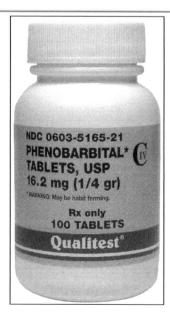

In North Carolina, the state in which I worked for most of my career, it has been the law that a drugstore cannot be open without a pharmacist on duty unless the pharmacy is barricaded in such a way that there is no access by the public. This is to prevent unauthorized persons from having access to the drugs in the pharmacy.

A pharmacist told me the following anecdote. He discovered one day that he mistakenly dispensed prednisone to someone instead of phenobarbital. It's easy to see how this can happen. Both of these are small white tablets. Prednisone is a powerful drug similar to cortisone. Phenobarbital is a totally unrelated drug, usually used (years ago) to prevent seizures. Taking the prednisone instead of the phenobarbital meant this customer could have had a seizure while, for example, driving a car. The results could have been disastrous.

In horror, this pharmacist told me that he locked the doors to the entire store and went to that person's home to retrieve the incorrect pills. I don't recall this pharmacist's description of the reaction from the customer when the pharmacist arrived at that customer's home. But I assume the customer must have been at least surprised. This pharmacist is a smooth talker so I assume he made up some innocuous reason for asking for the pills back.

Let me assure you that closing the entire store (as required by law if the pharmacy cannot be barricaded) is not a minor event. Closing the doors of the store in the middle of the day is a major violation of company policy. Nevertheless, being sued by a customer is even more highly frowned upon. If our supervisors found out about this incident, they would be unhappy that this pharmacist closed the store, but they would agree that he made the right decision under the circumstances.

2. I lied to a customer about my mistake.

Here is a mistake that I made myself which I lied my way out of. In 1976, I had been out of pharmacy school for about a year. I mistakenly filled a prescription for V-Cillin-K liquid instead of Keflex liquid. These are both antibiotics that were very popular at that time under their brand names. They are usually filled generically now. At that time, they were both packaged in boxes that were nearly identical: a white box with some green trim. The prescription was for a child.

For some reason, I happened to be looking back through the pile of prescriptions I had filled that morning and I happened to realize my error. I came upon a prescription in the pile that called for Keflex, but I realized that I had not dispensed any Keflex that morning. I remembered dispensing V-Cillin-K.

I called the child's mother and proceeded to lie to her. I made up the following story. I said that I happened to notice on the box in which the product was packaged that the date code indicated that the product was nearing its expiration. I told her that it was still good, that it was not out of date, but that I would feel more comfortable if she returned to the pharmacy so that I could give her a fresher bottle.

This was all a big lie. My error had nothing to do with expiration dates. I had simply dispensed the wrong drug.

As I had hoped, the customer was understanding and in fact seemed to appreciate my efforts to assure that her child was getting fresh medication. She seemed to be grateful and appreciative that I would go to these lengths to assure that the medication was fresh. As I said, this was all a big lie, a pretext to get her to bring the incorrect medication back. I had the correct medication ready when she returned and I think she was really proud of me for being so concerned that the medication was fresh. But it was all a big lie.

3. A pharmacist, terrified, called her husband and told him to go to a customer's house to get a prescription filled incorrectly.

A pharmacist told me this story: She had several prescriptions on the counter. One was for Mepergan Fortis, a powerful narcotic pain reliever. Another was for cephalexin 500 mg, an antibiotic. Both of these drugs are capsules that look nearly identical when viewed through the amber pill container. This pharmacist gave the customer Mepergan Fortis instead of the cephalexin. In describing this incident to me, she said that she had been interrupted by phone calls and various other distractions which resulted in her switching the medications. The customer had already left the pharmacy with the wrong medication when the pharmacist realized her mistake.

In absolute horror she called her husband who was at home. Knowing the customer's address from our computer, she told her husband to go to that person's house and retrieve the medication. She told me that she cried into the phone to her husband: "GO GET IT! GO GET IT!" Her voice broke as she relayed this story to me.

4. We'd like to ram that stopwatch up his ass!

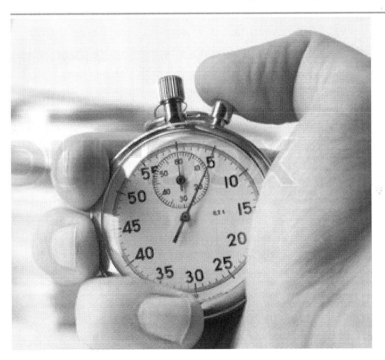

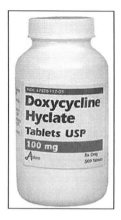 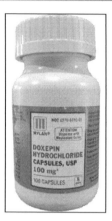

An error occurred when my partner dispensed the antibiotic doxycycline 100 mg instead of the antidepressant doxepin 100 mg. The circumstances surrounding this error are interesting. In 1993, my employer held what they called a contest to see whether pharmacists were following corporate procedures. Supervisors came around to each store with a clipboard and a list of procedures to see whether we were following guidelines. The chain said that the store with the highest score in each district would win a prize.

One of the parameters checked was the time it took the pharmacist to fill each prescription. Incredibly, each supervisor had a stopwatch. The supervisor reset the stopwatch with each prescription. When the pharmacist first touched the prescription, the supervisor started the stopwatch. When the pharmacist finally put the medication in the bag, the stopwatch was stopped. Other criteria checked were things like how many times the phone rang before the pharmacist answered, whether or not the pharmacist returned to any calls on hold every 30 seconds to tell the caller the status of his call, whether technicians wasted time chatting on the phone with friends, etc.

What happened in this case was that the pharmacist was so distressed by the experience of being timed with a stopwatch that he inadvertently dispensed the antibiotic doxycycline 100 mg instead of the antidepressant doxepin 100 mg. Let me emphasize that this so-called contest was held on actual prescriptions for actual customers in the middle of an actual business day. It was not held at some special contest site. The chain had the nerve to subject us to this stressful indignity as if it were no more disruptive of our work routine than a wart on our hand.

Enough pharmacists eventually complained so vociferously that management was forced to drop the stopwatch. But the rest of this "contest" (actually a productivity test) remained in subsequent stores that were tested. Most pharmacists say it was the most demeaning thing they've experienced since graduating from pharmacy school. I think it's an indication of the powerlessness of chain pharmacists, the wage-labor nature of our job, and the fact that pharmacy is now less a profession and more an assembly line. Like most workers in America, pharmacists today are piece-work, assembly line workers who are closely monitored.

5. My partner was sued for this error

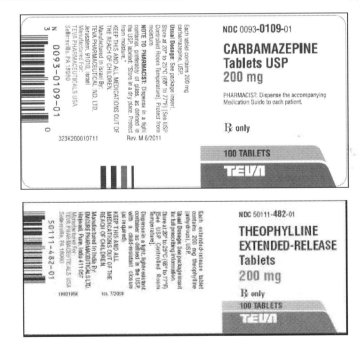

A local doctor called one day and said to me that one of his patients was in his office and "he's dying." The doctor said that we mistakenly dispensed carbamazepine 200 mg (an anti-seizure medication) instead of theophylline 200 mg (an anti-asthma medication). The doctor said that seizures were not one of the patient's medical conditions. The doctor said that the patient indeed has asthma and that it was out of control the last few days when he was taking the anti-seizure medication while expecting it to be the anti-asthma medication. Even though I don't know for sure, I suspect that the patient was sitting across the desk from the doctor and that the doctor made the call to me in the presence of the patient to emphasize to the patient that it was not the doctor's fault that the patient's asthma was out of control.

I said to the doctor, "Are you serious that the patient is dying?" The doctor's reply was that no, the patient wasn't dying, but that he was pretty damn mad for suffering with uncontrolled asthma for the last few days. The doctor, who has a reputation in town for frequently having an arrogant attitude, implied that the patient had grounds for a malpractice suit against us.

Further into the conversation (when it was clear that the patient would be okay), I asked the doctor the question that was uppermost on my mind from the beginning: "Which pharmacist's name is on the label?" The doctor was criticizing me as if I had filled the prescription and I didn't enjoy being on the receiving end of his anger if another pharmacist had filled the prescription. The law in my state requires us to put on the label at least the last name and first initial of the pharmacist who filled the prescription. The doctor read out my partner's name. I breathed a huge sigh of relief to myself. This took a little wind out of the doctor's sails, as it was apparent he was blaming the wrong person.

I called my partner at home and told him what had happened. My partner said that he didn't know whether he should call the patient and apologize because, by admitting error, the likelihood of a malpractice claim might increase. It turns out that my partner did call the patient and apologize. My partner says that the patient appreciated the apology. But it turns out that the patient sued my partner and our employer anyway. I don't know the dollar amount of the settlement given to the patient because lawsuits are not something that pharmacists like talking about. And I'm afraid that my partner would tell me, "It's none of your business."

The issue of whether pharmacists should admit an error and apologize to the customer is one of considerable controversy. In 1993, at a day-long meeting of about two dozen of the chain's pharmacists in the local district, our supervisors said that we should admit errors to customers and apologize. There was a great deal of discussion of this point. I have come to the conclusion that it was a corporate decision that the pharmacist responsible for the error should apologize to the customer.

During our lunch break that day, the half dozen pharmacists sitting around my table discussed this idea of admitting our error and apologizing to the customer. A couple of older pharmacists said they had never done it that way before and they didn't want to start now. They implied that the best way to handle errors was to try to obfuscate the whole thing either by lying or saying something to the customer like the drug is a generic equivalent or that it's the same drug from a different manufacturer. Of course, we tailor our smoke screen to the specific circumstances. If the customer is in danger, obviously we've got to take more direct action.

One of these older pharmacists said that most auto insurers recommend that policyholders not admit fault. I went home and checked my State Farm car insurance policy and, sure enough, on the back of my wallet card are these exact words: "Do not admit fault. Do not discuss the accident with anyone except State Farm or Police."

So why would my employer (one of the largest drug chains in the country) suggest that we admit fault to the customer and apologize? At our table, we concluded that the corporation was trying to protect itself by isolating us as the bad apple. In other words, we concluded that they were trying to isolate us on a limb and then, if necessary, cut off that limb. We figured that the chain would endeavor to get rid of us through various means if the case received widespread publicity in our community. As a result, most pharmacists I know are not eager to admit fault and apologize to customers.

How did this error occur?

It so happens that carbamazepine is the generic for Tegretol. In the alphabetical system that most pharmacies use to stock drugs, the generic product is stocked beside the brand name product. So, in this case the carbamazepine is stocked in the "T" section as is the theophylline. In the case of this particular pharmacy, the car-bamazepine was shelved directly above the theophylline.

There's nothing unusual about this. What was unusual was that we happened to stock the generic carbamazepine and the generic theophylline from the same generic manufacturer. It so happens that this manufacturer's containers all look alike. The size of the bottle, the color of the label, the color of the container, the printing on the bottle, etc., all look identical. The only difference, of course, is that the names of the pills in the bottles are different. Many manufacturers try to vary the size of the containers, the colors of the labels, etc., for this very reason, to make it easier for the hurried pharmacist to distinguish products quickly. What happened was that my partner inadvertently picked up the identical-looking bot-tle above the theophylline. The customer ended up getting car-bamazepine (for seizures) instead of theophylline (for asthma). As a consequence, my partner and our employer were sued.

6. A pharmacy gave my stepfather the wrong medication

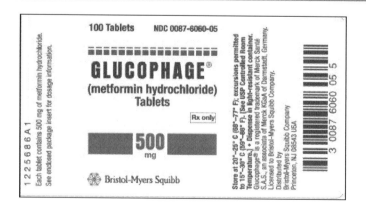

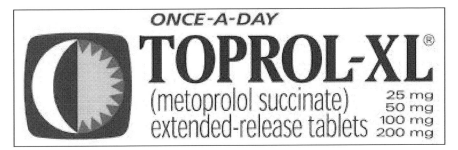

A pharmacy gave my stepfather a diabetes medicine (Glucophage) by mistake, instead of his blood pressure medicine (Toprol XL). My stepfather has never had diabetes.

In April of 1998, my stepfather was on Toprol XL for blood pressure. One morning, as he prepared to take one of his Toprol tablets, he said to me, "Why do some of these pills look different?" He proceeded to pour the contents of his prescription bottle onto the kitchen table.

I was amazed at what I saw. A scenario I know all-too-well was happening in my own family. It was instantly obviously that an error had been made by his pharmacy. The label indicated that the bottle contained Toprol XL, but it was clear that approximately half of the tablets in the bottle were not Toprol XL. I was initially unsure what the other tablets were. All the tablets were round and white but half of them were a little larger than the other half. Then I remembered that the other tablets looked like Glucophage 500 mg because of the markings BMS 500. (BMS stands for Bristol-Myers Squibb, the manufacturer.)

I told my stepfather that somehow the pharmacy had placed a diabetes medicine in the same bottle with his blood pressure medicine. He was not overly concerned but he was eager to go to the pharmacy to ask what had happened.

I told him that I would like to accompany him just as an observer, not mentioning to the pharmacist there that I, too, am a pharmacist. As we drove to the pharmacy (a large national chain), I told him to prepare for what I call the "minimization routine" in which the pharmacist downplays the significance of the error.

This pharmacy is one of the busiest community pharmacies I have ever seen, judging by the number of white coats (pharmacists, technicians, and cashiers) in the pharmacy. I counted thirteen. I figure they must do over 600 prescriptions per day based on the personnel levels I've seen in the pharmacies I've worked in. They may even do considerably more than that.

My stepfather asked for the pharmacist-in-charge. That pharmacist poured the contents of the bottle onto a tray and said simply "Hmm."

My stepfather asked the pharmacist "What are these other pills?"

The pharmacist could not identify the Glucophage 500 by seeing the imprint BMS 500 on the pills. Rather than show the pills to his coworkers (which is what I would have done), he proceeded to examine reference material that identifies pills by their markings (i.e., letters and numbers imprinted on the pill). He was finally able to determine that BMS stood for Bristol-Myers Squibb, so he called that manufacturer. He was told that BMS 500 is their diabetes medicine Glucophage.

The pharmacist told my stepfather, "This other medicine is Glucophage, a diabetes medicine." The pharmacist then asked my stepfather, "Have you ever had diabetes or been on Glucophage?"

My stepfather: "No."

The pharmacist: "Hmm. I don't know how this could have happened."

My stepfather: "What would have happened if I took those wrong pills?"

The pharmacist: "It may have lowered your sugar a little bit."

My stepfather: "Could that have hurt me?"

The pharmacist: "Only if you had taken a whole bunch of 'em."

The pharmacist then chose his words carefully, as I do in situations like this. He said, "Sorry for the inconvenience. We will refund the price of the prescription to you." The pharmacist then replaced the Glucophage with Toprol XL and gave my stepfather a slip for a refund.

My stepfather and I then proceeded to the refunds and exchanges counter in another part of this store. The pharmacy is only one department in this huge store. We had an authorization from the pharmacy for a refund of approximately thirty dollars.

On the way home from the store, I asked my stepfather how he felt about the situation. He wasn't very upset. He said, "Accidents happen. I'll only get mad if it happens again."

My stepfather is a very nice person and doesn't get upset easily yet I feel that his attitude about this incident reflects the attitude I see from customers whenever I have to explain (or explain away) an error. The public does not seem to understand the significance of these events. In most cases, no harm is done by our errors. But the possibility of an absolute catastrophe is much greater than you know.

Note that the pharmacist chose his words carefully by saying "I'm sorry for the inconvenience" rather than saying "I'm sorry for the error." We pharmacists try to avoid using the word "error," fearing a lawsuit. "Inconvenience" is a much less scary word than "error."

My employer, too, refunds the price of the prescription whenever there has been an error.

7. I erroneously typed "Take one tablet three times a day" on a sleeping pill prescription (Halcion). Sleeping pills are obviously taken at bedtime.

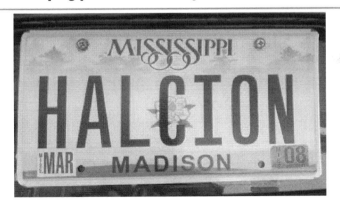

A short time after the sleeping pill Halcion was introduced onto the market, I received a prescription for this drug in which the doctor specified the directions "Take one tablet three times a day."

Obviously, sleeping pills are not taken three times a day. They are taken at bedtime.

Believe it or not, pharmacists may not necessarily be aware of the indications (approved uses) for a new drug or the number of times per day that it is usually administered. With so many new drugs being introduced these days (at least in part because the FDA is under pressure from Congress and the drug industry to relax standards for approvals—according to some critics), it becomes more difficult for pharmacists to keep up. We have a learning curve with each drug. And don't forget that there are a few thousand drugs on pharmacy shelves.

Of course, it is inexcusable that a pharmacist would dispense a drug for which he doesn't know the indications or how many times daily it's usually taken, but this is what actually happens sometimes in the real world. Certainly I was negligent in not checking the official prescribing information before I dispensed this drug. But the doctor made the original error and I didn't catch it.

Pharmacists are very busy people with very hectic lives and families to raise, etc. Finding the time to keep on top of the flood of new drugs is something to which we should give a high priority, but, in the real world, lots of drugs are dispensed in this country that pharmacists are not "on top of."

Part of the problem may be the circus atmosphere surrounding new drugs and pharmacists' feeling that drug companies are leading us around by the nose, forcing us to learn about their latest wonder drug.

Allow me to digress for a minute. It is a fact that a large fraction of the new drugs introduced each year are simply "me-too" or "copy-cat" drugs. For a detailed explanation of "me-too" drugs, see *The Truth About the Drug Companies* (NY: Random House, 2004) by Marcia Angell, M.D. Angell is a former editor-in-chief at *The New England Journal of Medicine*. In essence, each pharmaceutical company wants to have a "player" in a "hot" field (blood pressure, depression, cholesterol, type-2 diabetes, etc.), whether or not that player is any better than existing players. In many cases, the new drugs are no better and, in some cases, they're worse than existing drugs. The FDA does not require that new drugs be safer or more effective than existing drugs. New drugs must be sufficiently differ-ent to qualify for a patent. Drug companies want to get their share of any lucrative disease market. In my opinion, it is quite possible that pharmacists' skepticism toward the flood of copy-cat drugs contributes to a relaxed attitude toward learning about these new products. At least that attitude has affected me.

Back to the Halcion error. How was this error discovered? One day the physician who wrote the prescription called. I happened to be on duty at that time. He said something like "Somebody there typed 'three times a day' on a sleeping pill prescription I wrote." Apparently the patient had brought it to the doctor's attention.

Of course, this is an extremely uncomfortable situation for any pharmacist to be in. It's our worst nightmare. The pharmacist's immediate reaction is to hope that it may have been our partner or a fill-in pharmacist who filled the prescription. So, before we let the doctor chew us out, we delay things momentarily by saying something like "Let me pull the actual prescription from our files."

It turns out that my initials were on the prescription, so I was the pharmacist who had filled the prescription and made the error. But wait a minute! I see that the doctor specifically wrote "TID" on the prescription (the Latin abbreviation for "three times a day"). I said to the doctor, "I have your prescription in my hand and it clearly says 'TID'. You are welcome to stop by the pharmacy and examine it if you like."

The doctor's attitude softened. Somewhat surprisingly, he did not question the fact that he had mistakenly specified "TID." But he asked, "Why would you type 'three times a day' on a sleeping pill prescription?" I didn't have a good answer, but neither did he have a good answer for his mistake. So we were basically even (we had both screwed up) and the conversation then ended. Thank God.

There could have been tremendous liability involved if, for ex-ample, the patient didn't know this was a sleeping pill. A huge number of our customers are in a complete fog as to the precise purpose of each medication they swallow. So, if, for example, this customer had indeed taken it three times a day (not knowing it was a sleeping pill) and then he had been involved in a car accident, the potential liability for me and my employer could have been tremendous.

In this example, what percent of the fault belonged with me and what percent belonged with the physician? The doctor made a mistake and I didn't catch it. Luckily, as far as I know, the patient suffered no ill effects. But this could have been an absolute disaster.

8. "Is it even Claritin?"

In one store, a customer walked up to the pharmacy counter and said to me, "There are only fourteen tablets in this bottle but there's supposed to be thirty." The day before, another pharmacist had miscounted the tablets. The prescription was for Claritin, a non-sedating antihistamine used for allergy symptoms. (Claritin is now available without a prescription. At the time of this incident, it required a prescription.) This customer said that the pharmacist who dispensed the medication the day before was very busy: "He had four other customers waiting." The customer then asked me, "Is it even Claritin?"

When a customer asks something like "Is it even Claritin?" pharmacists know that we'd better have a good answer because we're talking to someone who knows enough to realize that pharmacists do indeed make mistakes. This is the type of question that pharmacists can't bullshit their way out of. A customer like this is essentially saying, "I trusted this pharmacist to fill my prescription correctly and I'm wondering if he did indeed fill it correctly."

Claritin is a very common-looking white pill. It is not a pill that is easily distinguished because of a distinctive color or shape. I went to our shelves and grabbed our stock bottle of Claritin, intending to show her that what we had in our stock bottle labeled Claritin was identical to what she had in her bottle. I asked her if she could read the numbers on the pills in her bottle. She said, "My eyesight isn't too good but it looks like 453 or 458." I was thankful that her eyesight was good enough to see that. I knew that I would be able to satisfy her since she was able to read the number. I showed her that the tablets in our stock bottle were numbered "458" and she seemed to be satisfied. Satisfying customers after an error is not always so easy, as the next anecdote will illustrate.

9. A customer goes ballistic because we forgot to tell him that a medication needed to be refrigerated and shaken before each use.

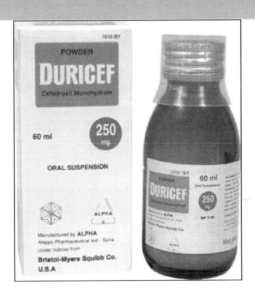

Here is an incident that was extremely uncomfortable for me. One morning a man approached the pharmacy and asked me to look in our computer and refill his mother's prescription for the antibiotic Duricef. This antibiotic was being used for a skin infection. He commented to me that since his mother had Alzheimer's disease, she needed the liquid form because she could not swallow capsules.

When I refilled the prescription and handed it to him, I told him to be sure to refrigerate it and to shake it well before each use. The man went ballistic. He told me that no one had ever told him to shake it or to refrigerate it. He emphasized that his mother had already finished two courses of this drug without shaking or refrigerating the container. He said that there were no SHAKE WELL or REFRIGERATE stickers on the bottle. He told me that the bottle had been kept on the kitchen table during both prior courses and that he had not shaken the bottle before giving her each dose. He asked me if the medication had lost its potency because it was not refrigerated. He wondered whether failing to refrigerate the drug was the reason it was not curing his mother's skin infection.

I decided to call the manufacturer, Bristol-Myers Squibb, while he was standing in front of me. I wanted to get a precise answer to his question and I wanted to show him that I took his concerns seriously. The person with whom I spoke at Bristol-Myers Squibb told me that their studies show that Duricef is stable at room temperature for ten days. What that means is that the active ingredient itself is stable for ten days. However, the person at Bristol-Myers Squibb was unable to guarantee that no microbial growth had taken place, contaminating the contents.

I told the customer that the manufacturer said it was probably still stable, but I did not tell him the second part of the message. I was afraid he would go into an absolute rampage if I told him about the possibility of contamination. He was already ballistic over the fact that we had failed to tell him that the medication was supposed to be refrigerated and that it needed to be shaken before each use.

He said he would call his doctor to see what harm may have occurred.

I gave him this refill at no charge. He told me that he felt that we should refund the price of the two previous courses. We did. Anything to please this man!!! I would have given him all the money in my wallet if I thought it would calm him down.

It appears that a pharmacy student had omitted a SHAKE WELL and REFRIGERATE sticker both times. The pharmacist with whom she was working evidently did not catch her omission. Upon my mentioning this incident to the pharmacy student later, she did not claim that she must have applied these stickers. The pharmacist-in-charge at this store said to her, "We've got to remember to put on those stickers!"

I was just filling in at this store so I don't know whether there were any further developments like a lawsuit. But the fact remains that I was placed in this extremely uncomfortable situation as a result of sloppy work done by others (i.e., the tech's omission of the stickers and the pharmacist's failure to catch that omission).

In my experience, when situations like this occur with a substitute pharmacist, that substitute pharmacist is sometimes blamed for not being able to defuse the situation quickly. Full-time pharmacists who have an assigned store (substitute pharmacists float between stores) sometimes seem to feel they can defuse any situation in their pharmacy in short order. So, despite my best efforts, I stood the chance of being accused (by the pharmacist for whom I was filling in) of doing a poor job in handling this irate customer.

10. A pharmacy student typed the wrong directions, instructing a customer to take four Lasix per day, rather than one per day as the doctor specified.

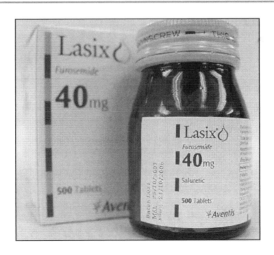

This error occurred when a pharmacy student typed the label directions for Lasix 40 mg (a diuretic): "Take one tablet 4 times a day." The student should have typed: "Take one tablet daily." The pharmacist who was on duty at that time was supposed to check this prescription, but that evidently did not happen. I blame the high volume of prescriptions done at this store, plus poor physician handwriting on the prescription, plus the use of Latin abbreviations.

The Latin abbreviation for "Take 1 tablet 4 times a day" is "1 qid." The Latin abbreviation for "Take 1 tablet daily" is "1 qd." If doctors would discontinue the practice of using Latin abbreviations on prescriptions and instead write out this stuff in plain English, there would be a lot fewer errors made by pharmacists who have difficulty reading doctors' handwriting.

When I was given this bottle of the diuretic Lasix to refill, I happened to look at the directions. That's something many or most pharmacists usually don't have time to do—we assume the directions are typed correctly initially. But for some reason I happened to look at the directions. What I noticed bothered me. I knew from experience that a smaller dose is far more commonly prescribed. I went to our prescription files and looked up the doctor's original prescription. Sure enough, it said, "Take one tablet daily" rather than what the pharmacy student typed on the label, "Take 1 tablet 4 times a day."

I then called my partner at home and told her what had happened. My partner hadn't caught the error made by our pharmacy student. My partner said to me, "Ask the customer how he's actually taking it. Maybe he's been on it before and maybe he knows he should just take one tablet daily instead of four times a day." So I asked the customer how he had been taking the Lasix. It turns out that this customer is a very nice man but he doesn't seem to be very intelligent. He laughed and said, "I noticed that the bottle said to take four a day but I knew that was wrong. I told my doctor and he said, 'Boy, they're really trying to dry you out!' [Diuretics like Lasix are used to remove excess fluid.] I've just been taking one a day."

Once again, I felt the weight of the world lifted from my shoulders. The customer did not know that our pharmacy student had screwed up, nor did the customer know that my partner had failed to catch the error. The customer never seemed to hold this error against us even though I certainly would have been upset and would tend to lose confidence in a pharmacist if a similar error had happened to me if I were the patient. And I'm surprised we never got an angry call from this customer's doctor.

11. A pharmacist told me that she discovered "at least a half dozen major errors" in a month. She said, "And I don't mean minor errors!"

I once worked briefly with a pharmacist who had only been licensed for three or four months. One day she told me that, soon after graduation from pharmacy school, she was placed in an extremely busy store in which she felt totally overwhelmed. She told me that in the month she worked there, she discovered "at least a half dozen major errors" that had been made by other pharmacists filling in at that store. Our district supervisor hadn't been able to find a permanent replacement for that store so there were a large number of pharmacists filling in there in the meantime. This young pharmacist told me, "And I don't mean minor errors!" She told me that she came to work early each day and left late and that she was still unable to handle the workload.

There are disagreements about what should be termed a "major error." "Major errors" do not necessarily mean "major harm." In fact, most major errors do not cause major harm. But some of them do. Getting Drug X instead of Drug Y at your drugstore can be a major mistake, but that doesn't necessarily mean that you will suffer major—or any—harm. If you get an anti-depressant like Prozac instead of an anti-arthritis drug like Celebrex, that is a major mistake by the pharmacy, but you are unlikely to suffer major harm.

12. A tech told me that a pharmacist she works with "doesn't check shit."

There's no doubt that the error rate among pharmacists spans the entire spectrum. Some pharmacists very rarely make mistakes. Other pharmacists scare me a great deal. The pharmacy tech at one store told me that one of the male pharmacists she works with "doesn't check shit." In other words, for example, once the pills are put in the bottle, this pharmacist doesn't usually look back a second time to see if they're the right pills or that the right directions are on the label, etc. She said that he makes lots of errors when he's talking to his new girlfriend on the phone. She said that he does things like putting medications for two completely unrelated people in the same bag.

I know this pharmacist and I can vouch for the fact that he does indeed make lots of errors. But so far none of the errors has been serious enough to jeopardize his job or reputation. From my perspective, he seems to think he can bullshit his way through anything in life—even a serious prescription error.

13. A pharmacist who was filling in for me dispensed the wrong eye drops to a child. As a result, the child's eye doctor was unable to perform an examination as planned.

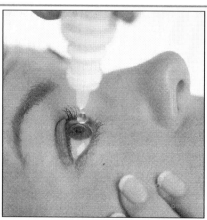

Less than a year after graduation from pharmacy school, I was working in a pharmacy in Summersville, West Virginia. This is a town with a population of only a few thousand. The pharmacy was open only from 9 AM to 5 PM so I was the only pharmacist assigned to this store. My days off were infrequent in this pharmacy, yet one day off is especially memorable. On that day a relief pharmacist had the misfortune of filling a child's prescription with the wrong eye drops. The eye drops were intended to prepare the child's eyes for an upcoming eye exam. The drops were to be applied in the morning on the day that the parents were to make an hour's drive to the child's eye doctor in Charleston, West Virginia. The eye drops that this relief pharmacist mistakenly dispensed did not pre-pare the child's eyes properly. As a result, the eye doctor was un-able to perform the exam as planned. This forced the parents to take off another day from work in order to make a second trip to Charleston.

As I said, I had been out of pharmacy school less than a year so I was unprepared for the task of handling this error. Even though I didn't make the error myself, I felt some responsibility because it happened in the store in which I was the only full-time pharmacist. I assumed that my employer (Rite Aid) would want me to try do anything I could to avoid a lawsuit.

It so happens that one of the technicians in that store had a very loose acquaintance with the parents of this child. I asked this technician to accompany me one evening to visit the family at their home. Luckily this technician has a very friendly personality and she's able to make conversation with people easily. I asked the tech to "do all the talking" herself because I was very uncomfortable with the entire situation. Even though I felt that visiting the parents at their home was a nice gesture, I dreaded it. I asked the tech to basically tell the parents that we were concerned about the error and that we regretted the hassle that it put them through, i.e., lost wages from taking time off from work to go a second time to the eye doctor in Charleston. My tech did what I felt was a great job in showing compassion for the family and regret for the error.

Over the years, I have learned that errors like this are so commonplace that having a pharmacist visit a family at home is highly unusual. But this was a small town and I feared that word would get around about this error and customers would be reluctant to have their prescriptions filled in this pharmacy.

During our visit the parents told me that they felt they deserved compensation for the ordeal, including travel expenses and lost wages. I was never told the dollar amount that was agreed upon, but I do know that my boss gave them a check.

14. Two people with the same name

At one store where I worked for a few years, my partner discovered that, to our dismay, there are two customers with the same rather uncommon name. I filled a prescription for Xanax for anxiety for one of these customers. The day before, my partner had filled a prescription for another customer with the same name. That prescription was for methocarbamol, a muscle relaxant. The next day, unknown to both of us, both customers' prescriptions were in the same bin, alphabetized by last name, ready to be picked up.

You guessed it. The prescription I filled for Xanax was picked up by the customer who was supposed to get the methocarbamol. My partner told me that this customer realized something was amiss when she got home and read the drug leaflet that we include with each prescription. It was only when she returned to the pharmacy with the wrong pills that my partner realized that there were two customers with the same name at this store. This was before we had computers which help us catch things like this.

Luckily, this customer seemed to be very understanding and there was no other fallout from this incident. My partner refunded the price of the incorrect medication and gave her the correct medication at no charge. This is company policy whenever a mistake is made.

15. Naproxen instead of Naprelan

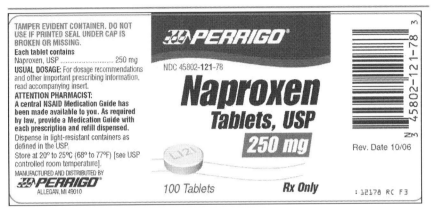

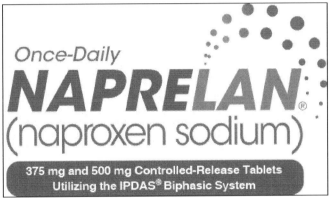

A customer called from home and asked, "Is my prescription for Naprelan ready?" I went over to the area where we keep finished prescriptions to check to see if there was a bag for this customer. Indeed there was, but the label on the bag stated naproxen, not Naprelan. These are two very similar drugs used for pain and inflammation. The difference is that naproxen is taken two (or more) times a day whereas Naprelan is taken once a day.

I told the customer on the phone that her prescription was ready and then hurried to correct the medication before she arrived at the store. This error was easy to fix. Had I first noticed the error when the customer was standing in front of me at the pharmacy, it would have taken a little quick thinking to make up an excuse to correct it without the customer realizing that I had discovered an error at that instant. I usually say something innocuous like "Hold on just a minute and let me check one thing." The customer is usually oblivious to what I'm doing because most customers seem to think that errors in the pharmacy are impossible. Quite wrong.

16. Switched drugs: Entex PSE and PCE 500

A tech filled two prescriptions as follows. One was for the antibiotic PCE 500 mg (erythromycin), taken twice a day. The other was for Entex PSE, a drug used for colds, also taken twice a day. The tech filled both prescriptions correctly in every detail except one. She put the PCE 500 in the Entex PSE bottle. And she put the Entex PSE in the PCE 500 bottle. So the medications that the patient would have received were correct but they were in the wrong bottles. In this case, it would likely have resulted in no harm since both tablets are taken twice a day.

17. Monopril instead of minoxidil

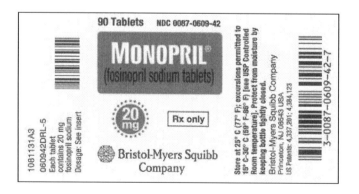

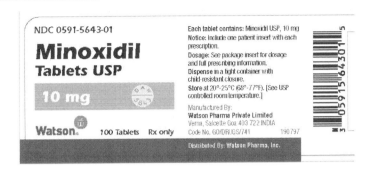

At one store where I worked, my partner dispensed Monopril on a prescription that called for minoxidil. Notice that both drug names look and sound somewhat alike. The customer brought back the bottle and asked, "Why do these pills look different from the ones I've been on?" I am not proud of this fact but I lied to this customer in explaining this error made by my partner. I told the customer that the unfamiliar pill was a generic equivalent for the drug the customer had been getting.

We pharmacists often feel that if no harm seems to have occurred, why should we tell the customer that, yes, we screwed up? Of course we correct the error but we don't necessarily admit to the customer what has happened.

In my twenty-five year career as a pharmacist, enforcement fluctuated regarding the policy that we report all errors to corporate headquarters. Sometimes pharmacists were strongly encouraged to report errors to management. At other times, we didn't hear much from our bosses about the need to report errors. Even when the policy of reporting errors was being tightly enforced, many (perhaps most) pharmacists didn't report errors. Pharmacists often felt that since the chain expected us to fill prescriptions so quickly, it was inevitable that mistakes would occur. It was kind of an "us versus them" (pharmacists versus management) attitude. The chains want us to fill prescriptions much more quickly than we're comfortable in doing, so why should we as pharmacists serve up our heads on a platter in our litigious society? Management screws us, so we're just getting even.

In this case with Monopril and minoxidil, both drugs are used for blood pressure. The customer seemed to be doing okay (admittedly a leap of faith on my part) so rather than open a huge can of worms by admitting my partner had given her the wrong drug, I lied to her. I did, of course, give her the correct pills in refilling the prescription.

It is situations like this that most pharmacists dread. Our attitude becomes: *What harm is done by lying ourselves out of a very embarrassing situation that could lead to a lawsuit? If management gave us adequate support staff, errors like this wouldn't happen nearly as often.*

18. A pharmacist was incredibly negligent in adding rubbing alcohol to a child's antibiotic rather than distilled water

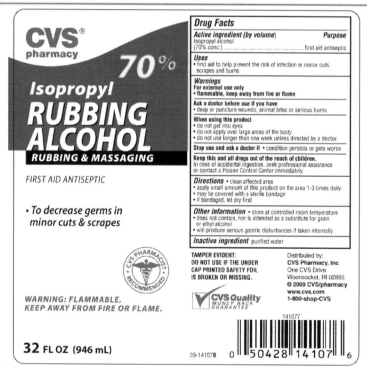

Rubbing alcohol is a very toxic substance if swallowed. Some pharmacists routinely use this substance as a disinfectant to clean their prescription counter. These pharmacists often transfer this rubbing alcohol from the manufacturer's stock container into a rubber squeeze container, thus making it easier to spray on the counter. Here's a brief story illustrating what can happen when a floater pharmacist fills in at a pharmacy for another pharmacist's day off (or for sick days, vacation days, jury duty, etc.).

Most children's antibiotics arrive at the pharmacy as a dry powder. When the pharmacist fills a prescription for such an antibiotic, we add distilled water and then shake the container to dissolve the powder and make a nice suspension. For convenience, some pharmacists transfer distilled water from gallon—or larger—containers to smaller containers that are much easier to handle.

I was working for Rite Aid in Hurricane, West Virginia. One day all the pharmacists at neighboring Rite Aid pharmacies were gossiping about how a local relief pharmacist had added rubbing alcohol to the dry powder rather than distilled water. The gossip among pharmacists regarded his incredible negligence in not first ascertaining the contents of the plastic squeeze bottle before adding it to the dry powder. This floater pharmacist assumed that the plastic squeeze container held distilled water. In fact, it contained rubbing alcohol.

Luckily the mother of the child for whom the antibiotic was intended immediately questioned the smell of the medication. Rubbing alcohol has a fairly strong and distinctive odor that should be easy to detect. The child's mother returned the medication to the drugstore before giving a dose to her child. So the child was not harmed in any way.

Though this incident is quite scary, like most errors it did not result in any discipline to the pharmacist responsible. I doubt that most employers would fire a pharmacist for such a mistake, even though our bosses might indeed feel that this pharmacist demonstrated spectacular stupidity in not first determining the contents of the squeeze bottle. This pharmacist simply assumed that it must contain distilled water.

For a better understanding of the potential seriousness of this incident, here's a snippet from *FDA Consumer* that discusses a FDA recall from a manufacturing plant in Puerto Rico. The plant's error is very similar to this pharmacist's mistake. The plant mistakenly attached labels indicating distilled water to containers that actually held rubbing alcohol. (Tom Cramer, "Recall retrieves rubbing alcohol labeled as distilled water," *FDA Consumer*, December 1991. http://findarticles.com/p/articles/mi_m1370/is_n10_v25/ai_11767821 Accessed Nov. 3, 2006)

Thousands of bottles labeled "Agua Destilada" (distilled water) were pulled from pharmacy shelves in Puerto Rico and the Virgin Islands after FDA investigators discovered that a number of the bottles contained rubbing alcohol, not distilled water. Five days after the labeling error was discovered, the manufacturing plant responsible was closed and has not reopened. The labeling mix-up could have killed or injured hundreds of children, since the distilled water was labeled for use in preparing infant formula and medicines. An infant can die after consuming formula containing less than half an ounce of rubbing alcohol. However, no injuries were reported in connection with the incident.

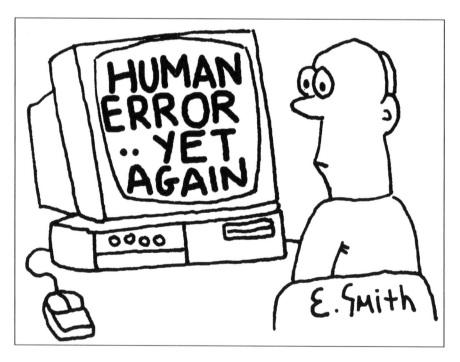

2

Other pharmacists' memorable misfills

A highly abbreviated version of this chapter was published as an editorial that I wrote for *Drug Topics* ("Memorable Misfills of a Retail Pharmacist," April 16, 2007, p. 44). With each editorial I write for this magazine, my e-mail address is included in case any readers care to comment. Several pharmacists e-mailed me with their own most memorable misfills. Here's a sample:

Pharmacist dispenses chili peppers instead of diabetes medication

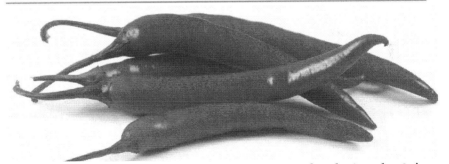

When I had my pharmacy in West Los Angeles during the 80's, filling 300 to 500 prescriptions per day in a heavily Jewish neighborhood, I had, as an employee pharmacist, one of the fastest and most accurate Rx fillers. I'll call him JT. He could clear the counter in a nanosecond. There was a hot dog stand connected to the outside of my building and JT had the habit of taking a 20 dram vial and filling it with chili peppers so he could snack on them while filling prescriptions. Anyway, JT worked every other day for me so one day, after he had worked, I received an absolutely frantic call from one of my best and oldest customers. She was sobbing, knowing that the story she was about to tell me would be hard to believe. She had picked up her prescription the day before. But when she went to take her prescribed medication that morning, she opened her 20 dram vial to find, not her medication, but eleven chili peppers. "How could this be?" she asked, her voice trembling, for she had paid a hefty price for her medications. At first, I could not believe her and was a bit dismissive. But all of a sudden, in the back of my mind, I remembered JT's habit of filling a vial with chili peppers. What could I say but to convince her that someone had broken into her house in the middle of the night, stole her diabetes medications and replaced it with chili peppers? It took almost an hour and one-half on the phone with her and in the meantime, her prescription was filled correctly and sent out. I was still on the phone with her when my delivery person arrived, and she was so thankful. I was her hero that day and I am ashamed.—[Pharmacist D. S.]

Pharmacist dispenses diet pill with directions "four times a day" instead of "once a day"

My most memorable error was on the typed sig [directions] on a Dexamyl Spansules prescription, a popular diet pill by SK&F (Dextroamphetamine/Amobarbital). Of course, the sig was one a day. I typed four times a day. Gadzooks. The poor woman didn't eat a thing for 2 days. She did not sleep either. When she came in, I confessed and made the correction. This was around 1968. She continued to trade with us. Acted as if nothing had happened.—[Pharmacist J. P.]

Customer requests repeat of pharmacist's mistake in dose of antidepressant

Back in 1988 in Puerto Rico a lady came to the pharmacy to get her Pamelor refilled for the third time. She left and then came back to tell me that I had given her the wrong medicine. I looked at it and I had indeed filled it correctly (Pamelor 10mg). She said "But the one you gave me last month was such and such color." We had given her 25mg Pamelor the previous month! I explained the filling error to her. She then looked at me and said "Look, I have not felt this good for a long time. You have got to misfill it again!" I explained to her that I could not do that. Later that week we got a call from her doctor for a new prescription for Pamelor 25mg!—[Pharmacist P. V.]

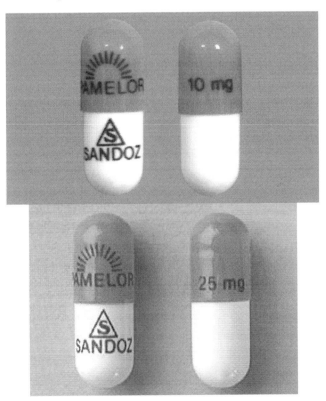

Pharmacist dispenses wrong type of alcohol, causing permanent scar on face of young lady

About 1957 when I was a young owner, I employed a much older pharmacist. He supplied isopropyl alcohol on a open call for rubbing alcohol. (Alcohol USP means ethyl alcohol.) The young lady squeezed a zit, dabbed on alcohol, took a nap, and woke up with a burn on the temple area the size of a quarter. My insurance adjuster said juries are very sympathetic to young ladies with scars but he would settle in such a manner that we would keep the customer. Six hundred dollars for plastic surgery did just that and the family remained patients for 42 more years. When I saw the girl, now a grandmother, in the Shop-Rite last year, the scar was still there.—Name withheld by request

Pharmacist dispenses gabapentin 600 mg instead of 100 mg

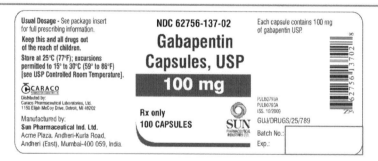

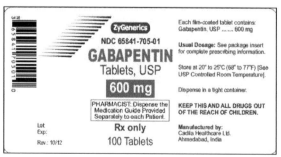

After my editorial titled "When efficiency is all that matters" appeared in Drug Topics *(February 2011, p. 56), I received an email from a Rite Aid pharmacist in Buffalo. In his email he discussed Rite Aid's new fifteen minute guarantee. Customers would be given a five dollar coupon if their prescriptions were not ready within fifteen minutes. This fifteen minute guarantee resulted in a tremendous amount of pharmacist anger directed at Rite Aid in the pharmacy blogosphere from pharmacists working in all settings, including Rite Aid pharmacists. This fifteen minute guarantee puts a tremendous amount of stress on pharmacists and techs, increasing the chance of a serious pharmacy mistake. This pharmacist and I subsequently exchanged a few emails. In one of those emails, I asked him whether he had ever made a serious pharmacy error. He replied:*

A few weeks ago you asked me if I had ever had a serious error. Ironic... Yesterday my DM [district manager] called to tell me I had dispensed a Rx for 100 mg gabapentin as 600 mg. [Gabapentin, the generic for Neurontin, is an antiseizure drug that is also used to treat various neuropathies/neuralgias. It is available in strengths from 100 mg to 800 mg.] I researched it and found that the tech had input [entered into the pharmacy computer] 600 mg and I, on checking, let it get by me. The lady took it for 2 weeks and is in the hospital being weaned off it. I feel like crap!! This is the scenario... It was in hour 10 of a 13 hour day. I had not eaten a thing all day. We had a stack of 35 baskets to input and did 398 Rx's that day. One pharmacist [on duty] all day. At the time of the error [there were only] one input tech and one cashier [on duty]. Put that in your book next to a picture of a pharmacist throwing up. That's my picture.

The other sick part is I tell my DM how much of my day had now been destroyed and she says, "Don't worry, you will get a call from our insurance company. Tell them what happened. I make calls like this all the time. You are not a repeat offender like many are." Didn't make me feel better but what a bunch of crap that is. Interestingly I had a conversation with her about 4 weeks ago about the $5 fiasco [coupon given to customers who have to wait more than fifteen minutes] and told her that someday it will cause a big problem and the story will end up on the front page of the local newspaper and at that point you can kiss Rite Aid business in Buffalo goodbye. I hope I am not that story!!—[Pharmacist in Buffalo]

Two errors posted on "The Student Doctor Network"

Hospital pharmacist misses neonatologist's error in dose of antibiotic vancomycin

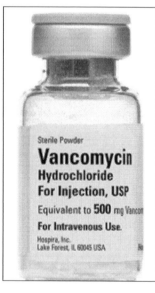

Sterile Powder

Vancomycin
Hydrochloride
For Injection, USP
Equivalent to **500** mg Vanco
For Intravenous Use.
Hospira, Inc.
Lake Forest, IL 60045 USA

I am an overnight pharmacist at a 450-bed hospital. It can get VERY busy. I only have one tech and the nursing staff at my hospital is horrible. I spend 90% of my night answering the most retarded questions. Anyhoo, I have been here a year and I made my first error. I received an antibiotic order from the nursery. The order was for vanco [vancomycin], Claforan and a TPN. I started working on it immediately. Checking doses, volumes, concentrations, etc. Within 2 minutes the nurse calls me, "We just scanned you an order that is super stat!!!! We need it right away!! Did you get it!?" I was slightly annoyed but understood the urgency. Obviously the call distracted me. I told the nurse we would have everything ready in 30 minutes. Three minutes later another nurse calls, "I know we already called you but this really needs to get up here sooner than 30 minutes. The doctor is standing right here, blah blah blah...." So now I am officially pissed and I told the nurse that this is the second interruption I have had trying to process this order. I kindly asked her to not call me anymore. I hung up and ironically I said to my tech "See, this is how mistakes happen!" Long story short, the neonatologist wrote for 100mg/kg of vanco, not 10mg/kg. I missed it too, with all the phone calls I probably bypassed the alert on the computer. The baby was fine when all was said and done but the part that gets me is that they didn't hang the drug until 2 hours later because there was no line access. I know this wasn't entirely my fault but I hate when stuff like this slips past me.

My hospital won't have CPOE [computerized physician order entry] until later this year. So everything is still paper. When I was informed of the error, my director was very explicit that she wasn't blaming me. I am very grateful that I work at an institution that doesn't believe in the "blame and shame" approach to handling errors. For my defense, I simply explained that the excessive phone calls from nursing, in this example and many others, needs to stop. One pharmacist can't process orders and pick up the phone every 2 minutes to be harassed by poorly trained nurses. I am surprised I haven't made any other errors in the past! **—Pharmacist, Miami Beach, Florida** (The Student Doctor Network, Accessed March 27, 2012 http://206.82.221.135/showthread.php?p=12314689)

Pharmacy student explains how patient received 40 mg of cholesterol-lowering drug lovastatin for three weeks—instead of 10 mg

NDC 54458-**982**-10

Lovastatin
Tablets USP

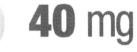

40 mg

Rx Only

See the accompanying drug information
sheet for full drug information

Depress tab and pull dosage card out
DO NOT SEPARATE FROM PLASTIC SHELL

My worst error resulted from me trusting the system too much. The days I'm scheduled, I'm the only intern/tech pulling and labeling meds. Usually, there are orders to be filled from 2-3 PM lying around along with the new admissions, so I end up filling about 150 orders in a 4 hour shift by myself. When I get into a groove of filling the orders, I have a tendency to overlook some things.

This particular error, the order was for a card of lovastatin 10 mg. I went to the box of lovastatin 10 mg cards, pulled it, labeled it, and threw it into the basket to be checked. It got checked and sent to the patient, and no one realized the error until 3 weeks later. The patient received lovastatin 40 mg instead of lovastatin 10 mg. The tech who makes all the cards and packs them onto the boxes on the shelves placed the 40 mg cards in the 10 mg box. **—Pharmacy student, Franklin Square, New York** (The Student Doctor Network, http://206.82.221.135/showthread.php?p=12314689 Accessed Mar. 27, 2012)

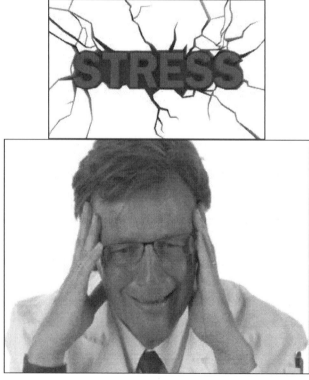

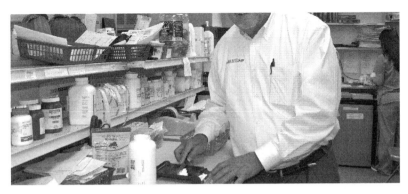

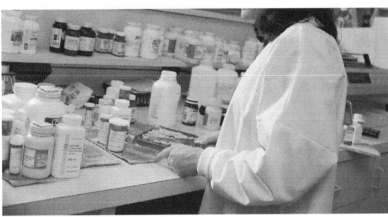

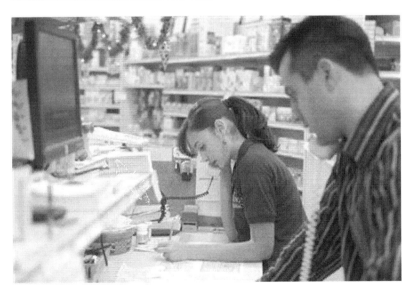

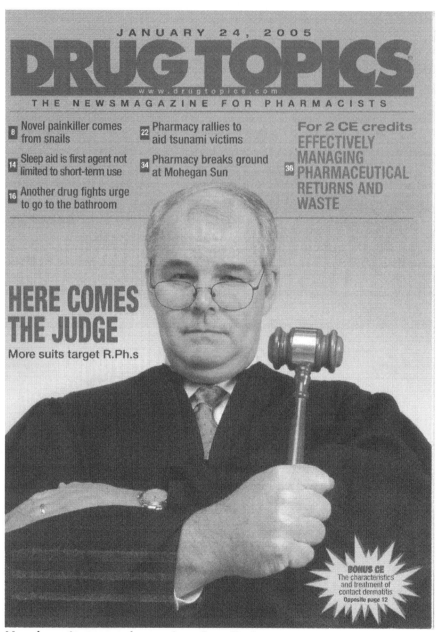

JANUARY 24, 2005

DRUG TOPICS

www.drugtopics.com

THE NEWSMAGAZINE FOR PHARMACISTS

HERE COMES THE JUDGE

More suits target R.Ph.s

BONUS CE
The characteristics and treatment of contact dermatitis
Opposite page 12

More lawsuits target pharmacists. *Drug Topics* cover story, Jan. 24, 2005

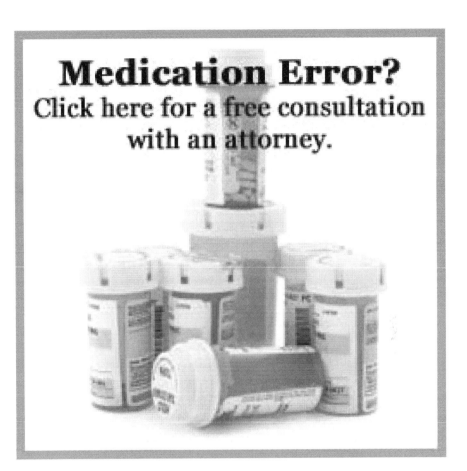

Medication Error?
Click here for a free consultation
with an attorney.

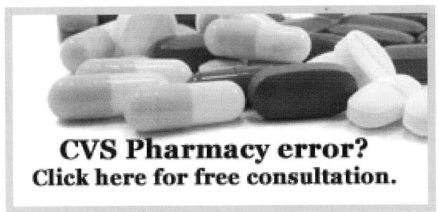

CVS Pharmacy error?
Click here for free consultation.

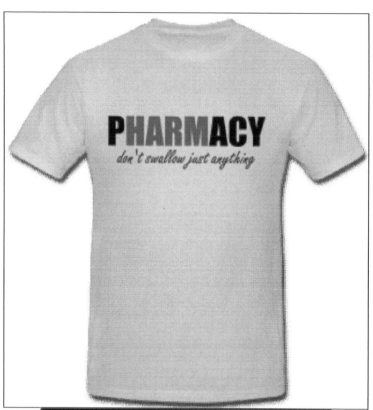

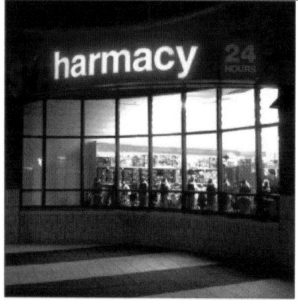

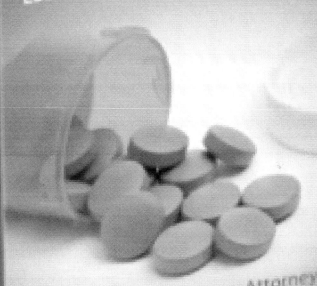

HOW TO MAKE PHARMACIES PAY FOR YOUR INJURIES CAUSED BY MEDICATION ERRORS

ESSENTIAL GUIDE FOR THE NON-LAWYER

David W. Hodges, Attorney

Galvin Kennedy, Attorney

PREVENTING MEDICATION ERRORS

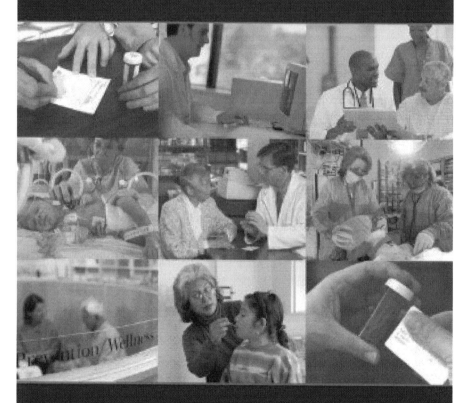

QUALITY CHASM SERIES

INSTITUTE OF MEDICINE
OF THE NATIONAL ACADEMIES

3

The hidden epidemic of pharmacy mistakes across America

Most people view the pharmacist's job as fairly straightforward, uneventful, and even boring. Doctors write prescriptions and pharmacists fill those prescriptions. What could be simpler? Too often, the reality is quite different. Due to competitive pressures in the marketplace, pharmacy has been transformed into a high-speed, high-stress, high-stakes enterprise in which powerful prescription drugs are just a blur on a hamburger assembly line. The big drugstore chains have embraced the McDonald's fast food model with disastrous consequences.

I quit pharmacy after twenty-five years because I was so fed up with slinging out prescriptions as fast as my hands and feet would allow. I am trying to expose the fact that mistakes are far more common in drugstores than patients and physicians realize. Powerful prescription drugs are dispensed across America in a system that is guaranteed to produce errors. The big chain drugstores don't want you to know that pharmacies are purposely understaffed to increase productivity and profitability.

A huge number of pharmacists are disillusioned with the profession and are not recommending pharmacy as a career for their children. A huge number of pharmacists say that they would never have chosen pharmacy as a career if they had known what conditions are like in what we sarcastically refer to as "McPharmacy." This is a reckless system that treats powerful and potentially deadly prescription drugs as if they were no different from any other consumer product in America. The big drugstore chains run their operations as if pharmacists were dispensing nothing more hazardous than a Big Mac at McDonald's or a Slurpee at 7-Eleven.

Many pharmacists feel that the chains have made the cold calculation that it is more profitable to sling out prescriptions at lighting speed and pay customers harmed by mistakes than it is to provide adequate staffing so that mistakes are a rarity rather than a predictable occurrence. Understaffing sometimes forces pharmacists to take educated guesses rather than call doctors to clarify illegible prescriptions. Understaffing sometimes causes pharmacists to override potentially significant drug interactions rather than phone the doctor who prescribed the drugs.

The chain drugstores' obsession with speed increases the occurrence of pharmacy mistakes. Pharmacists are under tremendous pressure to fill prescriptions at unsafe speeds. Drive-thru windows increase mistakes by creating the expectation among customers that prescriptions should be filled as quickly as McDonald's fills burger orders. It is a fact that the speed with which pharmacists fill prescriptions is one of the primary criteria used by chain management in determining whether pharmacists are doing a satisfactory job.

Pharmacists go home at night crossing their fingers and wondering whether all the prescriptions they filled (and supervised techs in filling) that day were filled properly. They say to themselves something like, "Mrs. Jones was in today but I don't even remember checking her prescriptions."

Pharmacists desperately hope that the public will become so enraged as to demand that the chains provide adequate staffing for the safe filling of prescriptions. Understaffing increases pharmacy profitability but it also increases the frequency of serious pharmacy mistakes. Don't allow yourself to become a pharmacy statistic. Let chain management know that the current system is entirely unacceptable. I can state with certainty that the public has no idea how common pharmacy mistakes are today.

As of today, I have written eighteen editorials for *Drug Topics*. I include my e-mail address (dmiller1952@aol.com) with each editorial in case any pharmacists care to comment. A huge number of pharmacists have pleaded with me to try to reach an audience beyond the pharmacists who read that magazine. Pharmacists desperately hope that the general public will be enraged by the common occurrence of pharmacy mistakes. Pharmacists desperately hope that the public will demand that safe staffing levels be given priority over the bottom line.

What would your reaction be if someone told you that there are **OVER FIFTY MILLION MISTAKES IN AMERICA'S PHARMACIES EACH YEAR?** Would you say that's impossible? The reality is that a large study of pharmacy mistakes estimates that "51.5 million errors occur during the filling of 3 billion prescriptions each year." (Eliz. Flynn, et. al., "National Observational Study of Prescription Dispensing Accuracy and Safety in 50 Pharmacies," *Journal of the American Pharmaceutical Assoc.*, March/April 2003, pp. 191-200) Some of the errors are trivial; others are deadly.

Margaret Mulligan, then the editor-in-chief at *Drug Topics*, wrote in the July 2009 issue, "While even one error is one too many, errors happen—to the tune of four errors per 250 scripts filled per day. The chance that a retail customer will receive an incorrectly filled prescription is approximately one in 30; the chance that an error will be clinically important is one in 1,000. How is this still happening in 2009?" (Margaret Mulligan, "System Breakdown: 4 Med Errors, 250 Scripts/Day," *Drug Topics*, July 2009, p. 22)

The following pages describe several very serious pharmacy mistakes that I found in various pharmacy magazines and web searches. Search Google for *pharmacy mistakes* and you will probably be shocked by what you discover. I have included over a dozen cases in which pharmacy mistakes appear to be the direct cause of patient deaths. The cases below are arranged by the size of the monetary award or settlement. I have arbitrarily placed the incidents involving patient deaths together near the middle of this chapter.

Carol Ukens, then a senior editor at *Drug Topics*, described three instances in which pharmacists killed themselves as a result of pharmacy mistakes. (Carol Ukens, "Compounding case leads to R.Ph. suicide," *Drug Topics*, May 6, 2002, pp. 44, 49)

A California pharmacist committed suicide in 2002 after a compounding error was blamed for three deaths. The pharmacist was not present when the error occurred in 2001, but he was a co-owner of the pharmacy where the compounding took place.

Jamey Phillip Sheets, 32, apparently could not accept the punishment meted out by the California pharmacy board for a fatal outbreak of meningitis from a drug compounded in the pharmacy he co-owned. A looming license suspension, five years on probation, and a hefty fine were more than the despondent pharmacist could bear. Late last month, he attached 500 mg of fentanyl patches to his neck and chest and lay down to die.

The Sheets suicide is not an isolated incident. For example, about a year ago, an Oregon pharmacist took her life after an error killed a patient. And about five years ago, a Kentucky pharmacist involved in a fatal error was on his way to the pharmacy board to surrender his license. Instead, he stopped his car and stepped in front of a semitrailer barreling down the Interstate.

Incidents involving pharmacy mistakes seem to be adequately reported by local newspapers and local television stations, but the national media have not, in my opinion, given this subject the coverage that it deserves. A noteworthy exception was a 16-minute segment on ABC News' 20/20 in which Brian Ross went undercover to report on pharmacy mistakes. The segment was titled, "Pharmacy Errors: Unreported Epidemic?" In my opinion that title accurately describes the problem except that the question mark should have been replaced by an exclamation point. [http://abcnews.go.com/Video/playerIndex?id=2997449 (June 13, 2007)]

Most of the legal cases described below involve mistakes made at drugstores. A few cases involve mistakes made at hospitals and nursing homes. Notice that the blood thinner Coumadin (warfarin) is involved in a large number of these cases with huge settlements. Since Coumadin is prescribed most commonly in the 5 mg tablet, if your doctor prescribes any dose other than 5 mg, be sure to double-check what strength you receive from your drugstore.

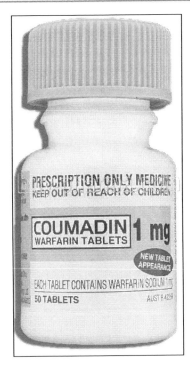

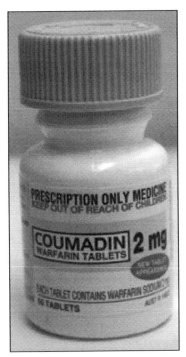

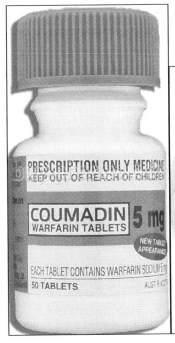

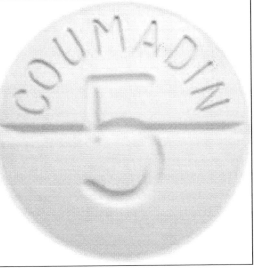

Oral drugs for Type II diabetes are also involved in many legal cases with huge settlements. Used improperly, Type II diabetes drugs (like glipizide, pictured below) can cause seriously low blood sugar levels, sometimes resulting in brain damage.

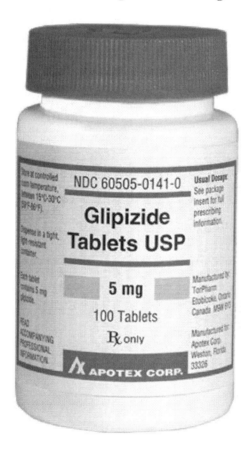

A study published in 2011 in *The New England Journal of Medicine* by Dr. Dan Budnitz found that blood thinners and diabetes drugs cause most emergency hospital visits for drug reactions among people over 65 in the United States. Most of the hospital emergency visits were for things like unintended overdoses, adverse effects, or allergic reactions. The study does not have a separate category for hospital emergency visits resulting from pharmacy mistakes. Nevertheless, the drugs that cause the most hospitalizations in the Budnitz study are quite similar to the drugs involved in huge awards in pharmacy mistake lawsuits. Anahad O'Connor describes the Budnitz study in *The New York Times*. (Anahad O'Connor, "Four Drugs Cause Most Hospitalizations in Older Adults," *The New York Times*, November 23, 2011 http://well.blogs.nytimes.com/2011/11/23/four-drugs-cause-most-hospitalizations-in-older-adults/):

Just four medications or medication groups—used alone or together—were responsible for two-thirds of emergency hospitalizations among older Americans, according to the report. At the top of the list was warfarin, also known as Coumadin, a blood thinner. It accounted for 33 percent of emergency hospital visits. Insulin injections were next on the list, accounting for 14 percent of emergency visits.

Aspirin, clopidogrel and other antiplatelet drugs that help prevent blood clotting were involved in 13 percent of emergency visits. And just behind them were diabetes drugs taken by mouth, called oral hypoglycemic agents, which were implicated in 11 percent of hospitalizations.

All these drugs are commonly prescribed to older adults, and they can be hard to use correctly. One problem they share is a narrow therapeutic index, meaning the line between an effective dose and a hazardous one is thin.

…Some require blood testing to adjust their doses, and a small dose can have a powerful effect. Blood sugar can be notoriously hard to control in people with diabetes, for example, and taking a slightly larger dose of insulin than needed can send a person into shock. Warfarin, meanwhile, is the classic example of a drug with a narrow margin between therapeutic and toxic doses, requiring regular blood monitoring, and it can interact with many other drugs and foods. …

One thing that stood out in the data, the researchers noted, was that none of the four drugs identified as frequent culprits are typically among the types of drugs labeled "high risk" for older adults by major health care groups. The medications that are usually designated high risk or "potentially inappropriate" are commonly used over-the-counter drugs like Benadryl, as well as Demerol and other powerful narcotic painkillers. And yet those drugs accounted for only about 8 percent of emergency hospitalizations among the elderly.

4

Lawsuits against pharmacists for major pharmacy mistakes

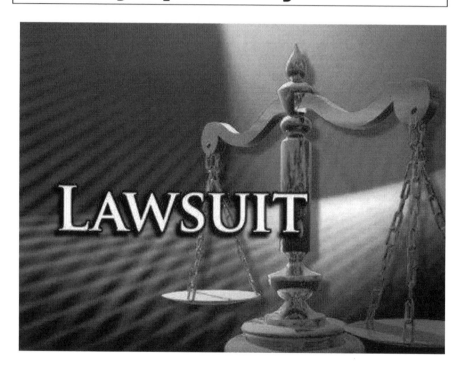

How do chain pharmacists react when they read about huge settlements in pharmacy mistake cases? In my experience, many chain pharmacists seem to react positively, figuring that the only thing that will get the attention of chain management is million dollar jury awards. I've heard several pharmacists comment something like, "Well I hope that the media coverage embarrasses the chains into providing adequate staffing so that pharmacy mistakes aren't inevitable."

[Please note: Throughout this book, brand name drugs are capitalized and generic names are in lower case.]

DEATH

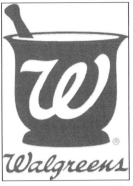

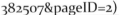

1. Walgreens pharmacist dispensed diabetes drug glipizide to Leonard Kulisek instead of gout drug allopurinol, leading to renal failure, stroke and death—$31.3 million award in Illinois

A Cook County, Illinois jury awarded $31.3 million to the estate of **Leonard Kulisek**, a Schaumburg man who died in 2002 after becoming ill the previous year when a Walgreens pharmacist gave him the wrong medication. Kulisek was supposed to pick up his gout medication but was given glipizide, a drug used to treat diabetes. The drug dropped his blood sugar to dangerously low levels and triggered a string of health problems, including a stroke in May 2001. ("Walgreens to appeal $31 million med-error award," *Drug Topics*, Nov. 6, 2006
http://www.drugtopics.com/drugtopics/article/articleDetail.jsp?id=382507&pageID=2)

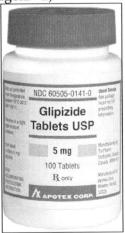

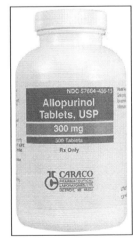

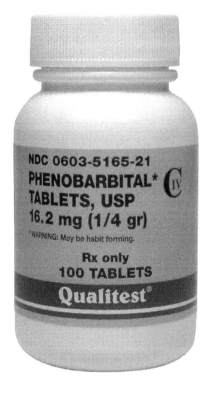

NDC 0603-5165-21
PHENOBARBITAL* C IV
TABLETS, USP
16.2 mg (1/4 gr)
*WARNING: May be habit forming.

Rx only
100 TABLETS
Qualitest®

2. Thrifty-Payless drugstore dispensed 100 mg of phenobarbital to <u>Bryn Cabanillas</u> instead of 15 mg prescribed dose— brain damage— $30.6 million award in California

A California jury awarded $30.6 million to the family of a girl who suffered brain damage following a phenobarbital dispensing error at a Thrifty Payless drugstore in Costa Mesa in 1994. The jury concluded that **Bryn Cabanillas** suffered brain damage after a Thrifty Payless drugstore dispensed 100 mg of phenobarbital instead of the 15 mg prescribed. The jury decided that the girl, who was born with cerebral palsy, should be paid $5.3 million for past damages and $25.3 million to cover medical costs and other living expenses during her projected 50-year lifespan. The panel found that the error took 20 years off her life. (Carol Ukens, "A jury awards $30 million in Rx error lawsuit," *Drug Topics*, August 3, 1998, p. 15)

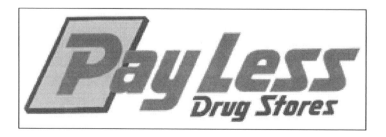

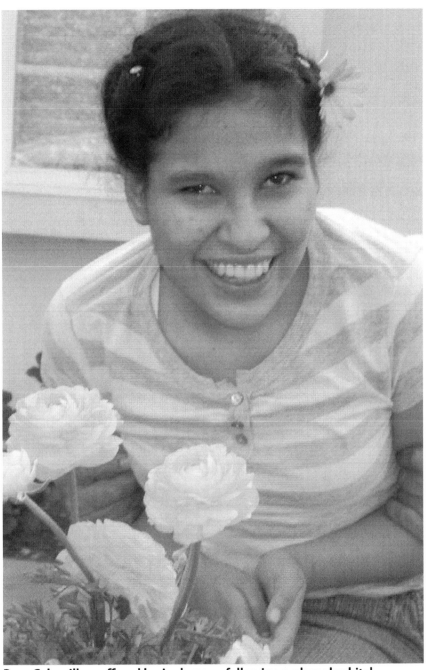

Bryn Cabanillas suffered brain damage following a phenobarbital dispending error at a California drugstore. The jury awarded $30.6 million.

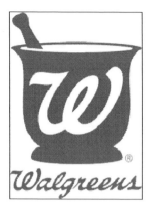

3. Walgreens dispensed blood thinner warfarin at 10 times the dose prescribed to <u>Beth Hippely</u>, causing cerebral hemorrhage—Teenage pharmacy technician's error—$25.8 million award in Florida

A jury awarded $25.8 million to the family of a cancer patient who was given a wrong prescription, had a stroke and died several years later, lawyers said on Aug. 17, 2007. **Beth Hippely** was prescribed warfarin, a blood thinner, in 2002 to treat breast cancer. The prescription filled at a Walgreens pharmacy was 10 times what her doctor prescribed, court documents said. The Polk County [Florida] Circuit Court jury found the prescription error caused a cerebral hemorrhage resulting in permanent bodily injury, disability and physical pain. The mother of three died in January 2007 at the age of 46. A 19-year-old pharmacy technician, with little training, misfilled the prescription, according to court documents. "Beth Hippely died unnecessarily because this tenfold overdose with warfarin by the pharmacy she trusted caused her cancer to come back with a vengeance and it interrupted all of her cancer treatments," her lawyer Chris Searcy said. (Associated Press, Bartow, Florida, Aug. 18, 2007,
http://www.cbsnews.com/stories/2007/08/18/business/main318097
9.shtml)

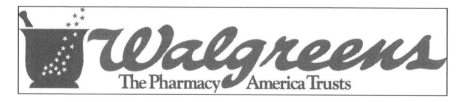

Walgreens Told to Pay $25.8 Million Over Teen Pharmacy Tech's Error
March 1, 2010
By AVNI PATEL and BRIAN ROSS
ABC News Chief Investigative Correspondent

http://abcnews.go.com/Blotter/walgreens-told-pay-285-mil-teen-pharmacy-techs/story?id=9977262

A Florida appeals court has upheld a $25.8 million judgment against Walgreens over an error by a teenage pharmacy technician that resulted in a mother of three receiving blood thinner pills with a dosage ten times greater than prescribed.

Beth Hippely of Lakeland, Florida, suffered a massive, crippling stroke after taking the pills and was forced to stop treatment for early stage breast cancer. She died in 2007, before the case went to trial.

The judgment against Walgreens was one of the largest ever because of a prescription error and the appeals court upheld it without comment last Friday.

The lawyer for the Hippely family, Karen Terry, said "justice has finally been served after eight years in which Walgreens has dragged out this litigation."

The case highlighted the use by major drug store chains of pharmacy technicians who in many states are not required to have a high school diploma.

In court testimony, the technician, Janelle Banks, said she had typed in "ten milligrams" on Hippely's prescription when it should have been one milligram.

Prior to working at Walgreens, the teen had worked at a movie theater where she made popcorn.

"If they don't change things they are going to continue to see judgments and maim people," said Terry, the Hippely family lawyer.

There is no minimum national standard for the training of pharmacy technicians who are supposed to work under the close supervision of licensed pharmacists.

'The Same Level of Training as Someone Working in Fast Food'

Walgreens would not comment on the Hippely case ruling, but said, in a statement, "We continuously work to improve quality, accuracy and service and we provide continuous training development programs for all pharmacy staff."

Critics say the major drug store chains have adopted a "fast food" culture to enhance profits, pushing pharmacists to oversee the prescriptions filled by as many as four or five technicians at a time.

"In fact, a lot of the people working in the pharmacy have about the same level of training as someone that would be working in fast food," said Trent Speckhals, an Atlanta lawyer now involved in a number of prescription error lawsuits.

"Forgetting to put your fries in the bag isn't going to lead to any harm, but obviously we're dealing with something much more serious with medicine," he said.

In a lawsuit he is bringing against Kroger's, Speckhals said pharmacy technicians complained of being overworked and afraid to take time to go to the bathroom.

There are no publicly available figures on the number of prescription errors in the country because pharmacies are not required under federal law to report prescription errors, even those resulting in serious injury or death. The actual error rates are treated by the big drug chains as closely held secrets, and they will not disclose even whether the number of errors has gone up or down over the years.

"I'm not aware of a public desire to know" the rates, said Edith Rosato, executive director of the National Chain Drug Store trade group.

The group has opposed calls for mandatory reporting of serious errors, but Rosato said, "If there was a requirement to report it, a federal requirement, our members would comply because they comply with the law."

Rosato said the chains strive "to put procedures in place, whether it's advancements in technician training, whether it's new technologies, that allow for verification of the prescription with the actual tablet in the bottle."

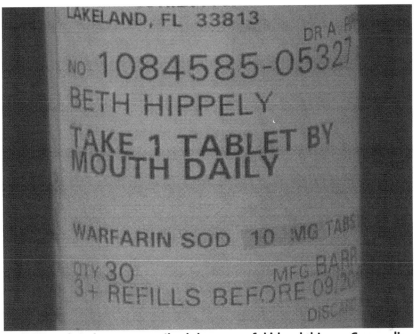

LAKELAND, FL 33813

DR A.

NO 1084585-0532

BETH HIPPELY

TAKE 1 TABLET BY
MOUTH DAILY

WARFARIN SOD 10 MG TABS

QTY 30   MFG BARR
3+ REFILLS BEFORE 09.20

DISC

Beth Hippely's doctor prescribed the powerful blood thinner Coumadin (warfarin) after she began chemotherapy for a treatable stage II breast cancer. But Walgreen's gave Beth pills that were ten times the prescribed dose. Walgreen's paid $25.8 million for this pharmacy mistake.

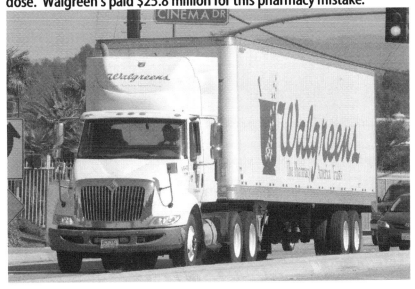

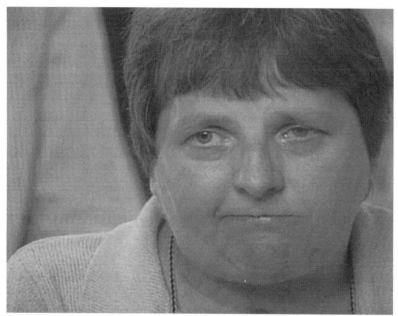

Beth Hippely was an active mother of three from Lakeland, Florida, who was left brain-damaged, disabled and unable to care for herself and her family after she suffered a stroke. A Walgreen's pharmacy technician, who was just a high school student at the time, gave her the wrong dosage for a prescribed blood thinner.

(*ABC News*, http://abcnews.go.com/Blotter/popup?id=2991778)

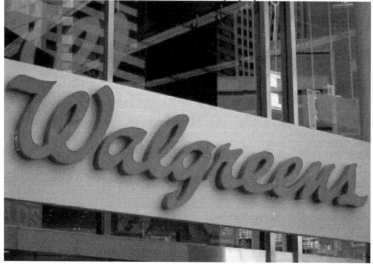

4. Walgreens dispensed adult diabetes drug glipizide to infant girl <u>Alexandra Gehrke</u> instead of anti-seizure drug phenobarbital— $21 million judgment in Illinois

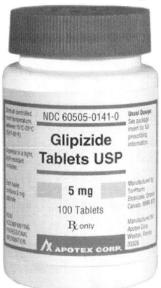
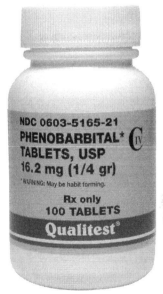

A prescription medicine Tracey Gehrke got from a Walgreens in Illinois was supposed to prevent seizures in her infant daughter, who had been born prematurely. The pharmacy instead filled **Alexandra Gehrke**'s prescription with an adult diabetes drug. A Cook County jury awarded $21 million to the Gehrke family, of Elgin. (Michael Higgins, "A $21 Million Judgment Against Walgreens in the Case of a Paralyzed Elgin Girl Points Up Potential Dangers in 3 Million Annual Pharmacy Errors," chicagotribune.com, August 11, 2004)

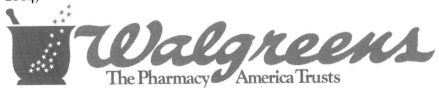

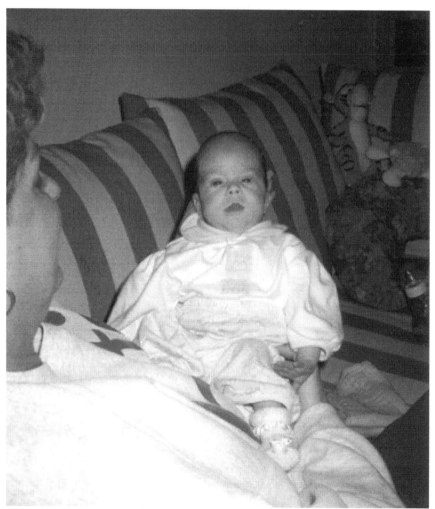

Alexandra Gehrke, seen here at seven months old, was given the wrong medicaton for seven weeks. Instead of preventing seizures in Alexandra, the medicine given to her mother by a Walgreen's pharmacist caused them, resulting in severe brain damage that doctors say will affect Alexandra for the rest of her life.

5. Pharmacist prepared contaminated chemotherapy for <u>Anton Weck</u>, causing paralysis—$18.5 million jury award in New Jersey

A New Jersey Superior court jury awarded $18.5 million to a man who was paralyzed from the waist down after he received contaminated chemotherapy treatment for leukemia. The jury found Eun Mi Jhun, the pharmacist who prepared the contaminated medication, responsible for the paralysis. The contaminated dose was injected into the spine of **Anton Weck** in 2001, resulting in his paralysis. Weck had previously been undergoing chemotherapy for three years and was receiving his final dose at the time he was paralyzed. (http://www.totalinjury.com/verdicts_medical_injury.asp)

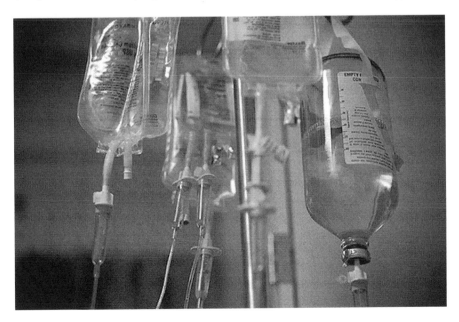

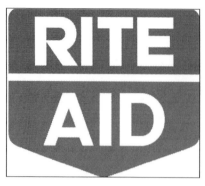

6. Rite Aid pharmacist dispensed adult diabetes drug Glynase to young girl instead of Ritalin— brain damage—$16 million award

A young girl who suffered brain damage as a result of a dispensing error by a Rite Aid pharmacist was awarded $16 million in damages under a jury verdict. Instead of Ritalin to treat the child's attention deficit disorder, the pharmacist dispensed Glynase—a drug used to reduce blood sugar levels in diabetics. ("Newsbites," *Drug Store News*, November 4, 1996, p. 15.)

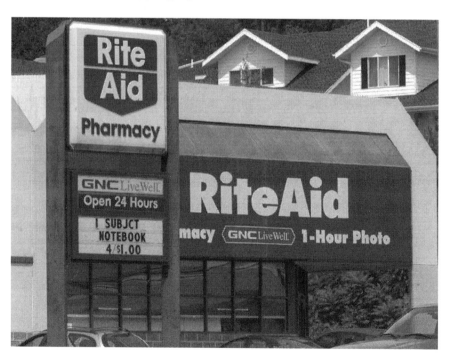

7. Pharmacy dispensed anti-asthma drug theophylline to nursing home patient instead of pain killer Darvocet— $15 million settlement

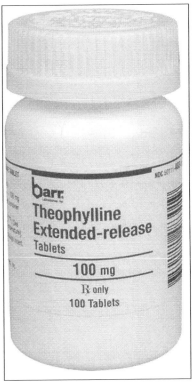

A pharmacist phoned a nursing home to inform the staff that the wrong drug had been sent to one of the home's patients. He explained that pharmacy technicians mistakenly filled a prescription for the pain killer Darvocet with the anti-asthma drug theophylline. The patient deteriorated, and he ultimately died. The patient's family sued, claiming the wrong drug caused seizures, a reversal in his recovery, and ultimately, his death. On the eve of the defendant's motion to dismiss the wrongful death action, the parties settled for $15 million. (Health Providers Service Organization—HPSO. (1999). Pharmacy. Medical Malpractice, Verdicts, Settlements, and Experts, 18(7), 41 http://www.hpso.com/newsletters/1-2000/pharm2.shtml#lesson)

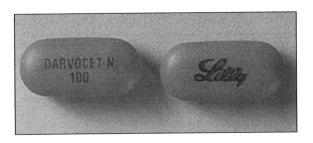

DEATH

8. <u>Genesis Burkett</u>, a six weeks old baby, died after a hospital pharmacy mistake caused a fatal dose of IV sodium chloride—$8.25 million settlement in Illinois

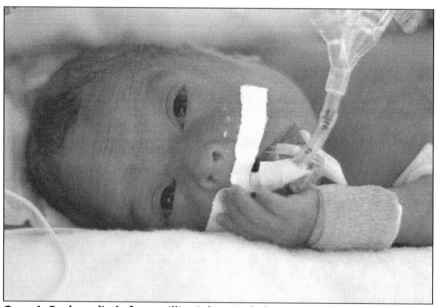

Genesis Burkett died after an Illinois hospital pharmacy error caused a fatal dose of IV sodium chloride. $8.25 Million settlement.

Born 15 weeks premature, **Genesis Burkett** survived despite weighing just 1 pound, 8 ounces. But the little boy couldn't survive a medication mistake made at a suburban hospital that gave him the wrong IV dosage and took his life when he was 40 days old. Advocate Lutheran General Hospital in Park Ridge has agreed to settle his par-

ents' wrongful-death lawsuit for $8.25 million—the largest such settlement ever in Illinois, according to the parents' lawyers. Fritzie and Cameron Burkett, of Chicago, are relieved the hospital acknowledged the error that killed their only child, their attorney said Thursday. "They're grateful the hospital recognized their significant loss," Patrick Salvi said. "They hope it never happens again." Genesis Burkett died at the hospital on Oct. 15, 2010, after receiving a fatal dose of sodium chloride in an IV administered to him after heart surgery. The suit claimed an error made by the hospital pharmacy resulted in Genesis getting a dose 60 times the amount that was prescribed by the boy's doctor, causing the infant to go into cardiac arrest and die. "The pharmacy made a critical mistake," Salvi said. A hospital investigation showed the mistake occurred because the dosage for the boy's IV "had been incorrectly entered into the machine that mixes IV solutions," Lutheran General spokesman Greg Alford said. Since his death, the hospital has changed procedures to prevent similar mistakes, according to Alford, who said, "We have taken comprehensive steps . . .to ensure this type of tragedy does not happen again." (Dan Rozek, "Couple whose baby died from wrong IV dose gets $8.25 million," *Chicago Sun Times*, April 5, 2012
http://www.suntimes.com/news/metro/11730830-418/couple-whose-baby-died-from-wrong-iv-dose-gets-825-million.html)

9. Thrift Drug pharmacist dispensed double the maximum allowable dose of Rocaltrol to <u>Michael Brown</u>— $8 million award in Pennsylvania

A Pittsburgh jury awarded **Michael Brown** $8 million in a drug error lawsuit against J. C. Penney, parent of Thrift Drug. The suit alleged that a Thrift pharmacist mistranscribed a telephone prescription for Rocaltrol, synthetic vitamin D. As a result, Brown, then 17, received a dosage that was double the maximum allowable. He went into hypercalcemic crisis and is totally disabled by seizures. ("Jury awards $8 million in drug error suit," *Drug Topics*, October 7, 1996, p. 7.)

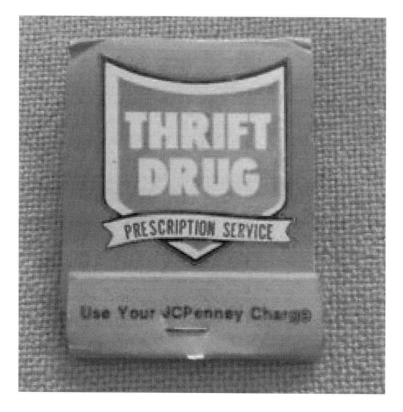

10. Pharmacy error causes kidney transplant patient <u>Tiffany Phillips</u> to take 1,250 mg of prednisone daily for 3 days, instead of 250 mg daily—loss of kidney—$7.7 million award in South Carolina—Eckerd and CVS settle

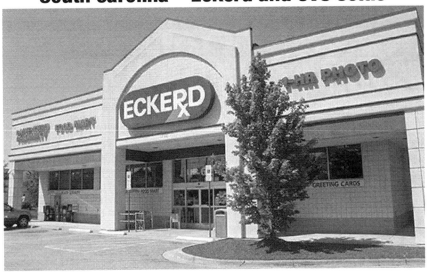

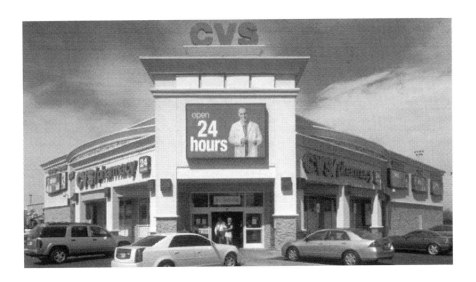

Late in 2006, a jury delivered a verdict ordering Eckerd Corporation to pay Ms. **Tiffany Phillips** $7.7 million for a pharmacy error which resulted in the loss of the young woman's new kidney. CVS, also a named defendant in the action, reached a confidential settlement with Phillips for an undisclosed amount. In 2002, plaintiff Tiffany Phillips went to the Eckerd pharmacy in Lancaster, South Carolina, to get a prescription filled for an anti-rejection drug (prednisone) in connection with a recent kidney transplant. The Lancaster Eckerd didn't have enough of the medication on site, so a pharmacy technician called a Lancaster CVS pharmacy to fill the entire prescription. However, an apparent miscommunication between the two stores occurred, resulting in Ms. Phillips being instructed to take 1250 milligrams a day of the drug for three days, over four times the intended amount of 250 milligrams. After taking the drug dispensed to her, Phillip's new kidney failed and she underwent a second kidney transplant. [*The Charlotte Observer*, Dec. 21, 2006, Page 1B. See also grossmanjustice.com (Law Offices of Scott. D. Grossman, LLC, Freehold, New Jersey, posted on March 28, 2007 by Scott Grossman), http://injurylaw.grossmanjustice.com/2007/03/articles/pharmacy-error/pharmacy-error-case-results-in-8-million-verdict/]

11. Pharmacy failed to dilute adult medication—Infant <u>Joey Rice</u> received massive overdose of high blood pressure drug enalaprilat—$7.1 million award in Massachusetts

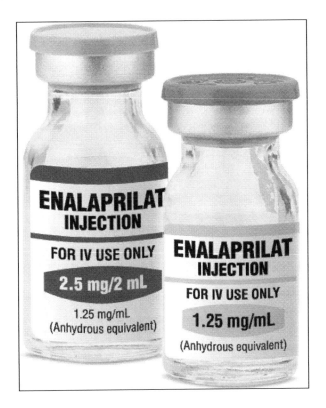

A Suffolk County, Mass. jury awarded $7.1 million in damages to the family of **Joey Rice**, a 4-year old Newton boy who, as a premature infant, received a massive overdose of the high blood pressure drug enalaprilat after pharmacists at Children's Hospital in Boston failed to dilute an adult medication. The dose had more than 100 times the proper amount. (Anne Barnard, "Family Awarded $7.1m for Overdose, *The Boston Globe*, March 28, 2002)

DEATH

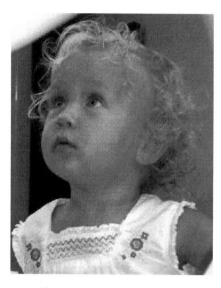

12. Death of <u>Emily Jerry</u>, two-year-old Ohio girl, after hospital pharmacy improperly compounded intravenous solution—$7 million settlement

An Ohio grand jury has indicted pharmacist Eric Cropp for manslaughter and reckless homicide in the death of a two-year-old child, which resulted from an improperly compounded IV solution. Both charges carry penalties of up to five years in prison. The medical error occurred in 2006 at Rainbow Babies & Children's Hospital where the child, **Emily Jerry**, was a patient undergoing chemotherapy. According to testimony presented before the Ohio board of pharmacy, the prescription for etoposide with a base solution of 0.9% sodium chloride was instead compounded by a technician with a base solution of 23.4% sodium chloride. Three days after receiving the medication, the child died. The grand jury declined to indict the technician, Katie Dudash. (Reid Paul, "Former pharmacist indicted for manslaughter after med error," *Drug Topics*, Sept. 17, 2007, p. 10. See also the Emily Jerry Foundation emilyjerryfoundation.org and http://emilyjerryfoundation.org/man-seeks-nationwide-law-after-toddlers-death/)

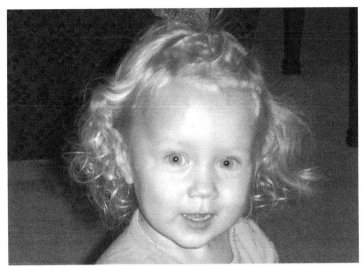

Emily Jerry was killed by a pharmacy error at age two.

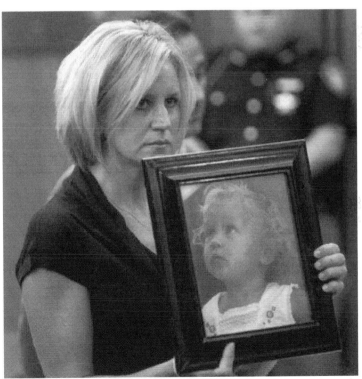

The mother of Emily Jerry holding a picture of her daughter who was killed by a pharmacy mistake.

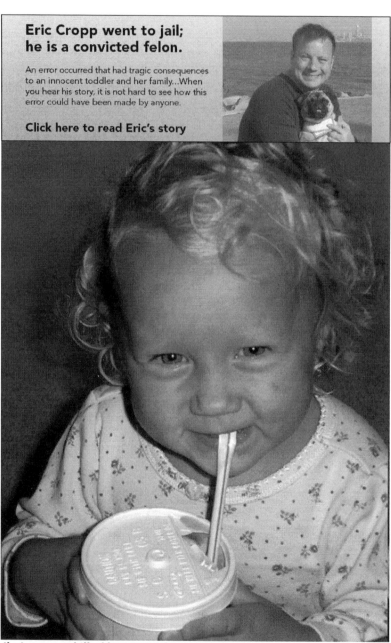

Eric Cropp went to jail; he is a convicted felon.

An error occurred that had tragic consequences to an innocent toddler and her family...When you hear his story, it is not hard to see how this error could have been made by anyone.

Click here to read Eric's story

Emily Jerry was killed by a mistake in which a hospital pharmacy incorrectly prepared an intravenous solution. Controversially, the pharmacist who was responsible for the error was sentenced to—and actually served–time in prison.

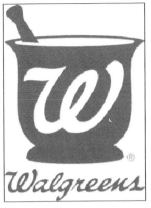

13. Walgreens dispensed female hormone Cycrin to <u>E. Nathan Johnson</u> rather than the prescribed blood thinner Coumadin—$6 million settlement in Florida

The insurance carrier for Walgreens agreed to pay $6 million to settle a dispensing error lawsuit in Daytona Beach, Fla. A Walgreens pharmacy dispensed Cycrin, a female hormone, to the plaintiff, **E. Nathan Johnson**, instead of the Coumadin prescribed. He took the wrong drug for eleven days before his wife discovered the error. Two days later, he suffered a stroke and subsequently a heart attack that left him in a coma. He now resides in a special care facility. "Walgreen settles Rx suit," *Drug Topics*, October 7, 1996, p. 7.)

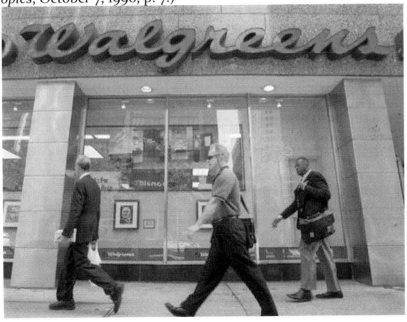

DEATH

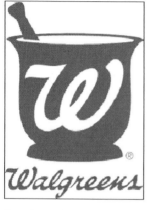

14. Thirty-one year-old high school wrestling coach Eric Warren dies from interaction between tramadol and methadone—Walgreens in Arizona—$6 million award

Most prescription errors don't cause major health problems, but the outcomes occasionally can be catastrophic. Walgreens has lost three trials involving deaths caused by drug mistakes since September 2006. Verdicts in the cases totaled more than $61 million. The cases include the 2002 death of Eric Warren, a 31-year-old Arizona high school wrestling coach. He died from an interaction between tramadol and methadone, painkillers dispensed at different times by a Walgreens pharmacy in Flagstaff, Ariz. A jury awarded his family $6 million in October 2007 after hearing evidence that Walgreens pharmacist Al Salembier neither warned Warren about the potential drug interaction nor double-checked the second prescription with his doctor. Walgreens is appealing the case. **(Kevin McCoy and Erik Brady, "Speed, High Volume Can Trigger Mistakes,"** *USA Today*, **February 11, 2008**
http://www.usatoday.com/money/industries/health/2008-02-11-prescrption-errors_N.htm   Accessed March 16, 2008)

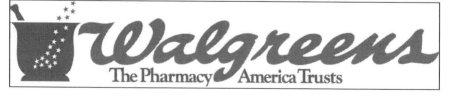

15. Pharmacy dispensed the synthetic thyroid hormone Synthroid .025 mg to 71-yr-old man instead of Synthroid .125 mg— $5 million settlement in Texas

A 71-year-old man was given a prescription for .125 mg Synthroid #100. His pharmacy filled it with .025 Synthroid #100. Due to the error, the patient suffered respiratory distress and weakness. The man sued and the case was settled for $5 million plus taxable costs. (Health Providers Service Organization—HPSO. Staff. 1998. Pharmacy. Medical Malpractice, Verdicts, Settlements, and Experts, 14(8), 54.
http://www.hpso.com/newsletters/6-99/pharm1.html#court)

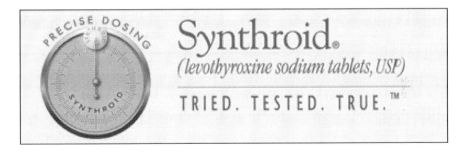

16. Amphotericin ordered for child with infection following appendectomy prepared in adult dosage, instead of child dosage–Cardiac arrest and renal failure—$3.85 million settlement includes $200,000 to child's sister, who witnessed cardiac arrest

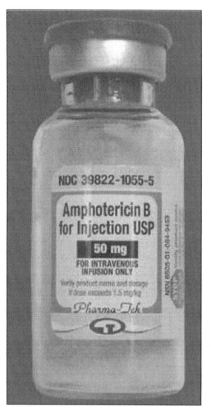

The plaintiff, age nine, was taken to a hospital in August 2006 due to an infection after the removal of her appendix. The antifungal drug, Amphotericin, was prescribed, but the hospital's pharmacy prepared an adult dose rather than one for a child. Shortly after taking the drug intravenously, the child went into cardiac arrest and renal failure with her seven year-old sister watching. She was resuscitated after being given blood transfusions and then transferred to another hospital for a six-week stay. The child suffers post-traumatic stress disorder, but has no physical sequella from the incident. According to a published account a $3.85 million settlement was reached, which included $200,000 to the sister who witnessed the arrest.

(April 2010 Legal Case Study, HPSO—Healthcare Providers Service Organization

http://www.hpso.com/case-studies/casestudy-article/328.jsp)

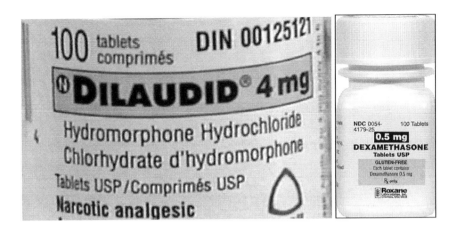

17. Dilaudid prescription filled with dexamethasone—Cushing's Syndrome and depression—$2.5 million verdict

The plaintiff had rheumatoid arthritis and obtained a prescription for Dilaudid from her physician in November 2006. She took it to the pharmacy to be filled. The plaintiff was dispensed dexamethasone. After a couple of weeks the plaintiff noted that her pain continued. She returned to the pharmacy and was told that the prescription was correct. She continued to have pain and went to her physician, who immediately realized the error. The plaintiff was referred to another physician who gave her a prescription to taper the dosage of the dexamethasone to wean her off gradually. The plaintiff, however, suffered depression, psychiatric disorders, brain damage, cognitive damage, exacerbation of her previous medical problems and Cushing's Syndrome. The plaintiff declined from an active lifestyle to wheelchair confinement. The plaintiff alleged negligence in dispensing the medication. The defendant admitted negligence, but disputed any long-term, permanent injuries. According to the *Jury Verdict Reporter,* a $2.5 million verdict was returned. (July 2010 Legal Case Study, HPSO—

http://www.hpso.com/case-studies/casestudy-article/331.jsp)

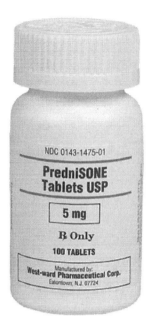

NDC 0143-1475-01

**PredniSONE
Tablets USP**

5 mg

℞ Only

100 TABLETS

Manufactured by:
West-ward Pharmaceutical Corp.
Eatontown, N.J. 07724

18. Pharmacy confusion caused patient to take 320 mg of prednisone daily for weeks instead of 80 mg daily—$2.5 million award in North Carolina

The defendant physician intended to prescribe an 80 mg daily dose of prednisone for the plaintiff's loss of kidney function. The pharmacist who received the prescription claimed that it indicated that 80 mg be taken 4 times a day, for a daily total of 320 mg. After receiving the first refill, the patient went to the emergency room and was diagnosed with thrush. He continued taking the 320 mg of prednisone daily for 23 days, until a follow-up visit with the physician revealed the dosage error. The plaintiff contracted a bacterial infection of the lungs and aspergillosis, a fungal infection of the brain, resulting in numerous operations and hospital stays. The plaintiff suffered permanent kidney failure and will require dialysis for the rest of his life. He sued the physician and the clinic for negligently writing the prescription and the pharmacy chain for negligence in dispensing the drug. Following the trial against the pharmacy chain, the jury awarded the plaintiff $2.5 million in compensatory damages. The appellate court upheld the verdict. (Larry M. Simonsmeier, JD, RPh, "The Dosage Was Too High, No Matter Where the Rx Was Filled," *Pharmacy Times,* December 2002 http://www.pharmacytimes.com/Article.cfm?Menu=1&ID=288   Accessed March 9, 2006)

19. Medication error in child with Urea Cycle Syndrome results in excessive blood ammonia levels and brain damage— $2.5 million settlement in New Jersey

At the age of two and four months, the child experienced severe hyperammonemia requiring hospitalization. The correct protocol was ordered, but prepared in an incorrect concentration by the hospital pharmacist. The patient's nurse then elevated an IV bag containing the prepared formula, but failed to compare the label on the bag (prepared by the pharmacist) with the written order from the physician. As a result, the patient received only twenty-five percent of the required medication over a period of nineteen hours. This under-medication situation resulted in escalating and dangerously high blood ammonia levels. When the error was discovered, the hospital failed to timely perform hemodialysis to remove the high levels of ammonia from the blood. The patient went into coma and was airlifted to another hospital for treatment. He suffered permanent brain injury as a result of the medication error. Eight years old at the time of settlement, the child is permanently disabled and has a seizure disorder. The case settled tor $2,500,000. ("Medication Error in Child With Urea Cycle Syndrome Results in Excessive Blood Ammonia Levels and Brain Damage—$2.5 Million Settlement in New Jersey," January 2003 Legal Case Study, Healthcare Providers Service Organization, http://www.hpso.com/case/cases_prof_index.php3?id=70&prof=Ph armacist Grecco v. Unnamed Hospital, Essex County, New Jersey, Superior Court)

DEATH

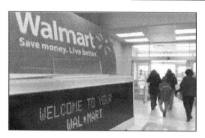

20. Death: Wal-Mart pharmacist dispensed Ziac instead of Zaroxolyn—$1.27 million award

The Arkansas Supreme Court upheld a $1.27 million jury award for a woman whose husband died after a Wal-Mart pharmacist gave him the wrong prescription medication, which he took for two and a half months before his death. Wal-Mart's lawyers had appealed the earlier verdict, saying there was insufficient evidence of the cause of his death and that the award to his widow and daughter was excessive. The man died in 1997 after a Wal-Mart R.Ph. in Arkansas filled his prescription for Zaroxolyn, a diuretic, with Ziac, a high blood pressure medication. The drug allowed fluid to accumulate in his body and caused severe weight gain. He died of congestive heart failure. ("Court upholds jury award in Wal-Mart death case," *Drug Topics,* July 14, 2003

http://www.drugtopics.com/be_core/d/templates/issue/show_article.jsp?styles heet=/be_core/d/stylesheets/xslt/view_free_pages.xsl&file-name=/be_core/d/online_only_content/free_pages/latehot.xml&showPoll=no)

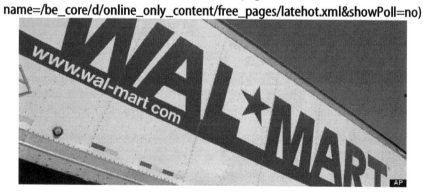

21. Pregnant woman's prescription for Medrol filled with dexamethasone— Child born with multiple problems— $1.1 million settlement

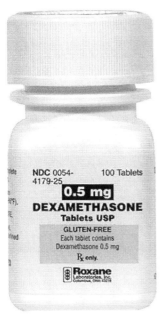

The plaintiff mother was prescribed Medrol in a two-milligram dose for a pulmonary problem in May 2005 when she was five months pregnant. The plaintiff claimed that the defendant's pharmacist filled the prescription with dexamethasone, which should not be taken during pregnancy and that the four-milligram dose was twenty times the normal amount for that drug. The woman's son was born prematurely, weighing two pounds and suffers from severe growth retardation, impaired speech, motor weakness and esophagitis as a result of the pharmacy error. The woman continued to take the wrong drug until March 2006, when her physician made an investigation after she developed swelling problems. The defendant claimed that the pharmacy error was caused by the woman's physician and that the child's problems were due to the mother's pre-eclampsia. According to a published account, a $1.1 million settlement was reached, most of which was placed into a structured settlement for the child. ("Pregnant woman's prescription for Medrol filled with dexamethasone—Child born with multiple problems—$1.1 million settlement," Health Providers Service Organization, January 2011 Legal Case Study, http://www.hpso.com/case-studies/casestudy-article/339.jsp)

22. K-Mart's label instructed <u>Alan Glock</u> to take 20 mg of blood thinner Coumadin daily instead of 5 mg daily—Overdose caused complications from hip surgery—$1.05 million Indiana verdict

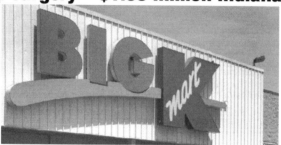

Dr. Alan Glock, then age fifty-nine, had been an orthopedic surgeon since the middle 1960's. In the fall of 1997, severe osteoarthritic changes necessitated a hip replacement which was performed on October 2, 1997 by Dr. Jeffrey Pierson. On October 5, 1997, Dr. Glock was discharged from the hospital with a prescription for Coumadin, a blood-thinning drug. He was advised to take one pill daily. The prescription was filled at K-Mart and store employees indicate Dr. Glock was advised to take one five milligram pill per day. Despite this warning, K-Mart's labeling instructed that the five milligram pills should be taken four times daily. As a result of the excessive Coumadin intake, the plaintiff's recovery from the hip surgery was prolonged for an additional three months, which otherwise would not have occurred. The plaintiff continues to report additional complex symptoms, all resulting from the overdose of Coumadin, and he has been unable to return to the practice of medicine. The problems include intra-cranial bleeding, with resulting vision and hearing problems, and a compartment syndrome in his hip. ("Instructions for Coumadin Written on Bottle Incorrectly—Overdose Causes Complications From Hip Surgery—$1,052,461 Verdict in Indiana," June 2002 Legal Case Study, Healthcare Providers Service Organization
http://www.hpso.com/case/cases_prof_index.php3?id=63&prof=Ph armacist Alan Glock and Carolyn Glock v. K-Mart, U.S. District Court, District of Indiana at Indianapolis, Case No.99 CV 1184)

23. Woman claims misfilling of anti-hypertension drug Toprol with anti-psychotic drug Zyprexa caused disabling stroke— $1 Million gross verdict in Louisiana

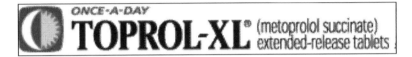

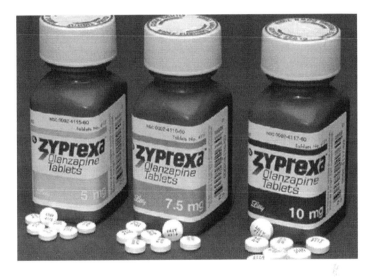

The plaintiff, age fifty-two at the time, had been under care for hypertension and was prescribed Toprol. The plaintiff then moved to out of state after severe weather in her home area. She returned to her home area in June 2006. In June 2006 the plaintiff was not feeling well and sought to transfer her Toprol prescription from her out of state pharmacy to a nearby local pharmacy location.

The plaintiff asked her son to pick it up for her and he used the drive-thru window to pick up the medication. The local pharmacy dispensed 20 milligram tablets of Zyprexa instead of Toprol. The 20 milligram tablets of Zyprexa is the maximum allowed dosage and is four times the drug's starting dosage. The plaintiff took one tablet that afternoon. Later that day she felt dizzy and nauseous. She laid down and asked for another Toprol pill.

A family friend with a background in nursing was present and recognized the medication as Zyprexa, not Toprol. The plaintiff went to an emergency room immediately. Her blood pressure was high and erratic, but was brought under control with administration of Toprol. The plaintiff was discharged early the next morning. The plaintiff then developed symptoms of arm numbness, nausea and vomiting. She went to another facility, where she was diagnosed as having suffered a stroke. The plaintiff was diagnosed with brain damage resulting in deficits for tasks associated with right cerebral hemisphere functioning. This includes cognitive disorder, major depressive disorder, residual left hemiparesis, as well as other deficits. The plaintiff is totally and permanently disabled and unable to live independently. The plaintiff had suffered two additional strokes in 2007 and 2008. The plaintiff maintained that the stroke was due to the ingestion of Zyprexa.

The local pharmacy admitted mis-filling the prescription, but claimed that the plaintiff and her son should have noticed that the wrong drug was dispensed. The defendant also claimed that the plaintiff's stroke was due to her underlying health problems, including diabetes, obesity, high cholesterol and high blood pressure. The defendant also claimed that the plaintiff had a long history of non-compliance with physician's instructions regarding medication and diet. The local pharmacy also maintained that the plaintiff had been prescribed Toprol in September 2005 with two refills, but no refill had occurred until the incident in question. The local pharmacy also maintained that the plaintiff had suffered another stroke prior to June 2006 which had never been diagnosed.

According to *Louisiana Jury Verdict Reporter* a jury found the local pharmacy sixty percent at fault, the plaintiff thirty percent at fault and the plaintiff's son five percent at fault. The jury awarded $1 million. ("Woman Claims Mis-Filling of Toprol With Zyprexa Caused Disabling Stroke—Local Pharmacy Claimed Woman Had Already Had an Undiagnosed Stroke—$1 Million Gross Verdict," . August 2013 Legal Case Study, Healthcare Providerss Service Organization, http://www.hpso.com/case-studies/casestudy-article/393.jsp)

24. Patient given three times prescribed dose of anti-seizure drug Dilantin for several days— Dilantin toxicity blamed for acceleration of dementia— $1 Million verdict in Alabama

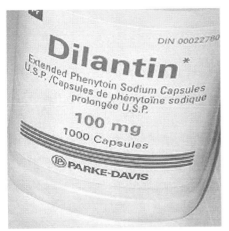

The plaintiff, a seventy-seven year-old man, alleged that the staff at the defendant Birmingham hospital overmedicated him with anti-seizure medication so severely in 1999 that his dementia was accelerated, and he suffered additional brain damage and damage to his sense of balance. He claimed that during a May 26 through June 1, 1999 hospitalization at Baptist Medical Center Montclair, after a fall at his home, he was given more than three times the dose of Dilantin than what his physician prescribed. Robert Ferguson testified that he was able to drive, hunt, fish, and walk on his own prior to the hospitalization. But the overdose left him with severely altered memory, and dependent on a cane and wheelchair. ("Nurse and Pharmacy Staff Err in Administering Treble Dose of Dilantin—Dilantin Toxicity Blamed for Acceleration of Dementia and Damage to Balance—$1 Million Verdict in Alabama," August 2003 Legal Case Study, Healthcare Providers Service Organization http://www.hpso.com/case/cases_prof_index.php3   Robert Ferguson v. Baptist Health System d/b/a Baptist Medical Center, Montclair. Jefferson County, Alabama.)

25. Plaintiff claims improper pharmacy directions caused him to ingest 100 mg of prednisone daily for 17 days (instead of for 5 days)—$1 Million settlement in New York

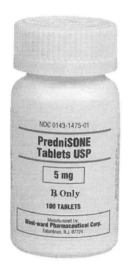

In January 1995, the defendants dispensed the steroid prednisone to the plaintiff, a thirty-six-year-old electrician. The plaintiff claimed that the defendants failed to properly label the prescription, which should have instructed him to ingest 100 milligrams of prednisone daily for five days only. The plaintiff ingested 100 milligrams for nearly seventeen days, and he then required additional prednisone for a gradual taper from the medication. The plaintiff claimed that defendants also altered the strength of the tablets prescribed—instead of dispensing fifty tablets, each containing ten milligrams, defendants dispensed fifty tablets, each containing fifty milligrams, resulting in the plaintiff ingesting an additional 1670 milligrams of prednisone than was intended by his oncologist. He subsequently developed avascular necrosis of the hips, which, he claimed, was a direct result of the excess medication ingested. The plaintiff requires bilateral hip replacements. According to The New York Jury Verdict Reporter, this action settled for $1,000,000 during trial. ("Improper Labeling of Prescription—Overdose of Prednisone—Bilateral Avascular Necrosis of the Hips—$1 Million New York Settlement," June 2000 Legal Case Study, http://www.hpso.com/case/cases_prof_index.php3?id=19&prof=Pharmacist   John and Rose Marie Oliver v. Evkin Pharmacy Corp., Ralph Ekstrand and Vincent Conte, Nassau County (NY) Supreme Court, Index No. 18963/97)

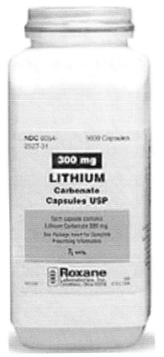

26. Pharmacy mistake results in patient taking 1800 mg of the bipolar disorder drug lithium daily (instead of the prescribed 900 mg daily)—Failure to notice signs of lithium toxicity lead to death—$1 Million settlement

A pharmacy error and the failure to notice signs and lithium toxicity lead to the death of 51 year-old woman. The decedent was a mentally retarded woman who died from lithium toxicity on May 13, 2002. She had been a resident at the defendant residential home from 1992 until her death in 2002. On April 13, 2002, the defendant pharmacy and pharmacist incorrectly filled the decedent's lithium prescription, dispensing lithium carbonate 300 mg capsules instead of the prescribed lithium carbonate 150 mg capsules. This mistake resulted in decedent consuming 1800 mg of lithium carbonate daily, instead of the prescribed 900 mg daily dosage, prior to her death. The case was settled for one million dollars during litigation with the pharmacy, pharmacist and residential home defendants. The case remains ongoing against the primary care physician and psychiatrist regarding failure to notice signs of lithium toxicity. ("$1M settlement for medication error, lithium toxicity," 2006 Medical Malpractice Settlement Report, Medical Malpractice Attorneys Lubin & Meyer PC, 100 City Hall Plaza, Boston, MA 02108, http://www.lubinandmeyer.com/cases/lithium.html)

DEATH

27. Death of cancer patient Lyle Ganske in Ohio—Pharmacist indicted for allegedly dispensing an overdose of chemotherapy drugs

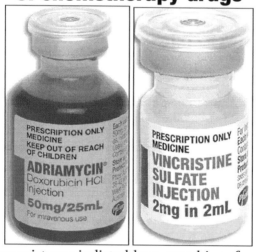

An Ohio pharmacist was indicted by a grand jury for allegedly dispensing an overdose of chemotherapy drugs that led to the death of a cancer patient. Daniel Scott, 41, a longtime pharmacist at Riverside Mercy Hospital in Toledo, was charged with one count of involuntary manslaughter in the death of **Lyle Ganske** on July 11, 2000. Prosecutors charged that Scott quadrupled the dosages of Adriamycin (doxorubicin HCl, Pharmacia) and vincristine he dispensed at the Riverside Mercy Home Pharmacy Services outpatient facility. The chemotherapy error was triggered when a nurse rewrote the physician's original order, said James Brazeau, an attorney who represented Scott before the pharmacy board. He said that the physician's order called for only one dose spread out over four days, but, in a phone call, a nurse indicated that the dose was to be "times four days," Brazeau said. The pharmacist interpreted that to mean a dose for each of four days. (Carol Ukens, "Ohio pharmacist indicted in Rx error death," *Drug Topics*, November 19, 2001, p. 22)

DEATH

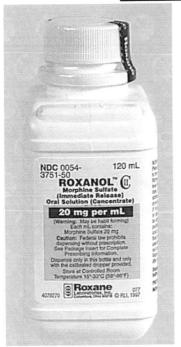

28. Death of 8-year-old Virginia girl <u>Megan Colleen McClave</u> after Demerol (meperidine) prescription filled with Roxanol (morphine)

Two days after getting her tonsils out, 8-year-old **Megan Colleen McClave** told her father in a raspy voice that her throat was aching. So Mike McClave went over to the kitchen cupboard and got out a bottle of prescription medicine he had filled at a local pharmacy. He mixed a couple of teaspoons into a glass of cherry-flavored 7-Up, remembering that Megan earlier had spit out the pain killer because it was bitter and "yucky." This time she slowly sipped about half the mixture. She felt sick and drowsy, but she watched a movie on television, made Jell-O with her dad and took a few more sips of the 7-Up mixture before crawling into bed for the night. The next morning, Megan never woke up. Because of a horrible mistake by a Newport News pharmacist, Megan was not given the standard pain-dulling medication her doctor had prescribed, but a powerful morphine-based compound typically used to comfort terminally ill cancer patients. ("Pharmacist's Mistake Costs 8-Year-Old Hampton Girl Her Life," *The Virginian-Pilot*, October 31, 1994, page B5, Source: Associated Press, Dateline: Hampton, Va.

http://scholar.lib.vt.edu/VA-news/VA-Pilot/issues/1994/vp941031/10310070.htm)

DEATH

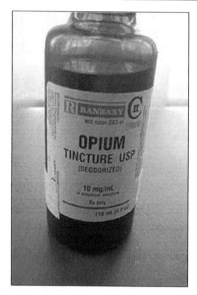

29. Death of Connecticut woman <u>Donna Marie Altieri</u>—Lawsuit filed alleging CVS caused fatal mix-up by dispensing opium tincture instead of paregoric. Opium tincture contains 25 times as much morphine as paregoric.

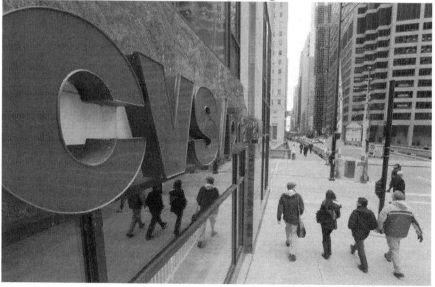

The family of a Connecticut woman filed a lawsuit alleging that she died because a community pharmacist dispensed opium tincture instead of camphorated opium tincture, which is commonly known as paregoric. **Donna Marie Altieri**'s physician wrote a prescription for one teaspoon of "tincture of opium camphorated" for her chronic diarrhea on June 15, 2001. The 51-year-old grandmother took the prescription to a CVS drugstore in Southington, where it was filled. However, the script was misfilled with opium tincture, which contains 25 times as much morphine as paregoric. The next day, she took one dose then complained of feeling weak, tired, and achy and went to sleep. She never woke up. An emergency room physician said Altieri probably died of a heart attack. One of her two sons found that hard to believe and became suspicious. He asked for an autopsy. Two months later, the coroner ruled her death was due to accidental morphine intoxication. (Carol Ukens, "Lawsuit alleges fatal paregoric mix-up," *Drug Topics*, March 18, 2002,

http://www.drugtopics.com/drugtopics/article/articleDetail.jsp?id=116571)

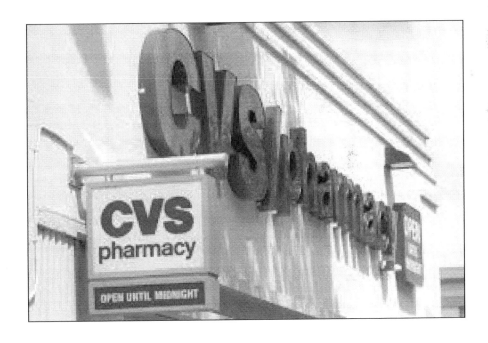

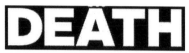

DEATH

30. Death of 5-year-old Virginia boy after 500 mg of imipramine dispensed (for bedwetting) instead of 100 mg

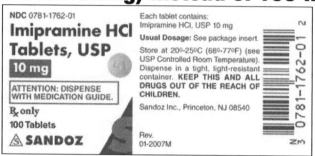

A five-year-old Virginia boy died as a result of an order entry and compounding error that was not caught by the usual check system. In this case, imipramine was dispensed in a concentration five times greater than prescribed. Imipramine is a tricyclic antidepressant used to treat adults, but it is also used to treat childhood enuresis (bedwetting). A technician entered the concentration into the computer as 50 mg/mL instead of 50 mg/5mL, along with the prescribed directions to give 2 teaspoonfuls at bedtime. He then mixed the solution using the incorrect concentration on the label and placed the prescription in a holding area to await a pharmacist's verification. The high workload made it impossible for the pharmacist to check the prescription right away. When the child's mother came in to pick up the prescription, the clerk was unaware that it had not been checked and gave it to the mother without telling a pharmacist. At bedtime, the mother gave the child two teaspoons of the drug (500 mg instead of the intended 100 mg) and found him dead the next morning. An autopsy confirmed imipramine poisoning. (Institute for Safe Medication Practices, "Tragic community pharmacy error—one year after owner talks about workload stresses to *NY Times*," August 23, 2000 http://www.ismp.org/MSAarticles/Tragic.html)

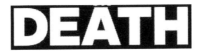

31. Death of man given wrong directions on insulin— Ten times the prescribed dose

The decedent went to the doctor to obtain some insulin for his diabetes. Several days after seeing the doctor, the decedent overdosed from the prescribed insulin. The decedent was in a coma in a nursing home and on a ventilator for two months prior to his death. The plaintiff claimed that the prescription given to the decedent was a different brand from what the decedent had been using. The plaintiff also claimed that the prescription was written for twenty units in the morning and ten units in the evening, but the pharmacy filled the prescription for 200 units in the morning and 100 units in the evening. (Healthcare Providers Service Organization, January 2007 Legal Case Study,
http://www.hpso.com/case/cases_prof_index.php3?id=118&prof=Pharmacist)

DEATH

32. Death of baby <u>Alyssa Shinn</u> after dose of zinc dispensed is one thousand times larger than neonatologist ordered at Las Vegas hospital

It was a simple miscalculation. Yet the error slipped through the hands of three pharmacists and several nurses at a Las Vegas hospital, leading to the death of a premature baby girl. The error leading to the death of three-week-old **Alyssa Shinn** on Nov. 9, 2006 certainly served as a wake-up call to Summerlin Hospital Medical Center, the facility where the mistake occurred. The breakdown that resulted in Alyssa Shinn's death began with the mishandling of the infant's prescription by hospital pharmacist Pamela Goff. In her testimony to the pharmacy board, Goff tearfully admitted she selected the wrong unit of zinc for the infant's TPN IV bag, choosing 330 mg rather than 330 mcg—a dose 1,000 times larger than Shinn's neonatologist had ordered. ("Infant death leads to changes at Las Vegas hospital," Michael Barbella, *Drug Topics*, Sept. 3, 2007, p. 18)

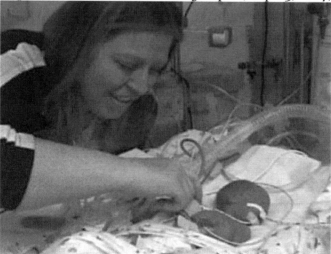

Three week old Alyssa Shinn died after receiving 1,000 times the dose of zinc ordered by a neonatologist at a Las Vegas hospital.

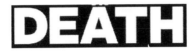

33. Death in Michigan is apparently caused by tenfold analgesic dosage error

Tenfold drug administration errors are common and pernicious in healthcare systems, but they could be almost entirely eliminated. They occur when a decimal placement is written incorrectly or mis-read. Decimal errors can result in a 10-fold, 100-fold, or even 1,000-fold overdose or underdose. Combine dosage danger with the fact that the cure can sometimes be worse than the dilemma, and you have the sad case of what appears to have happened at Botsford General Hospital in Farmington Hills, Mich. A recent lawsuit alleges that a hospital patient received a 10-fold overdose of an analgesic, which resulted in a dangerous drop in blood pressure. As a result of an attempt to treat that condition, the patient became paralyzed and died. But it was the decimal error that apparently killed him. (Martin Sipkoff, *Drug Topics*—Health-System Edition, Aug. 21, 2006 http://www.drugtopics.com/drugtopics/article/articleDetail.jsp?id=365727)

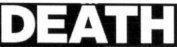

DEATH

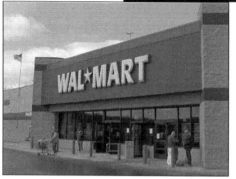

34. Death after Maryland Walmart allegedly dispensed wrong strength of Humulin to Keith Scofield—Walmart settles wrongful death suit due to insulin overdose

On December 13, 2005, **Keith Scofield** visited a Wal-Mart pharmacy in Frederick, Maryland, and ordered over-the-counter Humulin R (U-100). Instead, he was allegedly given Humulin R (U-500), a prescription drug that contains five times the insulin of the requested medication. He injected the insulin on December 20, 2005, lapsed into a diabetic coma, and died on January 2, 2006, according to a lawsuit filed by his family. The suit was settled during mediation without admission of liability or fault. (Linda von Wartburg, "Wal-Mart Settles Wrongful Death Suit Due to Insulin Overdose," *Diabetes Health*, Aug 7, 2007

http://www.diabeteshealth.com/read/2007/08/07/5361.html

Source: *Business Week*, July 2007)

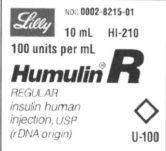

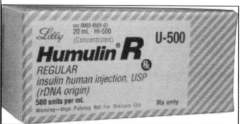

DEATH

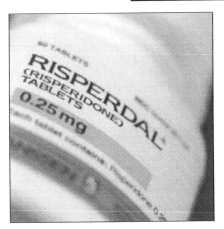

35. Pharmacy failed to dispense correct number of Risperdal tablets for psychosis— Child commits suicide due to lack of drug—$875,000 gross verdict

The decedent, age twelve, was discharged from the hospital in September 2002 with a diagnosis of psychosis no.5./schizophrenia. She was discharged with a prescription for a thirty-day supply of Risperdal, consisting of ninety .025 milligram tablets. Her mother filled the prescription on the day after discharge at a pharmacy. On the tenth day there was only one tablet remaining and the mother contacted the pharmacy about the shortage. The child went without medication for four days and committed suicide by hanging herself with a jump rope. A verdict for $875,000 was returned with the mother being found twenty-five percent contributorily negligent in not noticing any shortage earlier. ("Failure to Dispense Correct Number of Pills for Prescription for Risperdal—Child Commits Suicide Due to Lack of Drug—$875,000 Gross Verdict," September 2006 Legal Case Study, Healthcare Providers Service Organization, http://www.hpso.com/case/cases_prof_index.php3?id=114&prof=Pharmacist)

DEATH

36. Three-year-old <u>Sebastian Ferrero</u> dies after pharmacist prepares over ten times prescribed dose of arginine— $850,000 settlement in Florida

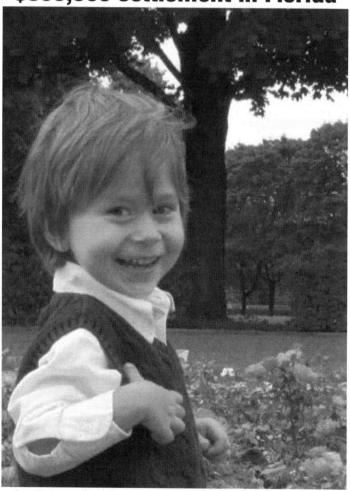

Sebastian Ferrero died from a pharmacy mistake at a Florida hospital.

ORLANDO, Fla. (AP)–Edna Irizarry, a pharmacist who filled a prescription that led to the death of a Florida boy, faced disciplinary action from the Florida Board of pharmacy for processing a prescription for 3-year-old **Sebastian Ferrero**, who died in October 2007. Ferrero died at a Shands hospital in Gainesville, two days after a routine test was supposed to help doctors determine why the boy's growth was below average. Instead of receiving the prescribed dose of 5.75 grams of the amino acid arginine, officials said the Shands Medical Outpatient Pharmacy gave him more than 60 grams. Hospital workers at Shands administered the arginine, and did not realize the dosing error even when the Ferreros asked them to check their son, who developed a headache and appeared to be in extreme pain. Shands admitted its errors caused Sebastian's death. Luisa Ferrero and her husband, Horst, received an $850,000 settlement from Shands Healthcare at the University of Florida. ("Pharmacist fined for role in 3-year-old's death." Sarah Larimer, Associated Press, Aug. 13, 2008
http://hosted.ap.org/dynamic/stories/F/FL_MEDICATION_ERROR
_FLOL-?SITE=FLTAM&SECTION=US

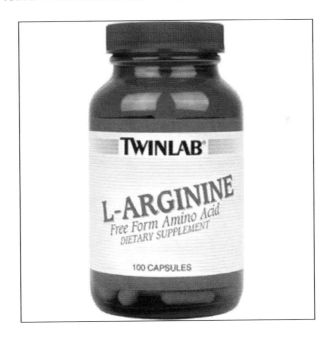

DEATH

37. Fatal overdose—K-Mart dispenses 5 mg of blood thinner Coumadin instead of 2 mg prescribed—$810,000 Illinois verdict

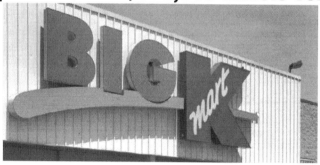

On May 30, 1995, a K-Mart pharmacy misfilled and mislabeled a prescription for decedent's blood thinner, dispensing five milligram pills instead of the two milligram pills for approximately one year, and the May 30 bottle in question was labeled as containing two milligram pills. Ingestion of the Coumadin overdose caused decedent, a seventy-six year old man, to develop an intracranial hemorrhage. On June 14 his wife found him soaked in blood which was coming from his mouth, rectum and ears. He was taken to St. James Hospital, where he died June 15, 1995. K-Mart contended decedent was contributorily negligent for failing to seek medical attention for blood in his urine on June 13, and that the effects of a Coumadin overdose could have been reversed in a matter of hours with no residual effects. According to the Cook County Jury Verdict Reporter, the jury returned a $900,000 verdict against K-Mart, reduced by ten percent to $810,000 for contributory negligence. (K-Mart Pharmacy Misfills Coumadin Prescription, Resulting In Fatal Overdose—$810,000 Illinois Verdict," August 1999 Legal Case Study, Healthcare Providers Service Organization, http://www.hpso.com/case/cases_prof_index.php3?id=17&prof=Pharmacist Estate of Ernest Van Hattem, deceased v. K-Mart Corp., d/b/a K-Mart Pharmacy No. 7289, Cook County (IL) Circuit Court, Case No. 95L-1322 1)

DEATH

38. Pharmacy fills tramadol (Ultram) prescription with Avinza—Death— $750,000 Settlement

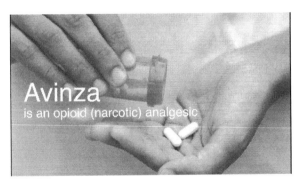

Avinza
is an opioid (narcotic) analgesic

The plaintiff's decedent, age seventy-four, took a prescription for tramadol to the pharmacy, but it was filled with high-dosage tablets of Avinza. She was found by her home health aide unconscious in December 2007. She was taken to a hospital, where she died of pneumonia a week later. The plaintiff claimed that the high level of opiates in her blood led to respiratory suppression and pneumonia. The pharmacy maintained that the Avinza did not cause the death, but that the decedent might have fallen following ingestion of the Avinza and that she had pneumonia before the accident. According to a published account, a $750,000 settlement was reached. ("Tramadol Filled With Avinza—Death—$750,000 Settlement," Healthcare Providers Service Organization, March 2011 Legal Case Study, http://www.hpso.com/case-studies/casestudy-article/341.jsp

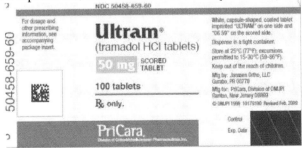

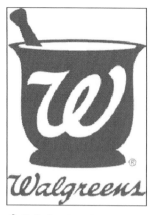

39. Walgreens mistakenly fills 1 grain thyroid prescription with 2 grains—Man develops increased circulation problems in leg—Below-knee amputation of leg—$691,179 net verdict in Colorado

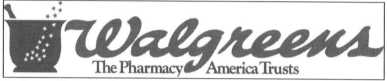

The plaintiff, age fifty-six, was diagnosed with severe peripheral vascular disease in his right leg in May 1996. The plaintiff had been on thyroid replacement hormone since 1970. In early November 1996 a Walgreen pharmacy mistakenly refilled the plaintiff's one-grain prescription with two-grain medication. The plaintiffs alleged that within one week of starting to take the double-dose medication, the plaintiff had symptoms of thyroid excess, including pain in the right leg and a sore on the right toe which would not heal. Testing in late December 1996 revealed that the plaintiff's blood flow was fifty-seven percent of normal, which was further reduced than testing done in April 1996. In early February 1997 the plaintiff had an arteriogram due to continued pain. The test results and tissue oxygen results were markedly low. The plaintiff was hospitalized in February 1997 and his right leg was amputated below the knee. While hospitalized, the hospital pharmacist discovered the medication error. The plaintiff claimed that the hormone excess caused the right leg to burn oxygen faster than it could be supplied and caused acceleration of the plaintiff's peripheral vascular disease and poor wound healing. The defendant admitted negligence in filling the prescription but denied that the error caused the amputation. The defendant claimed that the plaintiff lost his leg as a natural progression of his peripheral vascular disease and contended that the plaintiff did not properly follow the recommendations of his physicians. According to Jury Verdict Reporter of Colorado a $1,141,179 verdict was returned for the plaintiff and his wife was awarded $50,000. The judgment was reduced to $691,179 based on the applicability of the Health Care Availability Act. ("Thyroid Replacement Hormone Filled With Excessive Dosage—Man Develops Increased Circulation Problems in Leg--Below-Knee Amputation of Leg—$691,179 Net Verdict in Colorado," March 2005 Legal Case Study, Healthcare Providers Service Organization, http://www.hpso.com/case/cases_prof_index.php3?id=96&prof=Pharmacist)

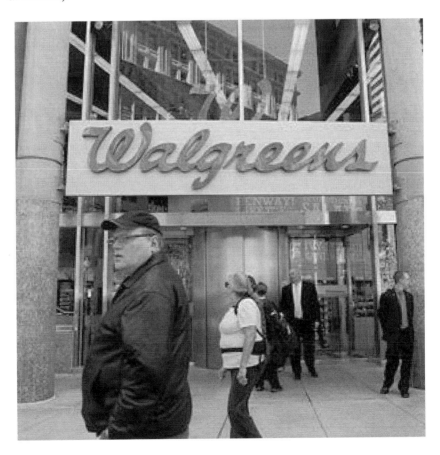

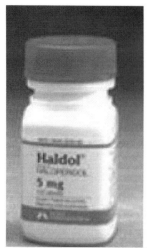

40. CVS pharmacy refilled Haldol prescription with ten times the correct dosage—Man with Tourette's Syndrome suffers overdose—Jury awards $383,300

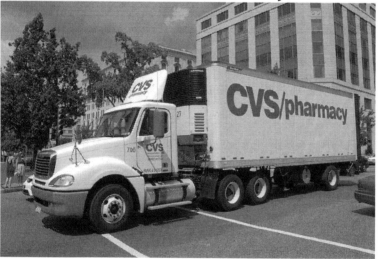

Plaintiff, a thirty-eight year old maintenance supervisor at the time of this incident on August 4, 1995, suffers from Tourette's syndrome. He claimed that defendant CVS store in Tottenville negligently filled his prescription of Haldol, and dispensed a refill that was ten times the correct dosage. Plaintiff testified that his prescription was for .5 milligrams of Haldol, to be taken four times a day as needed. He contended that defendant dispensed a refill of Haldol containing five milligram tablets. On September 1, 1995, plaintiff took three Haldol pills and suffered an overdose. He testified that he felt as if he was having a heart attack and then blacked

out. Plaintiff testified that as his neighbor was driving him to the hospital, he jumped out of the car and began rolling on the road shoulder screaming. Defendant CVS conceded liability after testing samples of the medication that it had dispensed, but contended that plaintiff was contributorily negligent in the manner in which he took the medication. Plaintiff argued that the medication that defendant dispensed was a generic brand and that the pills he took were the same color and shape as the correct dosage of Haldol. Plaintiff claimed he suffered post-traumatic stress disorder with depression, nightmares, and a sixty-pound weight loss. Plaintiff also claimed that his Tourette's syndrome has worsened. He testified that he now takes antidepressants and tranquilizers. According to The New York Jury Verdict Reporter, the jury awarded plaintiff $358,300, and plaintiff wife $25,000. ("Haldol Prescription Was Ten Times the Proper Dosage—Man With Tourette's Syndrome Suffers Overdose—Post-Traumatic Stress Disorder—New York Court Directs Verdict for Plaintiff on Liability—Jury Awards $383,300." November 2000 Legal Case Study, Healthcare Providers Service Organization,
http://www.hpso.com/case/cases_prof_index.php3?id=37&prof=Pharmacist Anthony and Toniann Davi v. Hook-Superx, Inc. d/b/a Revco Drug Center, n/k/a CVS Pharmacy, Richmond County, New York, Supreme Court, Index No. 12856/96)

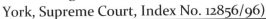

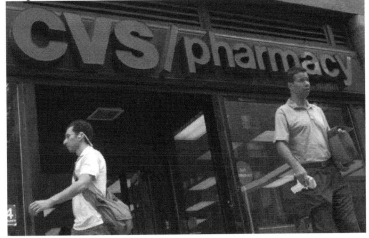

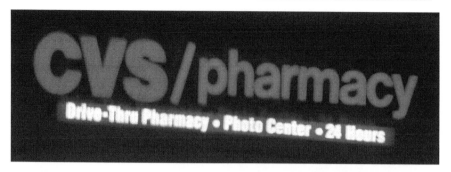

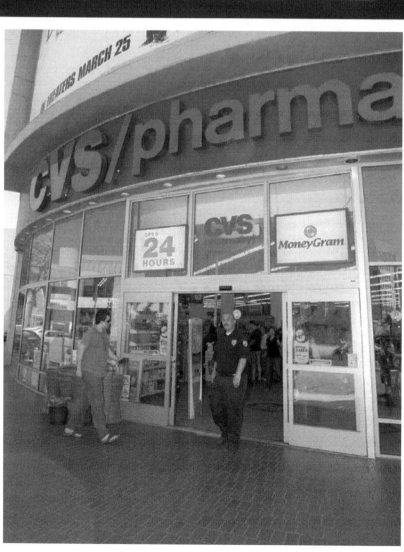

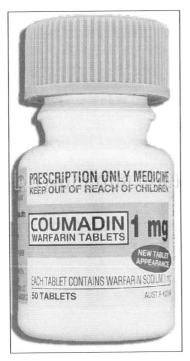

41. Pharmacy dispensed 5 mg of blood thinner Coumadin instead of 1 mg, resulting in stroke—Speech and right-side weakness necessitate move to nursing home— $374,400 net verdict

The plaintiff, age eighty-two, took a prescription for Coumadin to the pharmacy to be filled. The prescription was for one milligram pills, but she was dispensed five milligram pills. The plaintiff stopped taking the drug after noticing that the pills were the wrong color. A large black-purple hematoma then developed on her shoulder due to the excessive anti-coagulant. The plaintiff suffered a stroke twenty-three days after filling the prescription, causing her severe speech impairment and right-sided weakness. The plaintiff had been living independently in her own home, but had to reside in a nursing home after the stroke. The plaintiff's doctor's records indicated that he recommended that she resume taking Coumadin about a week after receiving the excessive dosage. The plaintiffs own notes stated that the physician had taken her off the anticoagulant, but warned her that she could suffer a stroke. The defendant pharmacy claimed that even though the prescription had been mistakenly filled, it was corrected soon thereafter and the physician's doctor was called. The defendants maintained that the stroke was not connected to the Coumadin and that it was due to the plaintiff's actions in failing to resume her

Coumadin once her condition was stabilized. According to a published account the jury found the pharmacy fifty-two percent at fault and assigned forty-eight percent fault to the plaintiff. The verdict was for $720,000, but the net amount was $374,400. ("Woman dispensed wrong pills for Coumadin prescription resulting in stroke—Speech and right-side weakness necessitate move to nursing home—$374,400 net verdict." Health Providers Service Organization, June 2011 Legal Case Study

http://www.hpso.com/case-studies/casestudy-article/349.jsp)

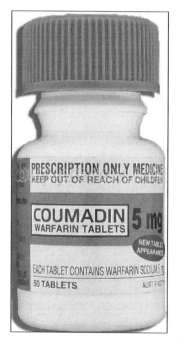

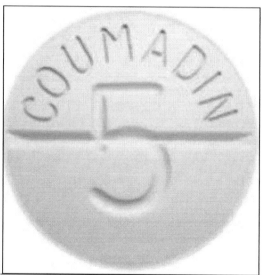

COUMADIN 5 mg

42. Prescription for the acid-reflux drug Prilosec filled with the anti-depressant Prozac—Infant hospitalized for five days—$350,000 verdict

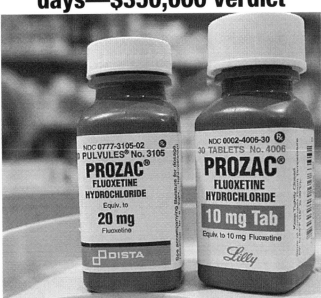

The plaintiff child, age eleven months, was treated by her pediatrician for stomach complaints and was prescribed Prilosec. Her physician called in the prescription to the defendant pharmacy. The prescription was filled with Prozac instead of Prilosec. The child became severely ill and was hospitalized for five days as a result of ingesting Prozac. The defendant admitted liability and the matter was tried on the issue of damages only. The plaintiffs alleged that the child suffered permanent injuries from the incident, while the defendant contended that the plaintiff made a good recovery. ("Prilosec Prescription Filled With Prozac—Infant Hospitalized for Five Days—$350,000 Verdict," June 2007 Legal Case Study, Healthcare Providers Service Organization
http://www.hpso.com/case/cases_prof_index.php3?id=124&prof=Pharmacist)

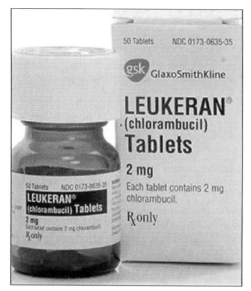

43. Leukeran dispensed instead of prescribed leucovorin—Man claims increased risk of developing leukemia—$350,000 settlement

The plaintiff, age sixty-five, was undergoing treatment for peripheral neuropathy which was causing foot pain. The physician prescribed leucovorin, which was intended to lessen the side effects the plaintiff was experiencing with his medication. The defendant pharmacy, however, dispensed the drug Leukeran, which is usually prescribed to treat certain leukemias or malignant lymphomas. Leukeran can lead to the development of leukemia in a cancer-free individual. The plaintiff took the drug for about eleven months, during which time he experienced severe flu-like symptoms and depression, leading him to retire from employment earlier than planned. The pharmacy's error was discovered when the plaintiff changed providers for his prescription medications and was dispensed the correct medication. After alerting his prescribing physician of the error, the plaintiff was referred to an oncologist, who advised him of the potential of Leukeran to cause leukemia. The plaintiff alleged negligence in dispensing the wrong drug and maintained that he had an increased risk for developing leukemia. According to a *Verdict Reporter*, a $350,000 settlement was reached. (April 2009 Legal Case Study, HPSO—Health Providers Service Organization, http://www.hpso.com/case-studies/article/260.jsp)

44. Prescription for ADHD drug Adderall filled with diabetes drug glipizide—Five year-old boy experiences seizures and severe hypoglycemia—$325,000 Massachusetts settlement

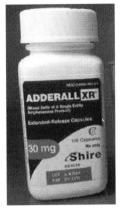

The plaintiff, a five year-old boy, was prescribed Adderall for ADHD (Attention-Deficit Hyperactivity Disorder). His aunt had an Adderall prescription for him filled at the defendant pharmacy and began administering the medication for the child the following day, according to posted dose instructions as labeled by the pharmacy. After three days, the plaintiff began to experience seizures and severe hypoglycemia. He was admitted to the hospital, where it was determined that the prescription, although labeled as Adderall, was actually filled incorrectly with glipizide, a glucose-lowering drug for diabetes. Liability was admitted and the case proceeded on the issue of damages only. The plaintiff alleged that, as a result of taking the wrong medication, he suffered a deterioration in his behavioral and cognitive functions. At the onset of seizures, he experienced tonic-clonic seizures with severe hypoglycemia. The defendant, however, contended the plaintiff's behavioral and cognitive difficulties were not related to taking the wrong medication, but were tied to residual effects of the pre-existing ADHD disorder, and the fact that he had been previously abandoned and abused. According to *Massachusetts, Connecticut, Rhode Island Verdict Reporter*, this case was settled for $325,000 (with half of the proceeds allocated to special needs trust, and the remaining half to be paid via a structured settlement with guaranteed payout of $410,000). ("Adderall Prescription Filled With Glipizide—Five Year-Old Boy Experiences Seizures and Severe Hypoglycemia—$325,000 Massachusetts Settlement," November 2004 Legal Case Study, Healthcare Providers Service Organization, http://www.hpso.com/case/cases_prof_inde)

45. Thrifty (Payless) pharmacist dispenses Calan instead of Lasix— Woman rushed in near-coma to emergency room—$305,000 award

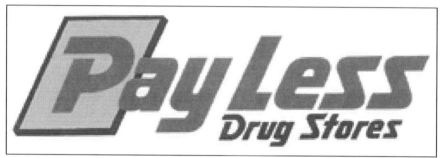

In February 1997, the plaintiff, a fifty year-old licensed vocational nurse who suffered from polymyositis—a chronic inflammatory disease of the muscle tissue-and hypertension, was hospitalized for one week with congestive heart failure. She was discharged on various medications, including the diuretic Lasix, and Calan, a calcium channel blocker used to treat hypertension. On April 27, 1997, the plaintiff's son picked up a prescription that was intended by her physician's prescription to be Lasix, filled for the plaintiff at the Thrifty Pharmacy in Long Beach, California. On May 1, 1997, the plaintiff's daughter found her mother in a near-coma condition. The plaintiff was rushed to the hospital, where she was diagnosed with pneumonia, hypoxia, congestive heart failure, and a polymyositis flare-up. She was hospitalized for five days. Shortly after discharge, she checked her medication and discovered Thrifty's error in filling the prescription. The plaintiff alleged that as a result of the pharmacy error, the pills she had taken from the bottle labeled Lasix were actually Calan. So, for four days she received no Lasix, and she received an apparent overdose of Calan. This medication mix-up caused the May 1997 health crisis, leading to her hospitalization, and this permanently aggravated her polymyositis, and may have caused brain damage with resulting cognitive deficits. The de-

fendant argued the plaintiff was given the correct medication and she was either confused or untruthful. All of the plaintiff's medical problems were attributable to natural causes and not to any alleged drug mix-up. The defendant maintained the plaintiff's claims of brain damage and/or cognitive defects were false. The jury awarded a gross damages verdict of $305,000. ("Lasix Prescription Filled With Calan—Woman Rushed In Near-Coma Condition to Emergency Room," July 2001 Legal Case Study, Healthcare Providers Service Organization
http://www.hpso.com/case/cases_prof_index.php3?id=49&prof=Pharmacist
Ivis Higgins v. Thrifty **Payless**/Rite Aid, Los Angeles County Superior Court Case No. NC 023 050)

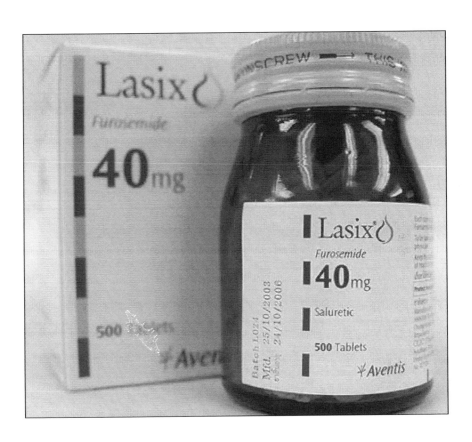

46. Eckerd Drug dispenses clonazepam instead of clonidine—$250,000 Pennsylvania settlement

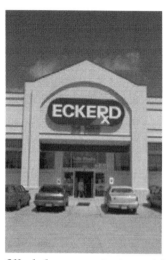

In Sloan v. Eckerd Drug (Pennsylvania), the patient went to her Eckerd pharmacy to fill a prescription for clonidine, a drug she used to control hypertension or high blood pressure. The pharmacy filled the prescription with clonazepam, a medicaiton which poses a risk of dependency. The patient took the medication for 3 weeks and experienced headaches, memory loss, and depression. She became addicted to the drug and required outpatient psychiatric treatment. She sued the pharmacy and her pharmacist and the case settled before trial for $250,000. (Attorney Dan Frith from the Frith Law Firm in Roanoke, Virginia, "Pharmacy Mistakes Kill," February 13, 2008. Accessed February 28, 2008.

http://roanoke.injuryboard.com/medical-malpractice/pharmacy-mistakes-kill.php?googleid=14934)

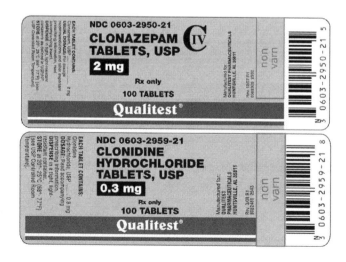

47. Pharmacy dispenses 50 microgram Fentanyl patches to a blind man, instead of the prescribed 25 microgram patches— Overdose blamed for worsening of sleep apnea—$200,000 settlement

The plaintiff, who is blind and uses a seeing-eye dog, brought a prescription for two boxes of 25 microgram Fentanyl patches to the defendant pharmacy. The pharmacy dispensed the plaintiff two boxes of 50 microgram Fentanyl patches. The plaintiff was unable to detect the dosage error before using the medication. The plaintiff applied the narcotic patches over the course of a week as prescribed and suffered a debilitating overdose. In addition to extreme discomfort, confusion, nausea and lethargy, the overdose caused permanent worsening of the plaintiffs sleep apnea, necessitating numerous sleep studies and supplemental oxygen therapy during sleep. The pharmacy admitted the error, but disputed the damages. A $200,000 settlement was reached, according to a published account. (March 2010 Legal Case Study, HPSO—Healthcare Providers Service Organization http://www.hpso.com/case-studies/casestudy-article/326.jsp)

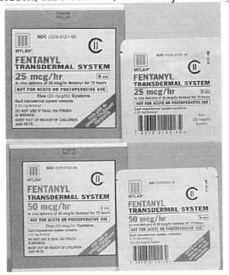

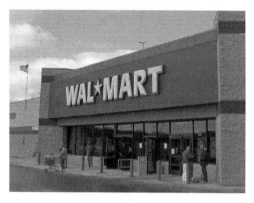

48. Wal-Mart pharmacist dispenses anti-fungal drug Grifulvin to 4-month old <u>Taylor Lang</u> rather than expectorant guiafenesin—$175,000 immediate settlement, plus agreement to pay for any future treatment

On November 4, 1998, the parents of **Taylor Lang** went to the Wal-Mart in Charleston, Missouri to have a prescription filled for their infant daughter. Their pediatrician had prescribed guaifenesin, an expectorant, for the infant, who had developed croup/cough. The pharmacist instead, by error, dispensed Grifulvin, an anti-fungal agent used to treat ringworm. After reading the medication literature included with the packaging, the parents called the pharmacy the next morning to verify that Taylor had been given the correct prescription. The pharmacist assured the Langs that the prescription was correct, and should be taken as directed, and that the information on a printed insert with a medication does not always reflect the purpose for which that medication was prescribed. Her explanation was that medications often have multiple uses. For twenty days, four month-old Taylor, who weighed thirteen pounds, was given doses of Grifulvin that would have been inappropriate even for a full-weight adult. She developed severe diarrhea, stomach cramps and pain, and general lethargy. When the mistake was finally verified, after the parents took the still-ill child along with the medication back to the pediatrician's office, Taylor was tested for liver damage, a potential side-effect of Grifulvin. Initially, Taylor had elevated liver enzymes, but a short time later, after the drug was withdrawn, her enzyme levels returned to normal. After four years of further development, she appears to have no permanent liver damage. The plaintiff alleged the Wal-Mart pharmacist departed from the standard of care in two instances—once when the incorrect medication was dispensed and secondly, when the pharmacist informed the parents by phone that Grifulvin was the correct drug, and to take it as directed on the labeling. The parties reached a settlement of $175,000, with an additional $500,000 available if Taylor should develop liver damage prior to age twenty. ("Wal-Mart Pharmacist Gave Four Month-Old Child Anti-Fungal Agent Rather Than Expectorant—Severe Diarrhea, Stomach Pain and Lethargy—Elevated Liver Enzymes—$175,000 Immediate Settlement, Plus Agreement to Pay for Future Treatment Provision in Missouri," Sept. 2004 Legal Case Study, Healthcare Providers Service Organization

http://www.hpso.com/case/cases_prof_index.php3)

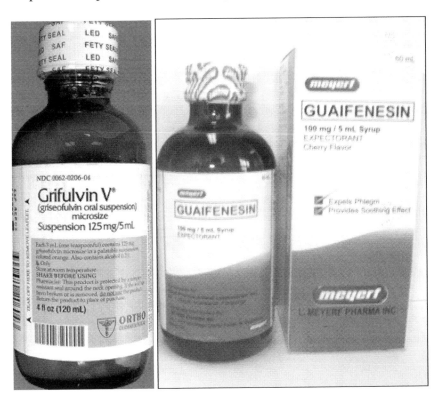

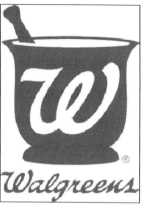

49. Lawsuit alleges Walgreens dispensed chemotherapy drug Matulane to pregnant woman instead of prenatal vitamin Materna, leading to miscarriage

Walgreen Co. has been sued by a Missouri woman and her husband who claim she had a miscarriage after a prescription for prenatal vitamins was filled with a chemotherapy drug carrying a similar brand name. Walgreens failed to properly supervise pharmacy personnel who dispensed the medicine to Chanda Givens instead of what her doctor prescribed, lawyers for Givens and her husband, Courtenay, said in a complaint filed in federal court in St. Louis. Givens had a miscarriage after taking the drug for less than a month. Givens received a prescription for Materna, a prenatal vitamin, on March 6, 2007. The pharmacist at her local Walgreens instead gave her Matulane, used to treat Hodgkin's disease. The drug is designed to interfere with the growth of cells by blocking their ability to split and reproduce, the complaint states. (Bloomberg News: "Suit: Chemo drug led to miscarriage," chicagotribune.com, October 19, 2007

www.chicagotribune.com/business/chi-fri_brief2_10190ct19,0,6644474.story)

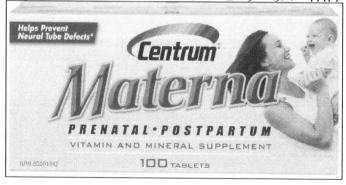

50. Pharmacist dispenses Arava (for arthritis) instead of Avapro (for hypertension)— Confidential settlement

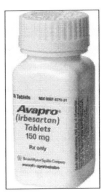

The plaintiff began to experience high blood pressure, weight loss, extreme headaches, uncontrollable diarrhea, blurred vision, and changes in her mental state in April 1999. Her treating physician was unable to diagnose the cause of her illness—and in particular could not understand why the patient's blood pressure medication which he had prescribed, Avapro, was no longer working. One month later, the plaintiff noticed that the contents of her medication bottle were listed as Arava—a rheumatoid arthritis drug. She telephoned the national pharmacy chain where she had picked up her prescription, but she was not able to speak to the pharmacist who filled the order. The plaintiff discovered that the night pharmacist who had filled the plaintiff's medication had misfilled forty-five prescriptions between June 1997 and November 2000 at that pharmacy. Other pharmacists at this same store averaged one error per year. The plaintiffs also discovered that the defendant pharmacist frequently worked ten-hour shifts seven nights in a row. After the error in this case became known to his supervisor, he was transferred to a different pharmacy in another town. But the regional supervisor did not tell his new on-site supervisor about his pattern of errors. The district supervisor also disclosed during discovery that she had never fired a pharmacist for incompetence, and she has been with the company since 1994. The plaintiffs also discovered that the pharmacy does not have a nationwide written policy requiring prescription misfills to be tracked. According to a published account, after the plaintiffs filed their negligence case in district court, a confidential settlement was reached shortly before trial. ("Overworked And Error-Prone Pharmacist Misfills Prescription— Confidential Settlement," June 2006 Legal Case Study, Healthcare Providers Service Organization)
http://www.hpso.com/case/cases_prof_index.php3?id=111&prof=Pharmacist)

51. Pharmacist dispenses Tobradex eye drops for one-month old infant instead of Tobrex—causing steroid-induced glaucoma

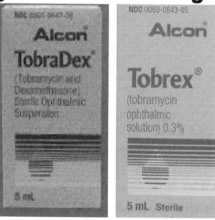

A pediatric ophthalmologist prescribed Tobrex (tobramycin) 0.3% ophthalmic drops for a one-month-old infant with a blocked tear duct (one drop 3 times a day to the left eye). The physician indicated this drug by checking off a space on a preprinted prescription order form which listed 12 different ophthalmic drops including Tobradex (tobramycin and dexamethasone) which appeared on the line above Tobrex. Somehow, the pharmacist misread the prescription order and erroneously dispensed Tobradex. Compounding the error, the pharmacist refilled the prescription with Tobradex when the initial supply was exhausted. When the infant's eye continued to worsen, the mother returned to the ophthalmologist. Under general anesthesia for a complete examination, the physician made a diagnosis of non-congenital, steroid-induced (dexamethasone) glaucoma. Surgery may be required. ("Child suffers glaucoma from inadvertent use of corticosteroid-containing eye drops," Institute for Safe Medication Practices, June 30, 1999 newsletter
http://www.ismp.org/Newsletters/acutecare/articles/19990630.asp?ptr=y)

52. Pill splitting leads to rhabdomyolysis and renal failure, setting stage for legal trouble

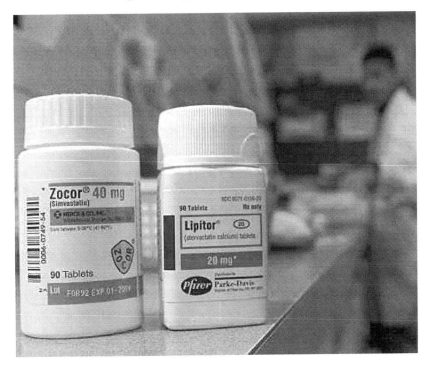

Patient compliance is always a tricky issue, but adding a complicated dosing regimen to the mix—such as pill splitting—can compound the problem, setting the stage for legal trouble. The following is a case illustrating the potential for medication errors with pill splitting.

A 59-year-old man who had undergone heart transplant was prescribed simvastatin (Zocor, Merck) at a dose of 20 mg. His cholesterol was slightly elevated (208 mg/dL), so the nurse practitioner increased his prescription for simvastatin from 20 mg to 40 mg at bedtime. When the patient took his simvastatin prescription to the pharmacy, the pharmacist filled it with an 80-mg tablet, with instructions for the patient to take one "half tablet at bedtime." The pharmacist did not contact the prescriber or the patient's clinic to divulge this information.

Six months later, the patient's cholesterol had risen slightly. He explained to the nurse practitioner that he was taking "half a tablet." She noted that the patient had previously been prescribed a 40-mg tablet and, thus, she assumed that he was taking 20 mg simvastatin as the half-tablet. The nurse practitioner told the patient to take "a whole tablet" from then on with the belief that he would then be taking 40 mg at bedtime. In actuality, the patient was now taking 80 mg per day—double the dose intended by the prescriber.

A few weeks later, the patient began to experience leg pain and was hospitalized. Physicians discovered that he had developed rhabdomyolysis, a serious muscle disease that can cause kidney failure. Fortunately, the patient survived the ensuing renal failure. The simvastatin was discontinued.

When confronted with the facts, the nurse practitioner and the lawyers for the clinic blamed the pharmacist for changing the prescription from a 40-mg tablet to one-half of an 80-mg tablet. They contended that the overdose, which led to the rhabdomyolysis, would not have occurred if the pharmacist had advised the nurse practitioner and the clinic of the dosage shift. The lawyers for the pharmacy (a managed care pharmacy group) defended the pill splitting, stating that it was a routine, cost-effective practice. The pharmacy denied any wrongdoing in the matter.

This case is about communication. The prescriber did not know that the pharmacy was changing the prescription to take advantage of pill splitting. The nurse practitioner assumed that the patient was taking a certain dose, without examining the prescription bottle and without calling the pharmacy to verify what dose he was taking. Such assumptions can cause serious health problems for the patient—and increased liability for the pharmacy. (James O'Donnell, PharmD, "Pill Splitting Leads to Rhabdomyolysis And Renal Failure, Setting Stage for Legal Trouble," *Pharmacy Practice News*, Issue: 2/2004, Volume: 31:02 http://www.pharmacypracticenews.com/index.asp?section_id=51&show=dept&issue_id=74&article_id=3515)

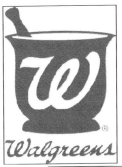

53. Walgreens pharmacist dispenses Risperdal instead of Pediapred— Baby permanently injured

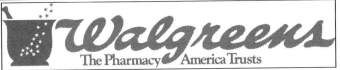

NEW PORT RICHEY, Florida—An alleged pharmacy mix-up that sent a 5-month-old to the emergency room and on to intensive care has prompted a negligence lawsuit against Walgreens and one of its pharmacists. The baby, adopted by plaintiffs Sandra and Charles Watts, was poisoned after ingesting "a potent psychotropic drug prescribed to adults for the treatment of schizophrenia," the lawsuit states. Identified in the lawsuit only by initials, the child spent five days in intensive care at All Children's Hospital in St. Petersburg with unspecified injuries following the incident Jan. 4, 2005, according to the lawsuit. According to the lawsuit, the incident began Jan. 3, 2005, when the 5-month-old was diagnosed with an upper respiratory infection and prescribed drugs including amoxicillin and the steroid Pediapred. When the Wattses took the handwritten prescriptions to the pharmacy at 7020 Massachusetts Ave. later that day, an employee asked for and noted the patient's date of birth, July 21, 2004, and then entered the prescriptions into the store's computer system, the lawsuit states. However, the employee entered Risperdal instead of Pediapred and "the computer generated a label in the minor's name listing Risperdal instead of Pediapred as the minor's prescribed medication," the lawsuit states. The next day, Sandra Watts administered the first dose of Risperdal before taking the baby to day care, the lawsuit states. Soon after, Watts got a call from day care personnel advising her the child was limp. A doctor at River's Edge Pediatrics, where the baby was a patient, quickly diagnosed the problem, and the child was rushed to

Community Hospital of New Port Richey and then to All Children's, the lawsuit states. The complaint does not detail the baby's injuries but states they are permanent. ("Walgreens Named In Prescription Lawsuit," David Sommer, *The Tampa Tribune*, May 13, 2007 http://pasco.tbo.com/pasco/MGBYTO5HM1F.html)

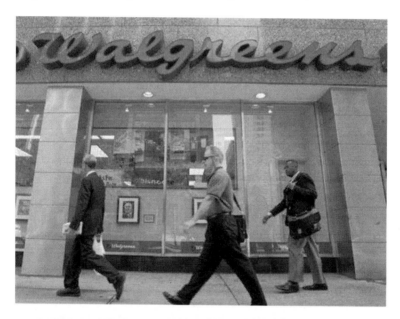

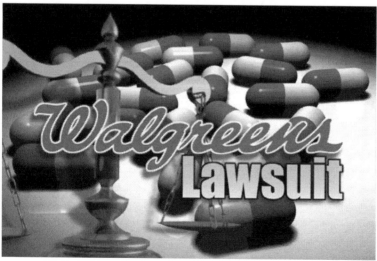

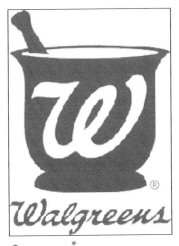

54. Walgreens mistake results in 5-year-old <u>Trey Jones</u> taking male hormone testosterone for 2 months rather than Inderal prescribed for hand tremors and hyperactivity

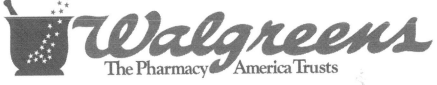

Walgreens

The Pharmacy America Trusts

Speed, high volume can trigger mistakes

R for errors

The prescription called for Inderal to control a little boy's tremors. A Walgreens pharmacy instead gave him Methitest, a steroid usually prescribed for older males. Five-year-old Trey Jones took the wrong medication for two months and began showing signs of early puberty. How do mistakes like this happen?

Family photo of Trey Jones

When Tabitha Jones picked up her stepson's medicine at a Walgreens store near Nashville in 2004, she had no way to know the pharmacy was so busy that its manager had asked for more staffing months earlier to "decrease the pharmacist's stress."

She also had no idea the drug Walgreens gave her that day was a steroid never intended for children and not the blood pressure drug prescribed to treat Trey Jones' hand tremors and hyperactivity. Walgreens refilled the prescription four times, eventually at double the adult dosage, before the error was caught. The 5-year-old not only went into premature puberty but also erupted in rages.

Trey's parents sued Walgreens, fearing the steroid could stunt the boy's growth or cause liver damage. "We don't know what could happen later on down the road," his father, Robert Jones Jr., said in a 2006 pretrial deposition.

Trey Jones ate three meals a day like a typical 5-year-old until he started taking Methitest, a synthetic hormone for older males whose bodies aren't producing enough testosterone. Afterward, he "would eat a plate full of food and come back and get seconds, and 10 minutes later, he would want thirds," his father, Robert, said in his deposition. The boy's wall-kicking rages made it difficult for him to focus on schoolwork. "You couldn't tell him to do anything," his father said.

Trey's hands continued to shake, so his doctor doubled the initial 10-milligram dose of Inderal. Walgreens again misfilled the prescription, this time with a higher dosage of the steroid. Trey began experiencing genital pain, his father said.

When Walgreens caught the error, the pharmacist told Tabitha Jones only to contact Trey's doctor, court records show. Trey's parents halted the steroid use soon afterward. Trey, now 8, gets regular growth and liver tests. Natasha Leibel, a Columbia University pediatric endocrinologist not involved with the case, says steroid use by a child "could, in theory, ... compromise adult height." Liver disease is a rarer effect of long-term use, she says.

Trey's parents filed a complaint with the Tennessee pharmacy board and sued Walgreens. Robert Jones knew the challenges would be hard but says keeping drug errors "from happening to someone else" was reason enough to fight.

Pretrial discovery in the Jones case showed the Springfield, Tenn., pharmacy where the errors began was busy: Trey's prescription was among 477 filled by two pharmacists on Sept. 30, 2004.

Months earlier, pharmacy manager Jill Brown had written in an internal report that the store had surpassed its goal of averaging 350 prescriptions a day and "could use a third pharmacist to ... decrease the pharmacist's stress." But she said in a pretrial deposition that Walgreens guidelines say a store must average 550 prescriptions a day to get a third pharmacist.

David Work, a former North Carolina Board of Pharmacy executive director tapped as an expert witness by the Jones family, wrote in a report filed in court that the store's prescription volume and staffing represented "a breach of Walgreens' (safety) obligation."

U.S. District Court Judge Aleta Trauger, who presided over the Jones case, wrote in a 2007 pretrial ruling, "Although the defendant denies that there is any connection between number of prescriptions processed per day and mistakes, common sense and at least one purported expert argue in favor of the opposite conclusion." Trauger said she would let a jury decide whether the prescription volume amounted to recklessness, a finding that could have exposed Walgreens to punitive damages.

But the case never went to trial. Walgreens acknowledged in a pretrial conference in March 2007 that it had violated the standard of care owed to Trey. The parties reached a late-December 2007 settlement that includes a confidentiality order barring Walgreens and Trey's family and attorneys from discussing the financial terms and other details.

Tennessee's pharmacy board conducted its own investigation. In 2005, it imposed a $500 fine on Walgreens pharmacist Avani Sindhal for violating state rules that require pharmacists to keep health and safety as their top concern. She said in a 2006 deposition that she thought Trey's prescription called for the steroid. Sindhal, who still works for Walgreens, also said she didn't recall seeing Trey's birth date on the prescription.

(Kevin McCoy and Erik Brady, "Speed, High Volume Can Trigger Mistakes," *USA Today*, February 11, 2008. Accessed March 16, 2008.
http://www.usatoday.com/money/industries/health/2008-02-11-prescription-errors_N.htm#uslPageReturn)

55. Safeway pharmacist accidentally gives abortion drug to pregnant <u>Mareena Silva</u> instead of antibiotic

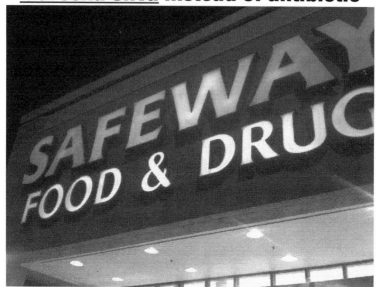

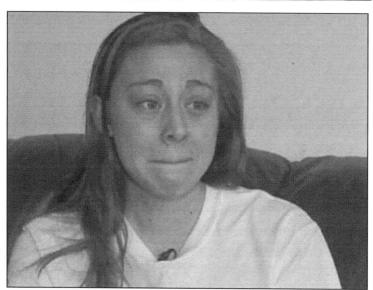

Mareena Silva received an abortion drug at Safeway by mistake instead of an antibiotic. She was pregnant at the time.

FORT LUPTON, Colo.—Having a baby should be a joyous time in one's life, but a 19-year-old Fort Lupton woman is filled with fear and uncertainty about her unborn child.

A pharmacist at a Fort Lupton Safeway at 1300 Dexter gave the wrong drug to the mother-to-be.

It's a potent drug that could harm or even kill her child.

"This will be our first baby. Yah, it'll be my first baby," says **Mareena Silva** and her boyfriend Christopher Castillo.

Silva is 6 weeks pregnant.

She was supposed to get antibiotics at the Safeway pharmacy, but the pharmacist accidentally gave her a prescription for another woman with a similar name.

"I didn't notice it didn't have my name on it because the lady's name is really similar to mine. It's Maria and mine is Mareena," she says. The two women share the same last name.

And that mistaken prescription was for methotrexate, a medication used to treat cancers.

The pharmacist told her to bring back the medicine. When she arrived, he told her to throw up the pill.

It had been about 25 minutes since she'd taken it.

"My doctor called immediately and said you need to get to an ambulance. I'm sending one to Safeway," she says.

Silva later learned methotrexate can cause birth defects in an unborn baby. She said that the drug is also used to cause abortions in troubled pregnancies.

The manufacturer warns that some people have died after taking this medication every day by accident.

"That's my biggest worry...is the baby being healthy and my baby surviving through this whole thing," says Silva.

Safeway's Public Affairs Director Kris Staaf released this statement:

We are "....very concerned about how this happened and we are conducting a full and complete investigation. Safeway has pharmacy systems and processes in place to prevent this kind of occurrence. We have a well-earned reputation for reliability and safely filling prescriptions and we will continue to work diligently to ensure our procedures and polices are being followed at each of our pharmacies."

"I'm angry. But there's not much I can do about it. I just wish I caught it sooner," says Silva.

The CU School of Pharmacy says it teaches its students to confirm with customers their street address or date of birth. That way, they make sure they are giving the right medicine to the right person. Silva says the pharmacist did not ask her these questions.

She says the pharmacist even told her the drug he was giving her was not good for a pregnant woman. And she said that's what the hospital prescribed. So, it must be okay.

"But I thought he was talking about the antibiotic," she says. Safeway says it is sorry for the mistake and it will pay for Silva's medical expenses.

(Tammy Vigil, "Pharmacist gives pregnant woman wrong prescription," KDVR-TV, Feb. 5, 2011,
http://www.kdvr.com/news/kdvr-pregnant-woman-giving-wrong-meds-20110204,0,5536174.story)

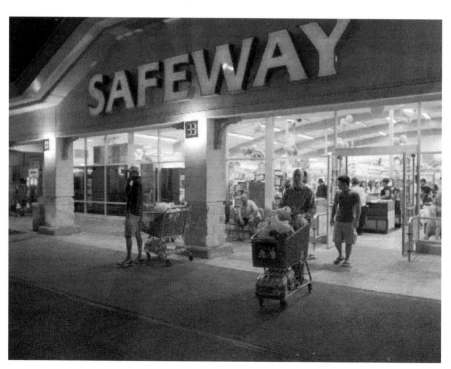

56. Thirteen prescriptions affected with CVS mix-up involving dispensing tamoxifen tablets (for breast cancer) to children instead of fluoride tablets (for prevention of tooth decay)

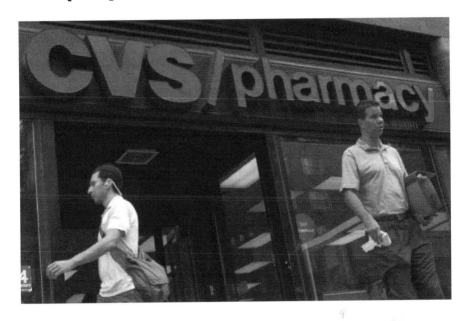

Between December 2011 and February 2012, a CVS pharmacy in Chatham, N.J., dispensed tamoxifen tablets instead of 0.5 mg chewable fluoride pills. The mix-up could have affected as many as 50 children, but only 13 prescriptions definitely were found to be affected, according to a CVS statement.

Michael J. DeAngelis, a spokesperson for CVS, stated that all families that could have received the wrong medication were contacted as soon as the mix-up was uncovered. "Fortunately, most of the families we spoke to informed us that their children did not receive any incorrect pills," he stated. "We will continue to follow up with families who believe that their children may have received incorrect medication. Thankfully, no negative effects have been reported."

DeAngelis said that the incident involved only a few tamoxifen pills mixed in with the fluoride tablets and that it was due to a "single medication restocking issue" at the Chatham pharmacy. The problem was brought to the pharmacy's attention by a parent, according to DeAngelis.

The consumer affairs division of New Jersey's attorney general's office has called for CVS to provide information on how the switch occurred, along with all communications about the problem. Company representatives will have to appear for questioning. CVS is conducting its own investigation. "We are also cooperating fully with the New Jersey attorney general's office," CVS's DeAngelis said. (Valerie DeBenedette, "CVS mix-up of tamoxifen, fluoride tablets affects 13 prescriptions," *Drug Topics*, March 7, 2012)

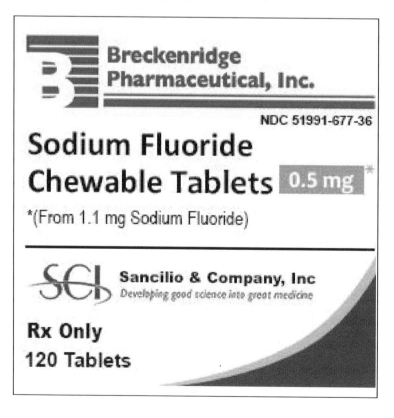

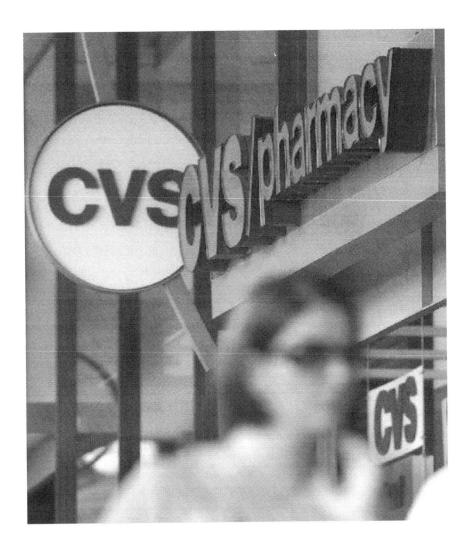

57. Lawyer says hospital patient <u>Elijah Goodwin</u> mistakenly injected with "extremely poisonous" green clothing dye instead of fluorescent dye used for angiograms

The attorney for **Elijah Goodwin** claims he was injected with a green dye normally used for dyeing clothing while at Northwestern Memorial Hospital in Chicago. Labeling the procedure as "a fiasco," the lawyer said he could not comprehend how no one in the operating room questioned the injection.

During a post-operative angiogram, doctors accidentally used "Brilliant Green dye" which is typically used to color silk, wool and other fabrics, according to the lawsuit. And moreover, this dye is "extremely poisonous." The hospital is alleged to have the dye in the pharmacy because it is "on occasion used in medicine as a topical anesthesia." The attorney said the consequences of the procedure were "really bad." These "really bad" consequences allegedly include: permanent damage to his lungs caused by permanent scarring, a seizure disorder that shuts down his kidneys for a time, and coughing spells in the middle of the night.

The lawyer said that "the drug they administered didn't have any FDA packaging" on it. The drug that the doctors wanted to use is called "IC Green," a florescent dye used in angiograms. According to the attorney, IC Green comes in powder form, while the chemical dye for coloring clothing comes in a liquid form. He concludes that "it was a really, really horrible mistake." (Atty. Stephen Alexander, "Lawyer Says Patient Injected With Green Clothing Dye," Technorati.com, April 8, 2012
http://technorati.com/women/article/lawyer-says-patient-injected-with-green/)

58. Utah teenager <u>Jessie Scott</u> in coma after Wal-Mart error involving oxycodone oral solution—He remains severely disabled years later as a result of the error

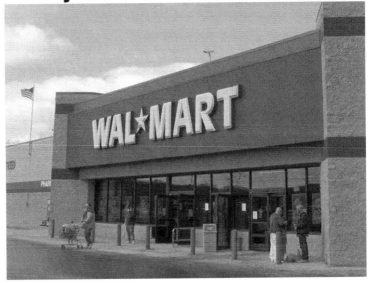

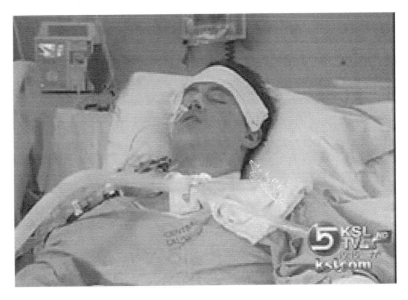

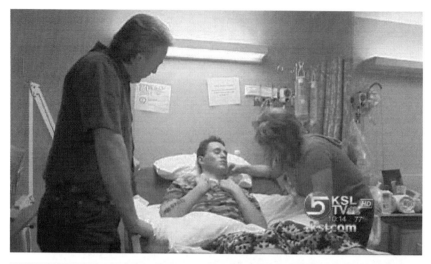

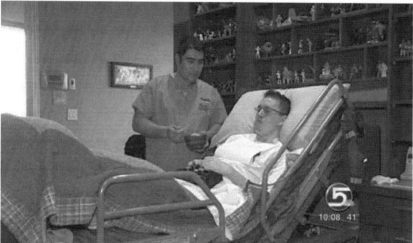

A teenager from Draper, Utah went into a coma because he was given the wrong dose of a pain medication. Eighteen-year-old **Jessie Scott** was given what was supposed to be a safe teaspoonful of the drug. Actually it was a potentially lethal dose.

At University Hospital, Wayne and Laurie Scott were told to gather their family.

"If you've got family, now's the time to call them up and let them pay their respects," Wayne Scott said. "So we made a bunch of calls, and the family responded."

Jessie's organs were failing. He was on a ventilator. One lung had collapsed. Physically and mentally, he was shutting down. All this happened within hours after he was given one teaspoon of pre-scribed oxycodone hydrochloride by his mother to help him sleep a bit and relieve pain from a strep throat.

But instead of five milligrams, attorney David Olsen says, "The dosage she gave was 20 times what was ordered. [It was] 100 milli-grams instead of five. That's because it was undiluted."

What Laurie had in her hands was a liquid concentrate that, ac-cording to Olsen, was supposed to have been diluted at the Wal-Mart pharmacy where the prescription was filled. The Scotts still can't believe it happened. Wayne Scott said, "This is obviously a horrible mistake."

Laurie Scott said, "This shouldn't have happened. It was need-less. It was senseless and it's changed lives forever, not just Jessie, but there are other people who love him and his future." Laurie trusted what she gave her son, what had been filled, was correct.

Wal-Mart Corporation issued the following statement to *KSL News:* "This is a very sad situation. Our thoughts are with this young man and his family."

Ed Yeates, "Teen in coma after wrong dose of medication," KSL TV (KSL.com), Salt Lake City, Utah, July 14th, 2008
http://www.ksl.com/index.php?nid=148&sid=3765921
See also, Ed Yeates, "Hope continues for victim of prescription over-dose," KSL-TV (KSL.com), Salt Lake City, Utah, May 9th, 2011
http://www.ksl.com/?nid=148&sid=15472010

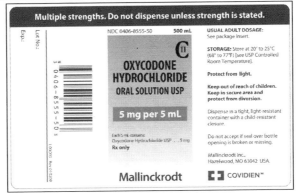

5

Serious errors involving drugs compounded by pharmacists

1. Compounding pharmacist prepares T3 capsules of varying dosages for Wilson's Syndrome patient, causing thyrotoxicosis—$650,000 settlement in North Carolina

The plaintiff, age forty-five, had a history of cardiac palpitations and shortness of breath. She presented to a physician seeking medical treatment for weight loss. The physician diagnosed her with Wilson's Syndrome, a disorder of peripheral conversion of thyroxin to T3 and ordered thyroid studies.

Though he initially ruled out Wilson's Syndrome, the physician reconsidered based on the plaintiff running an average temperature below 98.6. The physician prescribed T3, to be prepared by the defendant compounding pharmacist. The plaintiff began taking the T3, and four days later began suffering thyrotoxicosis, with symptoms of tachycardia, lightheadedness, insomnia, and itching.

Analysis of the T3 capsules prepared by the defendant pharmacist revealed wildly varying dosages between capsules, with some containing thousands of times the prescribed dosage. The plaintiff continued to experience tachycardia and shortness of breath after being discharged, and was later diagnosed with post traumatic stress disorder.

According to published accounts, the case settled for $650,000. ("Forty-Five Year-Old Female Patient Roe v. Roe Pharmacist, M.D. unknown." Healthcare Providers Service Organization, September 2005 Legal Case Study, Accessed March 9, 2006 http://www.hpso.com/case/cases_prof_index.php3?id=102&prof=Ph armacist)

---

2. Colchicine compounded by Texas pharmacy leads to three deaths

The Oct. 12, 2007 issue of *Morbidity & Mortality Weekly Report* (*MMWR*) describes three deaths attributed to a Texas compounding pharmacy error resulting from an eightfold overdose in patients seeking off-label treatment with IV colchicine for back pain. Toxicology reports showed the colchicine vials contained 4 mg/ml instead of the 0.5 mg/ml indicated on the label; therefore, the intended 2-mg dose was actually 16 mg. Bonnel et. al. (*J Emerg Med*, 2002) showed that deaths have been reported with cumulative doses of colchicine as low as 5.5 mg. According to *MMWR*, the deaths underscore the potentially fatal ramifications of errors by compounding pharmacies, which generally are not subject to the same oversight and manufacturing practices as pharmaceutical manufacturers. In response to the incident, the Texas State Board of Pharmacy, in cooperation with the FDA, issued a recall of all colchicine that had been sold or produced by the compounding pharmacy within the past year.
["*MMWR* reports on colchicine deaths due to compounding error: Three deaths determined to be result of colchicine toxicity," October 15, 2007, *Drug Topics* (Daily News) www.drugtopics.com/drugtopics/article/articleDetail.jsp?id=465163]

---

3. California pharmacist commits suicide after three deaths and thirteen hospitalizations blamed on compounded betamethasone

A California pharmacist committed suicide in 2002 after a compounding error was blamed for three deaths. The pharmacist was not present when the error occurred in 2001, but he was a co-owner of the pharmacy where the compounding took place. (Carol Ukens,

"Compounding case leads to R.Ph. suicide," *Drug Topics*, May 6, 2002, pp. 44, 49)

Jamey Phillip Sheets, 32, apparently could not accept the punishment meted out by the California pharmacy board for a fatal outbreak of meningitis from a drug compounded in the pharmacy he co-owned. A looming license suspension, five years on probation, and a hefty fine were more than the despondent pharmacist could bear. Late last month, he attached 500 mg of fentanyl patches to his neck and chest and lay down to die. ...

The downward spiral that ended in Sheets' suicide began May 2001 when a meningitis outbreak was traced to betamethasone compounded in a pharmacy he co-owned. The contaminated drug mixed in Doc's Pharmacy in Walnut Creek was blamed for three deaths and 13 hospitalizations.

The meningitis outbreak triggered a heavy media barrage and public outrage aimed at the pharmacy and the practice of compounding. And that put the pharmacy board under heavy pressure to discipline those responsible for the contamination. ...

The Sheets suicide is not an isolated incident. For example, about a year ago, an Oregon pharmacist took her life after an error killed a patient. And about five years ago, a Kentucky pharmacist involved in a fatal error was on his way to the pharmacy board to surrender his license. Instead, he stopped his car and stepped in front of a semitrailer barreling down the Interstate. These cases underscore the results of a federal study that found that pharmacists have the second-highest suicide rate in the country (*Drug Topics*, Nov. 6, 1995).

---

4. Injectable methylprednisolone compounded by pharmacists in southeastern state allegedly results in patients contracting fungal meningitis and some deaths

---

The injectable dosage form of methylprednisolone was discontinued by a manufacturer, and several medical practices contacted the pharmacy to inquire whether it could compound the product for their use. The pharmacists in a southeastern state responded to this request, preparing more than 1000 vials. Patients who received the injections contracted fungal meningitis, and some died—allegedly as a result of using the medication. The state board of pharmacy conducted an investigation and concluded that a fungus mold linked to spinal meningitis was in the product. (James L. Fink III, B.S.Pharm., J.D., "Pharmacy Law: Liability Coverage for Contaminated Compounds," *Pharmacy Times*, published online Nov. 1, 2008)

5. Five-year-old with attention-deficit hyperactivity disorder given 1000-fold overdose of clonidine as result of compounding error in which *milligrams* substituted for *micrograms*

A 5-year-old child who weighed 17.5 kg received 50 mg of clonidine. The amount ingested was confirmed by analysis of the suspension administered (clonidine HCl 9.78 mg/mL). To our knowledge, this represents the largest ingestion in a child and the largest ingestion on a milligram per kilogram basis in the medical literature. The child's initial presentation included hyperventilation, an unusual feature of clonidine toxicity. The child was discharged without sequela 42 hours after admission. A serum concentration of clonidine 17 hours postingestion was 64 ng/mL, the highest reported to date in a pediatric patient. The intoxication was traced to a pharmacy compounding error in which milligrams were substituted for micrograms. Increased prescribing of clonidine in young children coupled with the requirement to compound clonidine in a suspension and the narrow therapeutic index suggests that the frequency of severe ingestions in children will increase in the future. (M.J. Romano and A. Dinh, "A 1000-fold overdose of clonidine caused by a compounding error in a 5-year-old child with attention-deficit/hyperactivity disorder," *Pediatrics*, 2001 Aug; 108(2): 471-2. PMID: 11483818)

6. Florida pharmacy incorrectly compounded supplement given to 21 polo horses that died prior to championship match

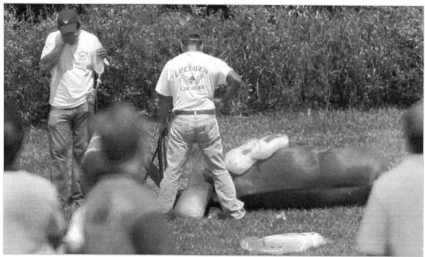

Twenty-one polo horses were killed by a pharmacy compounding error.

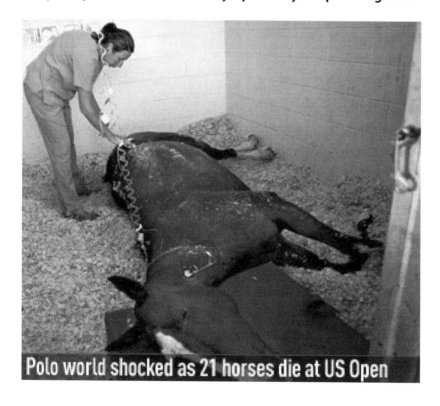

Polo world shocked as 21 horses die at US Open

WEST PALM BEACH, Fla.—An official at a Florida pharmacy said Thursday the business incorrectly prepared a supplement given to 21 polo horses that died over the weekend while preparing to play in a championship match.

Jennifer Beckett of Franck's Pharmacy in Ocala, Fla., told *The Associated Press* in a statement that the business conducted an internal investigation that found "the strength of an ingredient in the medication was incorrect." The statement did not say what the ingredient was.

Beckett, who's the pharmacy's chief operating officer, said the pharmacy is cooperating with an investigation by state authorities and the Food and Drug Administration.

The horses from the Venezuelan-owned Lechuza polo team began crumpling to the ground shortly before Sunday's U.S. Open match was supposed to begin, shocking a crowd of well-heeled spectators at the International Polo Club Palm Beach in Wellington.

"On an order from a veterinarian, Franck's Pharmacy prepared medication that was used to treat the 21 horses on the Lechuza Polo team," Beckett said. "As soon as we learned of the tragic incident, we conducted an internal investigation."

She said the report has been given to state authorities.

Lechuza also issued a statement to AP acknowledging that a Florida veterinarian wrote the prescription for the pharmacy to create a compound similar to Biodyl, a French-made supplement that includes vitamins and minerals and is not approved for use in the United States.

"Only horses treated with the compound became sick and died within 3 hours of treatment," Lechuza said in the statement. "Other horses that were not treated remain healthy and normal."

Lechuza also said it was cooperating with authorities that include the State Department of Agriculture and Consumer Services and the Palm Beach County Sheriff's Office.

Biodyl contains a combination of vitamin B12, a form of selenium called sodium selenite and other minerals. It is made in France by Duluth, Ga.-based animal pharmaceutical firm Merial

Ltd. and can be given to horses to help with exhaustion. It is widely used abroad, but not approved in the U.S.

Compound pharmacies can, among other things, add flavor, make substances into a powder or liquid or remove a certain compound that may have an adverse reaction in different animal species. Only in limited circumstances can they legally recreate a drug that is not approved in the U.S., according to the FDA.

Necropsies of the 21 horses found internal bleeding, some in the lungs, but offered no definitive clues to the cause of death.

FDA spokeswoman Siobhan DeLancey said compounding pharmacies cannot legally recreate existing drugs or supplements under patent. In most cases, they are also not allowed to recreate a medication that is not approved for use in the U.S.

On its Web site, the FDA says it generally defers to "state authorities regarding the day-to-day regulation of compounding by veterinarians and pharmacists."

However, the agency says it would "seriously consider enforcement action" if a pharmacy breaks federal law in compounding medications. It isn't yet clear Franck's broke the law. (Brian Skoloff, "Pharmacy Takes Blame in Horses Deaths," *Associated Press*, Apr. 22, 2009 http://news.aol.com/article/horses-die-before-polo-match/435339)

---

7. Tainted ophthalmic solutions from Florida compounding lab left at least 33 people with fungal eye infections

While Franck's Compounding Lab insisted that the source of the tainted ophthalmic solutions that left at least 33 people with fungal eye infections has been fixed, the fallout may be just beginning.

Franck's business manager Stephen Floyd said that the company has "taken appropriate corrective action and now have this issue behind us."

But some say the compounding lab is likely to face serious sanctions from state and federal officials just three years after another mistake by the lab killed 21 prized polo horses.

"You can understand a mistake happening once, but this particular pharmacy has had a series of missteps along the way," said Paul Doering, professor emeritus at the University of Florida School of Pharmacy. "I hate to sound holier than thou, but there is no room for error in the pharmacy business, and this is two huge mistakes for them. I was kind of dumbfounded that this was happening again."

Doering said the state Board of Pharmacy is likely to take "definitive action" against Paul Franck, the owner of the compounding lab, and may even seek to suspend or revoke Franck's pharmacy license.

The tainted products included a dye and a steroid used in eye surgeries. At least 23 of the 33 people who were treated with the products in seven states suffered eye infections that caused vision loss. Twenty four required further surgery.

In the 2009 case, Franck's was cited by the state Department of Health for numerous violations of Florida law covering pharmacies. The state alleged that the lack of experience of Franck's staff contributed to the error in mixing the supplement. A staffer erroneously mixed a high, fatal dosage of selenium into the supplement. [Carlos E. Medina, "Trouble ahead for Franck's?—Second drug controversy in three years could spell problems for Ocala compounding lab," Gainesville.com (The Gainesville Sun), May 4, 2012
http://www.gainesville.com/article/20120504/ARTICLES/120509758?tc=ar]

---

8. Death of 5-year-old Virginia boy after pharmacy technician compounded imipramine solution for bedwetting at five times the dose prescribed by physician

A five-year old Virginia boy died as a result of an order entry and medication compounding error that was not caught by the usual verification process. In this case, imipramine was dispensed in a concentration five times greater than prescribed. Imipramine is a tricyclic antidepressant used to treat adults, but it is also used to threat childhood enuresis (bedwetting). An extemporaneous solution was to be prepared at this pharmacy that specialized in compounded prescriptions since a liquid formulation was not commercially available. A pharmacy technician incorrectly entered the concentration of the prescribed solution into the computer as 50 mg/ml instead of 50 mg/5ml, along with the prescribed directions to give two teaspoonsful at bedtime. He then proceeded to prepare the solution using the incorrect concentration on the label rather than the concentration indicated on the prescription. When the compound was completed, the technician placed it in a holding area to await a pharmacist's verification. At this time, one of the two pharmacists on duty was at lunch and the high workload of the pharmacy made it difficult for the pharmacist to check the prescription right away. When the child's mother returned to pick up the prescription, the cash register clerk retrieved the prescription from the holding area without telling a pharmacist, and gave it to the mother, unaware that it had not yet been checked. At bedtime, the mother administered two teaspoonsful of the drug (500 mg instead of the intended 100 mg) to the child. When she went to wake him the next morning, the child was dead. An autopsy confirmed imipramine poisoning. (Institute for Safe Medication Practices, "Safety Can Not Be Sacrificed For Speed," *North Carolina Board of Pharmacy Newsletter*—National Pharmacy Compliance News, April 2006, p. 2.)

---

9. At least 48 deaths—Fungal contamination of compounded steroid medication—New England Compounding Center

New England Compounding Center (NECC) Meningitis Outbreak
Location: United States (23 States)
Cause: Fungal contamination of steroid medication
Deaths: 48
Injuries: 720
Litigation: 400+ lawsuits filed against NECC
http://en.wikipedia.org/wiki/New_England_Compounding_Center
_meningitis_outbreak Accessed August 24, 2013

In October 2012, an outbreak of fungal meningitis was reported in the United States. The U.S. Centers for Disease Control and Prevention (CDC) traced the outbreak to fungal contamination in three lots of medication used for epidural steroid injections. The medication was packaged and marketed by the New England Compounding Center (NECC), a compounding pharmacy in Framingham, Massachusetts. Doses from these three lots had been distributed to 75 medical facilities in 23 states, and doses had been administered to approximately 14,000 patients after May 21 and before September 24, 2012. Patients began reporting symptoms in late August, but because of the unusual nature of the infection, clinicians did not begin to realize that the cases had a common cause until late September. Infections other than meningitis were also associated with this outbreak, which spanned 19 states. As of March 10, 2013, 48 people had died and 720 were being treated for persistent fungal infections. In November 2012, it was reported that some patients recovering from meningitis were experiencing secondary infections at the injection site. Although no cases of infection were reported to be associated with any other lots of medication, all lots of all medications distributed by NECC were recalled in separate actions by NECC and regulators. Subsequent analysis identified some contamination in other lots.

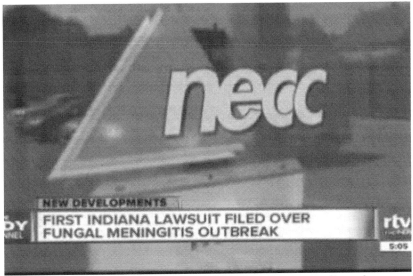

New England Compounding Center (NECC) , a compounding pharmacy in Framingham, Massachusetts.

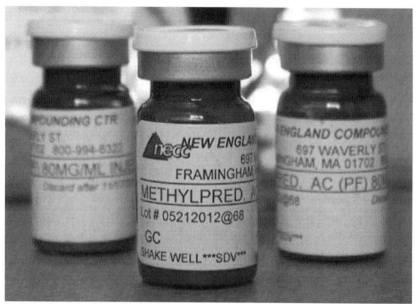

Methylprednisolone, used for sterile epidural injections, compounded by New England Compounding Center

---

10. Clonidine compounded at ten times intended dose— Prescribed for anxiety and hyperactivity in 5-year old— $240,000 settlement

---

The plaintiff, age five, had been prescribed clonidine to help with her anxiety and hyperactivity. Her mother picked up a refill of the prescription at the defendant's pharmacy and gave the plaintiff her usual dosage of the liquid suspension at bedtime, as was usual.

Within thirty minutes of taking the medication, the plaintiff had a seizure. The mother rushed her to a nearby emergency room. The child was intubated and ultimately diagnosed with a clonidine overdose. She was hospitalized for eleven days. The plaintiff made a complete recovery with no lingering side-effects.

The mother had saved the bottle of medication that was given to her by the defendant pharmacy, despite the pharmacy's attempt to have her return the medicine to them. The medication dispensed was analyzed and found to contain over ten times the concentration of the active drug prescribed for the plaintiff and what was noted on the label for the medication.

The plaintiff's expert opined that the defendant pharmacy had made a compounding error which had led to the overdose.

A $240,000 settlement was reached without the filing of a lawsuit.

"Error in Compounding Clonidine for Child Blamed for Overdose - Complete Recovery After Eleven-Day Hospitalization - $240,000 Settlement," Healthcare Providers Service Organization (HPSO), June 2013 Legal Case Study, http://www.hpso.com/case-studies/casestudy-article/388.jsp

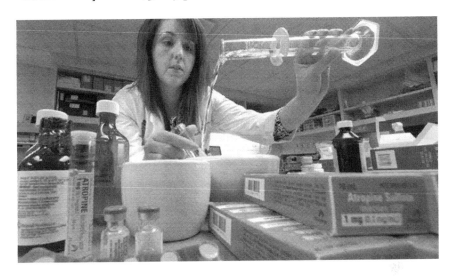

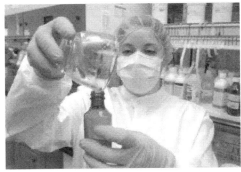

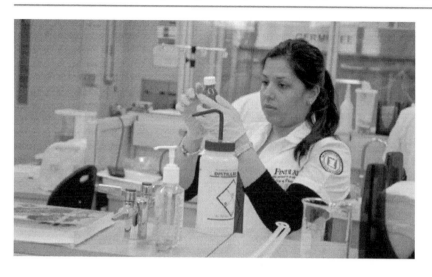

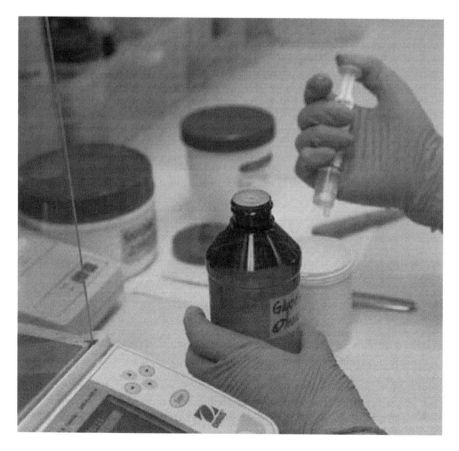

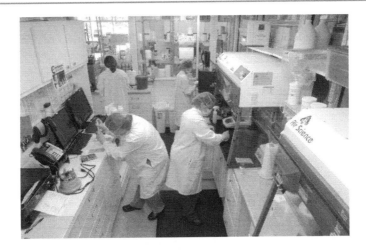

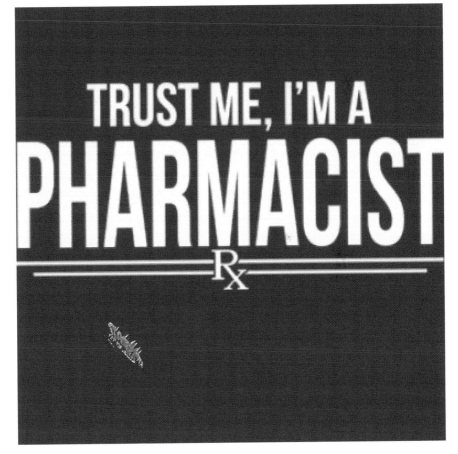

6

How do customers react when they discover pharmacy mistakes?

Even though many mistakes remain undiscovered, customers do sometimes detect the pharmacist's error. One day a lady handed me her prescription container and told me that I refilled her prescription with the wrong drug. Sure enough, the day before I had given her the wrong antidepressant. I dispensed Paxil 20 mg instead of Prozac 20 mg. She looked at me with an expression implying that I was a sloppy or incompetent pharmacist, that I should be ashamed of myself, and that the community would be better off if I worked somewhere else. She did not know that I try extremely hard to be accurate. I think it would be fair to say that I made fewer errors during my 25-year career than most pharmacists. I assume she would not have been impressed if I had tried to assure her about my error rate. Auto accidents, for example, are statistically uncommon, but if you are involved in one, statistics are of little comfort. This customer knew nothing of my deep concern for accuracy. Her expression made me feel an inch tall. She seemed to wonder how I still had a license to be a pharmacist.

This incident occurred over fifteen years ago, but it is seared deeply into my brain. Immediately after the incident occurred, I asked myself how I could have made this mistake. Most likely, this error occurred because both drug names begin with the letter "P", both drugs are in the same class of antidepressants known as SSRI's, and both are available in 20 mg. strengths. Apparently my subconscious verified several relevant factors, but obviously not all. Fatigue, workload, and distractions may also have played a role.

One of the biggest surprises for me during my career as a pharmacist is that most customers do not become angry when they discover a pharmacy mistake. Most customers return to the pharmacy oblivious to the fact that the error implies a complete breakdown in the pharmacy. The number one job of the pharmacist is to dispense the right drug to the right customer. I would probably lose confidence in a pharmacist if he dispensed the wrong drug to me or a member of my family. Most customers seem to be much more forgiving or else they don't understand the significance of pharmacy errors. Most customers don't realize that pharmacist errors can be anywhere from trivial to fatal.

Here are two examples from Complaints.com and one from ComplaintNow.com in which pharmacy customers did indeed understand the significance of pharmacy mistakes.

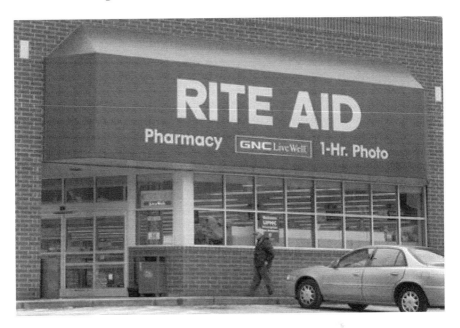

Today I submitted a prescription to my usual **Rite-Aid Pharmacy** in Concord NH. The prescription was for 200mg of Serzone. I picked up the prescription just in time to pop one of the pills in which I was an hour behind in taking. Serzone is a mild anti-depressant anxiety drug.

As I was ready to put the pill in my mouth, I noticed it looked nothing like the Serzone pills I had been taking in the past.

It was stamped with Seroquel. I thought that was strange. Was it a generic for Serzone, or did my therapist change my drug without telling me? I called the pharmacy and the girl who answered said Seroquel worked the very same way and did not seem to think there was a mistake.

I asked her to go check the original prescription, because I didn't trust her untrained opinion.

Sure enough! They gave me the wrong drug.

She said again that they work very much the same. On further investigation on the net, I found that they are two very different drugs! Seroquel is a drug to treat schizophrenia! With some serious side effects. I can't believe they did this.

I almost started to take this drug. I see now how people die from pharmacists' sloppiness. There is a lesson to be learned here.

—Rebecca Spencer, "Rite-Aid Pharmacy in Concord, New Hampshire— Prescription filled with wrong drug," Complaints.com, Feb. 1, 2002 http://www.complaints.com/february2002/complaintoftheday.february2.5.htm   (Accessed August 16, 2005)

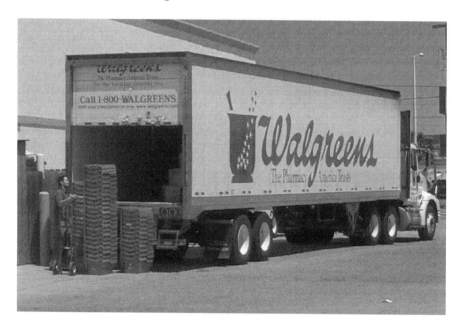

After a recent trip to a **Walgreen's** store, I feel compelled to tell you how unhappy I was with the pharmacy. Let me tell you why I was dissatisfied.

I have been to the store twice to have a prescription filled and both times they were filled incorrectly.

The first time was a dosage error. The second time was the wrong medication. While the medication given was not life threatening, it frightens me to think that if this has happened to me 100% of the time, how many other people are walking out of Walgreen's with an incorrect prescription?

The next customer may be a heart patient. Will someone have to die before this is taken seriously?

I am a new customer of Walgreen's. As a result of this experience, I definitely will not shop there again. Since word of mouth is the most effective form of advertising, I definitely will also tell others about this experience.

I hope Walgreen's is committed to customer service and I am confident they will want to resolve this issue quickly and thoroughly.

Again, you can be sure my dissatisfaction will be voiced to others.

—Rod Faulkner, "Pharmay Error: Walgreen's," Complaints.com, Dec. 2, 2000 (Accessed August 16, 2005)
http://www.complaints.com/complaintofthedaydecember32000.11.htm

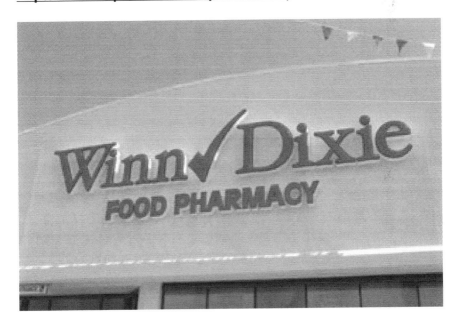

The pharmacy at my local **Winn Dixie** filled the prescription for my 5 day old 7 week premature twins wrong. They had the dosage way too high to where if I would have given it to them, it would have caused them to quit breathing. I have actually spoken to the DM [district manager] for the pharmacy and he said that he got all the proper paperwork filed and turned it over to the legal dept, and that they would be in contact with me. That was over a week ago and I still have not heard anything. I understand that they don't see the gravity of the situation. They feel like I caught their mistake so no harm came to my infant, but I feel differently. I was on medication and recovering from a C-section. What if I had been resting and my husband or someone had went to give them the medicine and just read the directions on the bottle!!! I am very upset over this matter.

—Chelle1205, ComplaintNow.com, Apr. 13, 2012
http://www.complaintnow.com/Winn-Dixie-Stores-Inc./complaint/complaints/thread/print/160147/173959

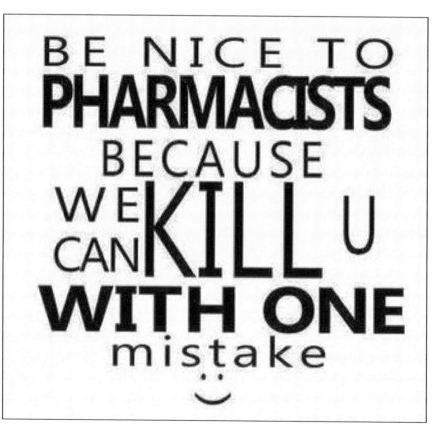

7

How to protect yourself from serious pharmacy mistakes

There are several practical things that pharmacy customers can do to protect themselves from harm.

In the last few years, several websites have become available that greatly simplify the process of identifying tablets and capsules, whether they are brand name drugs or generics. Search Google for pill identifier and you will find several websites such as **1) drugs.com, 2) rxlist.com, 3) healthline.com, 4) healthtools.aarp.org, and 5) webmd.com.**

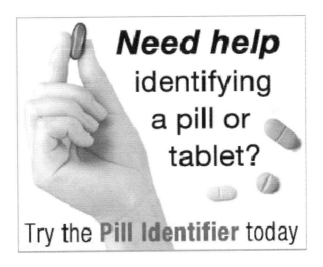

Need help identifying a pill or tablet?

Try the **Pill Identifier** today

Identifying your tablets or capsules on these websites is usually surprisingly simple. All you have to do is enter the numbers or letters or words that are stamped or imprinted on your pills. I

grabbed several different pills at random to see how accurate the
the drugs.com website is in identifying pills. I entered the numbers, letters, and words into the appropriate fields and was quickly
given the precisely correct identity for each pill. Here is the information I entered and the results.

54 543	Correctly identified as Roxicet
SP 4220	Correctly identified as Niferex-150
Endo 602	Correctly identified as Endocet
INV 276 10	Correctly identified as prochlorperazine 10 mg
M 15	Correctly identified as generic Lomotil
Watson 349	Correctly identified as generic Vicodin
KU 108	Correctly identified as generic Levbid
MP 85	Correctly identified as generic Septra DS
OC 20	Correctly identified as Oxycontin 20 mg

Even though all of these pills were identified quickly and accurately, obviously these pill identifier websites have no way of determining whether the pills in your bottles are actually what your
doctor prescribed. For example, many drugstores print a short
physical description of your pill on the prescription label or on an
"auxiliary" label attached to the side of the vial. These descriptions
can be very helpful in verifying that the pills in your bottle match
the brand or generic name on the label. But keep in mind that if
your pharmacist or tech misreads your doctor's handwriting and
enters the wrong drug into the computer, you may have an accurate
description of the wrong pill.

In the last few years, several websites have become available
that offer free drug interaction checkers. Search Google for drug
interaction checker. On most of these websites, you can enter up
to a dozen or more drugs and receive very helpful information
about potential drug interactions.

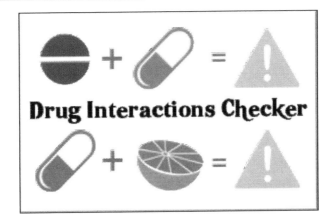

A few years ago, *USA Today* reported the case of a 31-year-old high school wrestling coach who died from an interaction between tramadol and methadone, painkillers dispensed at different times by a pharmacy in Flagstaff, Arizona. A jury awarded the patient's family six million dollars after hearing evidence that the pharmacist neither warned the patient about the potential drug interaction nor double-checked the second prescription with his doctor. (Kevin McCoy and Erik Brady, "Speed, High Volume Can Trigger Mistakes," *USA Today*, Feb. 11, 2008)

In this tragic case, if the patient had used one of the online drug interaction checkers available today, he would have seen that the **AARP.org** checker labels this interaction as "severe." He would have seen that the **medscape.com** checker describes this interaction with the words "serious" and "monitor closely." He would have seen that the **drugs.com** checker states "Comcommitant use of tramadol and other opoids should be avoided in general."

If the size, shape, or color of your pills change when you have your prescriptions refilled, call your pharmacist and ask why. In most cases, the answer is that you have received a generic made by a different company. But that is not always the case.

William Winsley, executive director of the Ohio State Board of Pharmacy, comments on this tendency to freely use the "It must be a generic" explanation ("Are All Drug Errors System Errors?" *Drug Topics*, April 15, 2002, pp. 18, 20). He says that several cases of severe patient harm have resulted from using this explanation too freely:

When a patient calls the pharmacy and asks if the medication he just received is correct since it has a different color or shape than what he was expecting, the prudent pharmacist reviews the prescription, the patient record, and asks for the color, shape, and identifying marks on the dosage form received by the patient. In several cases this board [the Ohio State Board of Pharmacy] has dealt with, the pharmacist did none of these steps. Instead, he told the patient that the dosage form must have been a generic equivalent and should be safe to take. Several cases of severe patient harm have resulted, followed by board hearings, due primarily to the pharmacist's carelessness.

Pharmacy customers need to become actively involved in learning as much as they can about the drugs their doctors prescribe. With so many potent pills on the market today, you cannot afford to be a passive consumer. Passivity is a dangerous posture in our medical system that seems to value speed over accuracy and quantity over quality.

In the following chapters, you will learn in much greater detail about the infinite number of things that can go deadly wrong at the drugstore, and practical things you can do to protect yourself.

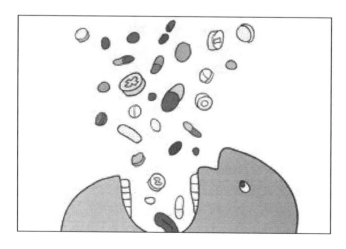

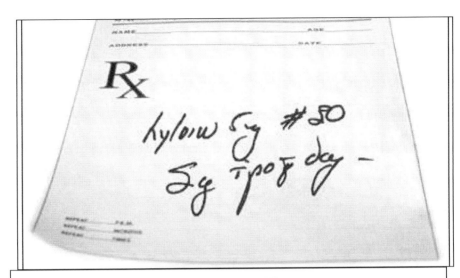

PART II

ILLEGIBLE HANDWRITING

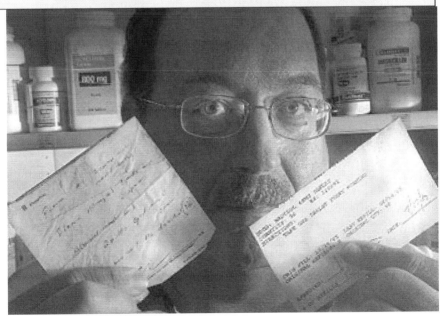

8

Why doctors' handwriting is no laughing matter

You've heard all the jokes about physicians' illegible handwriting. I challenge you to name another activity in our society in which such critical information is conveyed in such a reckless manner. There's no question that illegible handwriting causes some people to get the wrong drug, the wrong dose, and/or the wrong directions. A hurried pharmacist is forced to occasionally make educated guesses. By the time the pharmacist gets through the busy phone number to the receptionist or nurse, or by the time he locates a doctor who is away from his office or has gone home for the day, the pharmacist is causing other customers to get upset from having to wait.

When a pharmacist calls a doctor's office and talks to the doctor himself, the doctor's tone often implies something like "What kind of a pharmacist are you that you can't read prescriptions?" If the drug name and directions are bad, the signature is even worse. I have had prescriptions in which not only were the drug or directions unclear but it was impossible to identify which doctor, among several in the group practice, actually wrote the prescription. Calling the office then becomes a demeaning experience because I don't even know which doctor's office to request the receptionist connect me with. One time I ended up describing the doctor's signature to the nurse-receptionist as we tried to figure out which doctor had actually written the prescription. I had to be pleasant because obviously it's taboo to be rude to doctors (and their staff) but I usually feel like saying "Why can't that guy write like someone who got past the first grade?"

Physicians are not people who inherently write poorly. They did not have courses in medical school on how to write poorly. In my opinion, illegible handwriting is an expression of ego, a statement of the doctor's position in the power hierarchy of modern medicine. Illegible handwriting is an ongoing affirmation of medicine's dominance over pharmacy.

Imagine this scenario: Say a physician were to be sued for malpractice and the judge were to tell the doctor, "Write out your defense in your own handwriting." In this imaginary scenario, I bet that the physician's handwriting would be perfectly legible.

When a pharmacist receives a prescription that is not entirely plain, his attitude is often, "If the doctor doesn't care enough to write plainly and if he doesn't show me enough respect to write plainly, why should I show more than an equal amount of concern for the prescription?" This is the attitude that frequently contributes to the possibility that the pharmacist will make an educated guess rather than call the doctor's office.

An illegible prescription can mean only one thing: the doctor doesn't really care enough to ensure that there is absolutely no chance of an error in reading the prescription. In one town in which I worked, a pediatrician known for his arrogance called my partner and chewed her out for mentioning to a child's parents that the tetracycline he was prescribing could leave their child's teeth permanently discolored with a very unattractive gray tint. Yet this physician has some of the most illegible handwriting in town. After my partner told me about this, I wanted to call the doctor and say that if he cared so much about the well-being of his patients, why couldn't he write legibly enough to make sure that his patients got what he wanted. It is my feeling that his illegible handwriting says something about his basic concern for his patients.

When my father was discharged from a hospital several years ago, his physician handed him a prescription. I was standing next to my father and looked at the prescription as the doctor momentarily turned away. A few seconds later, I asked the doctor "Do you want...?" I was immediately interrupted by the doctor who said, "Don't worry about it. The pharmacist can read it." I felt like saying, "I've been a pharmacist for twenty-five years and I can't read it." But that would have upset my father who prefers to avoid confrontations. As it turned out, the pharmacist in my father's home town filled the prescription with what we both guessed was the proper medication. It made sense from the diagnosis. It was one of those borderline prescriptions where we were right at the edge of uncertainty. An extra millimeter and the doctor would have been phoned.

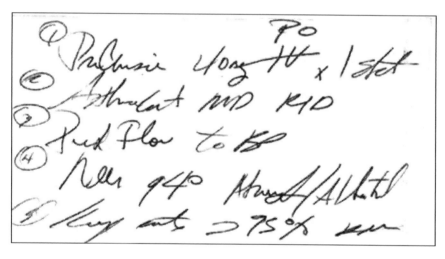

9

Has there been a deliberate effort to create a mystery around the handwritten prescription?

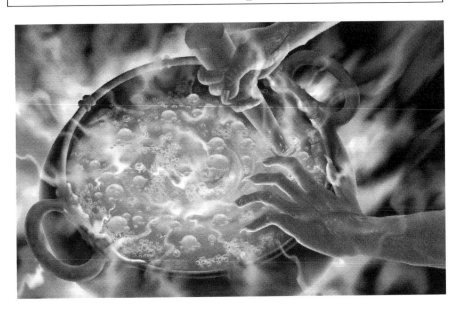

It never ceases to amaze me the way in which customers laugh and smile when I tell them that I can't read their doctor's handwriting. They seem to have the feeling that a prescription is a statement of the doctor's intellectual brilliance and that "Wow, it's so brilliant that even the pharmacist can't read it!" Instead, customers should be repulsed by illegible handwriting. If customers only knew the endless opportunities for disaster that can result from a poorly written prescription, they would demand that doctors write legibly.

I often feel that an illegible prescription is part of the mystique that physicians intentionally cultivate for themselves. It's part of the placebo effect inherent in the doctor's prescription. Several years ago, *FDA Consumer* published an article that said that, historically, physicians intentionally cultivated such a mystery around the prescription. Ask pharmacists whether they feel this effort to create mystery has ended. Prescriptions were originally made up of all kinds of symbols and Latin to intentionally create a mystery. There was, in fact, a conspiracy.

In an effort to keep the knowledge of medicine and pharmacy from the general public, physicians used strange alchemic symbols to designate the materials and processes to be used in compounding medications. "The effect on the appearance of the prescription may be readily imagined," one medical historian has written, "and it is evident that the physician succeeded perfectly in making his preparation a mystery to the patient." Keeping the patient in the dark and creating an aura of mystery and magic are precisely the reasons given by medical historians to explain the use of Latin in prescription writing as late as 1900.

Ask any pharmacist whether he believes this ended in 1900. Latin abbreviations are in common use today even though, in most cases, an English abbreviation could be written just as quickly. It is obvious that this deliberate effort to create a mystery is still very much alive today.

According to another issue of *FDA Consumer* (March 1979, p. 12), English physicians were forbidden to teach their patients about medicines four hundred years ago: "Back in 1555 England's Royal College of Physicians advised the profession thus: 'Let no physician teach the public about medicines or even tell them the names of medicines...'." The article goes on to say "That attitude persists to some extent to this day, but change is coming." I can only say that change is not coming very fast. In my opinion, the creation of mystery is still a large part of the prescription.

Illegible handwriting combined with Latin abbreviations facilitate the creation of a fog of mystery surrounding the prescription. Patients are endlessly impressed that doctors use Latin abbreviations. In reality, most doctors use fewer than a dozen Latin abbreviations in their practices. The average prescription contains maybe two or three of these abbreviations, such as: *po* (by mouth), *qd* (daily), *bid* (twice a day), *tid* (three times a day), *qid* (four times a day), *ac* (before meals), *pc* (after meals), *q4h* (every 4 hours), and *hs* (at bedtime). Doctors and pharmacists certainly do not need to be able to read formal Latin as such. We simply need to know a few dozen Latin abbreviations. In less than an hour, most people could memorize (or at least become familiar with) all the Latin abbreviations used in prescriptions.

Jesse Vivian, a pharmacist, attorney, and professor at Wayne State University College of Pharmacy, writes: "Practitioners of any vocation in any sector of the universe have communication short-cuts, abbreviations, and foreign phrases or languages that are known only to those inside the occupation. In fact, there is a notion that professionals intentionally use words or phrases that are unknown to the general populace as a mechanism of keeping lay people from getting to know too much about any given profession." ("In Pari Delicto," *U.S. Pharmacist*, January 2007, p. 88)

Doctors have been slow in adopting computers in their prescribing and for transmitting these prescriptions to pharmacies. If the use of computers by doctors becomes routine at some point and the handwritten prescription becomes history, I wonder whether this will contribute to a cultural shift in medicine. Will the demise of doctors' illegible scrawl eliminate the feeling of mystery and aura that has been such an important part of the handwritten prescription for so long? Have doctors been slow in embracing electronic prescribing partly because they have known intuitively that the mystique created by their illegible handwriting is a powerful tool in their armamentarium? Handing a patient an illegibly written prescription is certainly more awe-inspiring than telling the patient "I'm going to transmit the prescription to the pharmacy." When the prescription leaves the realm of mystery and enters the realm of commerce as a simple commodity, the magical and placebo aspects of the process are diminished. There is more magic when a prescription comes directly from the hands of a god than from a computer.

Should we as pharmacists welcome the predicted demise of the handwritten prescription and the magical/mystical aura associated with it? Should we view this as a sign of medicine's embrace of science and rejection of snake oil? Every pharmacist knows that the placebo effect can be powerful. Placebos can lessen pain, lower blood pressure, ease depression, etc. Should the placebo effect be ridiculed? Is it dishonest for a health professional to marshal whatever recuperative powers he can? When prescribing a drug, a doctor may say to the patient, "This is a highly effective drug." Such comments have been shown to increase the likelihood that the patient will experience benefits from the drug. On the other hand, when a doctor says to the patient, "I'm not sure whether this drug will work, but let's give it a try," the likelihood of patient benefit is diminished. This is the power of suggestion. The placebo effect is closely associated with the ritual involved in prescribing drugs. It's part of the whole authoritarian figure, white coat, dangling stethoscope persona that doctors intentionally cultivate.

Our customers seem to think that their doctor's handwritten prescription is far more than a simple note telling the pharmacist what drug to dispense, in what quantity, with what directions, etc. Many of our customers view the prescription as a personalized directive from a god. Of course, doctors do little to dissuade their patients from viewing them as gods.

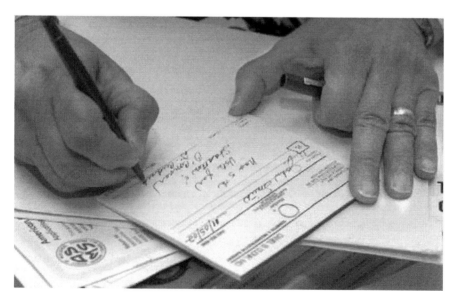

10

Two lawsuits resulting from doctors' illegible handwriting

Illegible handwriting has been a sore spot with pharmacists for many years. It seems that whenever a pharmacist misreads an illegible prescription and consequently dispenses the wrong drug, the pharmacist gets all the blame. But things may be changing. Physicians were named in two lawsuits in the late 1990s because of illegible handwriting.

An illegible prescription that allegedly triggered a fatal medication error resulted in a physician being named as a defendant in a liability lawsuit in Texas. (Carol Ukens, "Fatal Vision, "*Drug Topics*, Sept. 1, 1997, p. 32) A lawsuit was filed against a cardiologist, a pharmacist, and a chain pharmacy in Odessa, Texas, on behalf of the widow and three children of a man who died following the medication error.

The suit alleged, in effect, that the cardiologist who wrote the illegible prescription handed the pharmacist a loaded gun. The pharmacist then pulled the trigger by failing to contact the prescriber and by failing to catch an excessive dosage.

The case began when a man in his 40s was discharged from the hospital by the cardiologist who had been treating him for heart problems. The physician wrote a prescription for the anti-angina drug Isordil. The suit alleged that when presented with the illegible prescription, the pharmacist made no attempt to contact the physician for clarification. The pharmacist read the prescription as the antihypertensive drug Plendil. The patient took the medication for one day. The following morning he suffered a heart attack, and he died several days later.

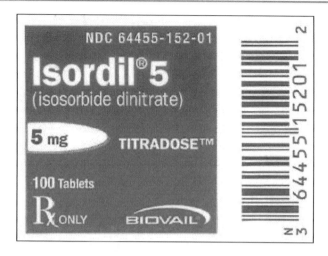

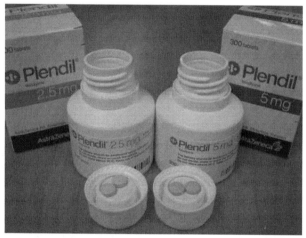

The plaintiff's attorney, Kent Buckingham, said, "The physician screwed up by writing illegibly. The pharmacist screwed up by not calling."

The pharmacist was named in the suit because he did not question the illegible prescription or the high dose of Plendil. The pharmacy was named in the suit because it failed to incorporate controls that could have prevented the error. For example, the pharmacy computer did not catch the excessive dose. And the physician was named in the suit for writing illegibly. According to the Institute for Safe Medication Practices, naming physicians in dispensing error lawsuits has been uncommon. ("Handwriting on the wall?" ISMP Medication Safety Alert, Institute for Safe Medication Practices, July 16, 1997)

On October 14, 1999 the jury found the physician liable for poor penmanship. The cardiologist, Albertson's pharmacy, and the pharmacist were ordered to pay $450,000 to the relatives of the deceased man. The physician was ordered to pay $225,000. Albertson's and the pharmacist were ordered to pay the other $225,000, but the pharmacy settled with the plaintiffs earlier for an undisclosed amount without admitting fault. ("Jury Punishes Poor Rx Penmanship," *Drug Topics*, November 1, 1999, p. 8)

I had hoped that this jury award would send a message to the medical profession that doctors need to learn basic penmanship. Alas, nothing has changed. But I am sure that pharmacists continue to hope that physicians are held accountable for their handwriting. Common sense says that it is almost impossible that this error would have occurred if the prescription had been typewritten or generated by a computer.

In a New York case, a plaintiff sought to recover damages from a pharmacy and pharmacist after ingesting the antihypertensive drug Dynacirc, which was erroneously dispensed instead of the prescribed antibiotic Dynacin. Subsequently, the pharmacy and pharmacist filed a suit against the prescriber, alleging negligence based on the physician's failure to write the prescription clearly and legibly. The pharmacy was found liable for the damages resulting from the dispensing error, and its attempt to shift liability to the physician failed. (Larry M. Simonsmeier, "Pharmacy Blames Physician's Handwriting," *Pharmacy Times*, June 1997, p. 21)

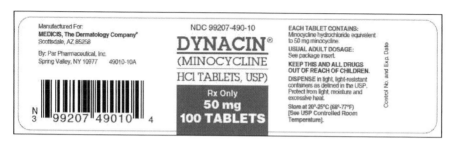

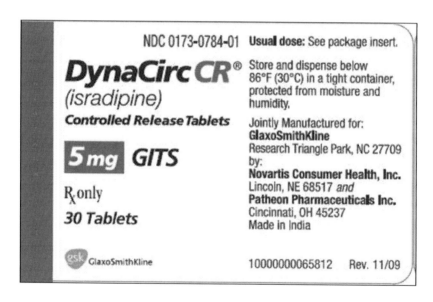

Who should be liable when an injury results from a prescription error allegedly caused by physicians' poor handwriting? Pharmacists are usually irate when they are held liable for misreading a poorly written prescription, while the physician goes blameless.

I propose that all patients who receive poorly legible prescriptions tell their doctors that they are concerned that the pharmacist will have difficulty reading it. If enough people begin doing this, doctors will get the message. The public should be offended by prescriptions that are poorly legible. Patients should request that each letter in each word is plainly written and that each number is plainly written. Doctors cannot justify their poor handwriting. If the public demands it, physicians will be forced to take more time with their handwriting, or, better yet, adopt computer-based prescribing and computer link-ups with community pharmacies.

Illegible handwriting wastes too much time. It wastes the pharmacist's time having to decipher the scrawl. It wastes the doctor's staff's time when the pharmacist calls. It wastes the doctor's time resolving the confusion. And, of course, it inconveniences our (frequently impatient) customers.

The magazine *Pharmacy Times* has a regular section each month titled "Can You Read These Rx's?" I have noticed that some pharmacists approach this section (and illegible handwriting in general) as a fun game. Rather than be amused or entertained or challenged by poorly written prescriptions, pharmacists should be offended. The stakes are simply too high.

Here are a few more things that I wish the public would encourage their doctors to do, in order to cut down on errors from poorly written prescriptions. I wish doctors would always write the purpose of the medication on the prescription. For example, doctors should write, "Take one tablet daily for blood pressure" rather than "Take one tablet daily." This helps both the pharmacist and patient verify that the right medication is being dispensed.

Doctors should write out instructions rather than use abbreviations. For example, they should write "daily" rather than "QD." "QD" is too easily interpreted as QID (four times a day). Several years ago, a pharmacy intern at our store typed "Take one tablet four times a day" on a prescription for the diuretic Lasix for which the doctor had written "1 QD" (one tablet daily). We didn't discover the error until the customer returned for a refill. In this case, no harm occurred because the customer had been taking this drug for several months. We asked him about it and he said, "Yeah, I saw your directions, but I knew I was just supposed to take one a day. I mentioned it to my doctor and he said, 'Wow, they're really trying to dry you out!'" In other circumstances, the results could have been disastrous.

11

Nurses have as much trouble as pharmacists reading doctors' handwriting

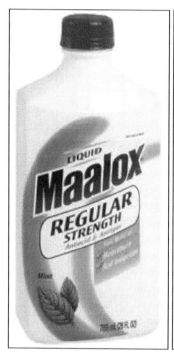
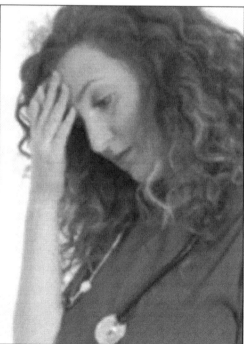

Nurses, like pharmacists, have trouble reading doctors' handwriting. Both nurses and pharmacists are often reluctant to check with the doctor, often because of the doctor's attitude. Here is an anecdote from a caring physician, David Hilfiker, M.D., that accurately describes the trouble illegible handwriting can cause (*Healing the Wounds: A Physician Looks at His Work*, New York: Pantheon, 1985, pp. 156-157).

Angie (I don't even know her last name) lays her own work aside and starts to copy the orders for Mrs. Dimmerling. "Who the hell does he think he is?" she mutters to herself. "I can hardly read this." I continue to write, but I'm listening, almost without knowing it, to Angie's angry comments to herself.

"Beth," Angie says as she walks over to an older nurse on the other side of the nurses' station, I can't even read this. What's Oberdorfer want here?"

"Hmm. I'm not sure. Looks like two teaspoons of Maalox every two hours."

"Yeah, I guess you're right. Two teaspoons. Wait a minute! Oberdorfer never orders two teaspoons of antacid. Remember him getting on that poor intern for not ordering enough? He said you always order at least two tablespoons. Remember him quoting that Journal article about antacid efficacy? He can't have meant two teaspoons."

"Yeah, but he sure didn't write two tablespoons. That's got to be two teaspoons. Why don't you page him and ask."

"Oh, sure, page Oberdorfer and tell him he blew it. 'Dr. Oberdorfer,'" Angie mimics herself in a singsong Southern drawl, "'I think you just made a mistake. You didn't really mean two teaspoons of Maalox, did you?' Come on, Beth, remember when Tricia tried to correct him? He just laid into her and ripped her apart. He wrote 'two teaspoons' and Mrs. Dimmerling's getting two teaspoons."

"I suppose so. It won't hurt Mrs. Dimmerling any, and maybe it'll teach Oberdorfer a lesson. I wouldn't count on that, though."

Angie and Beth return to their work and I try to return to mine. I can hardly believe what I've just heard.

12

I can't read this prescription... Is this doctor prescribing Pediaprofen? Pediapred? Pediazole?

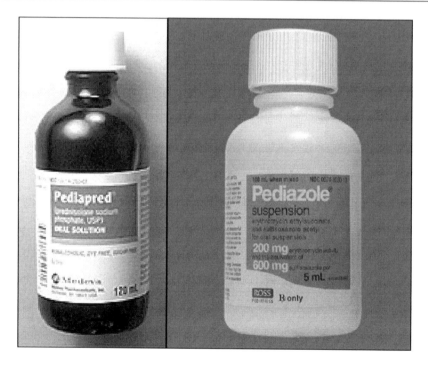

Several years ago I received a poorly legible prescription from a local doctor. It was a Saturday morning when a lady brought in a prescription for her young son. I couldn't tell whether the doctor wanted Pediaprofen or Pediapred. The directions were clearly written: "Take 2 teaspoonsful every 12 hours." I called the doctor's office and got his answering service. I was told that this doctor was not on call this weekend. His partner was on call. The doctor who had actually written this prescription a couple of days earlier was at the beach this weekend. I asked the answering service to have the on-call partner call me at the pharmacy.

An hour or so later, the partner finally called. I explained the situation to him. I said, "It looks like either Pediaprofen or Pediapred." Then the doctor asked me, "How old is the child?" We had the child's age in the computer from a previous visit. Based solely on the child's age and his partner's directions, the doctor determined that the prescription couldn't be for Pediaprofen. He concluded that it had to be Pediapred. So he said, "Make it Pediapred."

It turns out that the customer was not coming back until later in the day, so I kept the prescription on the counter and kept looking at it. I was uncomfortable with the way that the partner had come to his decision without checking the patient's records.

About three hours later (the child's mother still hadn't come back), I looked at the prescription again and, eureka! it occurred to me: It's not Pediapred or Pediaprofen. It's Pediazole!!!

So I double-checked the recommended dosage for Pediazole. The *Physicians' Desk Reference* says that Pediazole should be given three or four times per day, not every twelve hours as the doctor had clearly written.

I called the doctor's on-call partner and told him that I thought the prescription was not for Pediaprofen or Pediapred. I said it looks like Pediazole. The doctor then said that I should fax the prescription to their office—where he would be in an hour—so that he could look at it. He told me that he also wanted to show his partner how much of a problem this illegible handwriting was causing.

We get a ton of prescriptions from these two doctors so I didn't want to make either of them mad at us. So I said jokingly that I wished he wouldn't make his partner mad at us for this incident. (I know from past experience that the out-of-town partner can be a first class jerk.) He said, "If he gets mad, that's his problem." Hopefully, my joking eased the tension in this situation because the partner with whom I was speaking was becoming mildly irritated over the situation.

I faxed the prescription to their office. About three hours later, having received no return call, I called their office and asked whether he received my fax. He said, "Yeah, and it looks like Pediazole." This made him look negligent for jumping to the conclusion earlier that the prescription was for Pediapred.

The doctor asked whether I had the mother's phone number handy because he wanted to call her to see exactly what the child's problem was in order to determine which drug had been prescribed. I gave the doctor the patient's home phone number. A few minutes later, the doctor called back and said that he had spoken with the child's mother and that, based on the child's symptoms, the prescription had to be for Pediazole even though he couldn't figure out why his partner had prescribed it every twelve hours.

In summary, this is what happened. I initially called this doctor and told him that his partner apparently was prescribing either Pediaprofen or Pediapred. The partner jumped to the conclusion that the prescription had to be for Pediapred. It turns out that it was neither. It was for Pediazole.

Situations such as this occur far too frequently. It's time that pharmacists take a stand and it's time that the public realizes the absurdity of jokes about doctors' illegible handwriting. Illegible handwriting is no laughing matter.

Note: Just because all three of these drug names start with *pedia* doesn't mean they're used for the same thing. They certainly are not. They are all entirely different. Pediaprofen (now, Children's Motrin) is used for pain, fever, and inflammation. Pediapred is a prednisone-like drug that is used for a long list of disorders (endocrine, rheumatic, collagen, skin, allergies, respiratory, blood disorders, cancers, etc.). Pediazole is an antibiotic. *Pedia* in each case stands for "pediatric." What these three drugs do have in common is that they're all used in kids.

13

Do male doctors write less legibly than female doctors?

The existence of physicians' poor penmanship has been acknowledged for a long time. But I have never heard anyone ask the obvious question: *"Why* do physicians write so poorly?" Probably the most frequently cited explanation is that doctors are very busy people. But this explanation isn't very convincing because lots of people in our society are very busy. Is illegible handwriting proportional to how busy one is, or are there other considerations?

A study in the *British Medical Journal* [Berwick DM and Winick-off, DE, "The truth about doctors' illegible handwriting: a prospective study," *BMJ* 1996 Dec 21-28;313(7072):1657-8] found that significantly lower legibility than average was associated with being an executive and being male, rather than being a doctor per se.

It might be interesting to ask pharmacists whether they feel that female physicians are less likely to have illegible handwriting. What percent of calls to doctors' offices for prescription clarification are to female physicians? As I look back on my career as a pharmacist, my impression is that calls to doctors' offices to clarify illegible handwriting are overwhelmingly to male doctors.

Of course, it would be wrong to associate illegible handwriting completely with ego. One of the most arrogant physicians in one town I used to work in had absolutely beautiful handwriting. I never recall having any difficulty in reading his prescriptions. Yet, whenever he called the pharmacy, it was clear that he expected us to genuflect to him. We were only pharmacists and he was the doctor and God help us if we forgot that.

In fairness to doctors, it occurs to me that there are lots of pharmacists who also write poorly. Is poor handwriting by pharmacists any less dangerous than poor handwriting by doctors? I can recall many instances in which I have had questions about a phoned-in prescription that was transcribed by another pharmacist. It wouldn't be so bad if all pharmacists filled all their "doctor phone-ins" themselves before they leave their shift. However, in many instances, pharmacists leave a pile of these "doctor phone-ins" for the pharmacist on the next shift. But there is a significant difference here. When the illegible handwriting is from another pharmacist, I can usually contact that pharmacist more easily than a doctor. And the pharmacist's attitude is usually more understanding and less arrogant, so I am less reluctant to call the pharmacist.

Do male doctors write less legibly than female doctors?

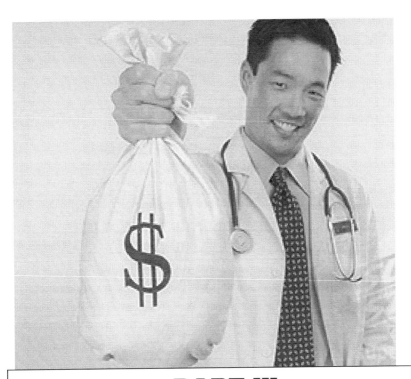

PART III

DOCTORS

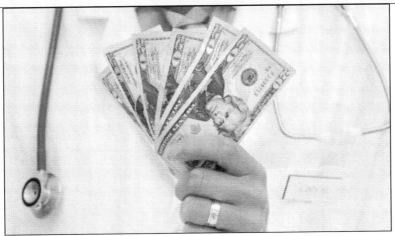

14

Mistakes when doctors talk too fast on the phone

I once worked with a pharmacist who had recently graduated from pharmacy school. He had been licensed for only a few weeks. One day he made the comment to me that he was sometimes having difficulty keeping up with doctors when they phoned in prescriptions. This pharmacist asked me if I knew any way to slow the doctors down. In the real world, telling the doctors "Slow down!" is not a great option. Doctors are busy people who seem to do everything in a hurry, including speaking with pharmacists.

This young pharmacist has a very legitimate concern. Doctors often phone the pharmacy with anywhere from one to five prescriptions for a single patient. The pharmacist must write down the patient's name, the drug name, the number of pills, how often the pills are to be taken (once a day, three times a day, every 4 hours, etc.), and the number of refills. Each piece of info is critically important, so pharmacists are rightfully concerned with writing down everything accurately. The more prescriptions the doctor phones in, the greater the chances that pharmacists will write down something incorrectly.

Early in my career, I, too, experienced this problem with speedy doctors. On more than one occasion, I had to call back to the doctor's office and ask the receptionist/nurse/office manager, "Dr. Smith just called me with a prescription for Bob Williams and I'm not sure how many Vicodin he wants Mr. Williams to have. Could you ask Dr. Smith?" Obviously this is an uncomfortable conversation and it is time consuming.

Some pharmacists think they can remember the doctor's instructions as if somehow our brain records everything and lets us mentally rewind and replay the phone conversation after the doctor has hung up. But most pharmacists do try to write down everything as the doctor speaks, rather than rely on our memory. Sometimes I write down the info so quickly that I can't decipher my own handwriting after the doctor has hung up.

You ask: Why not read each prescription back to the doctor? Reading everything back to the doctor when the doctor finishes is a good idea but it is sometimes quite uncomfortable because the doctor's impatience is palpable. Reading everything back to the doctor might imply that I am a rookie pharmacist who's not confident and competent in my job. Pharmacists sometimes like to impress doctors by our ability to keep up with them. An experienced pharmacist doesn't have to ask the doctor to repeat anything. After writing down everything the doctors says, the experienced pharmacist immediately says to the doctor simply "Thank you." We as pharmacists are saying to the doctor: *Doctor, you think you're good at what you do. Well I'm just as good at what I do.*

In answering this young pharmacist's question regarding a method to slow down doctors on the phone, I told him what worked for me: "To slow the doctor down, every few seconds I interject an *okay* into the conversation. Sometimes I say *okay* quickly. Other times I drag out my *okay* for as long as I can. The pharmacist needs a way to break the doctor's stride when he's off to the races. Only a doctor who's a first class jerk will run over your *okays*. Inserting the word *okay* forces the doctor to pause momentarily or else appear to be a complete asshole who's totally unconcerned with avoiding mistakes."

Clearly, most phone calls from doctors are not what I would describe as being at a leisurely pace. I once witnessed a pharmacist answer the phone line reserved for incoming calls from doctors (our so-called "doctors' line"). After a few moments, the pharmacist said, "Doctor, can you hold on for a second? You caught me with my pants down." The pharmacist couldn't find a pen or pre-scription pad to write down the doctor's prescription. This could be viewed as a friendly and human way to ask the doctor to wait for a few seconds, but I admit I felt a little uncomfortable hearing the pharmacist express it that way.

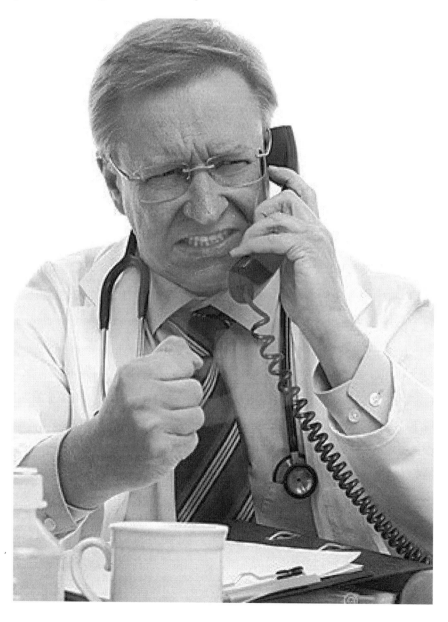

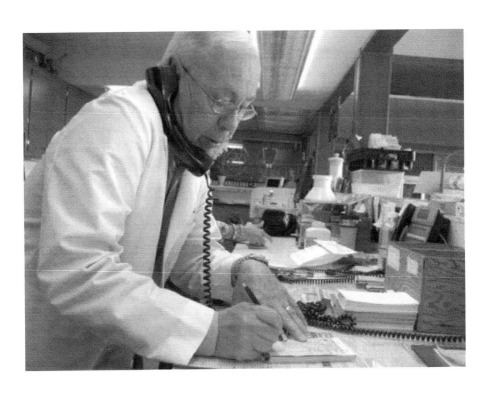

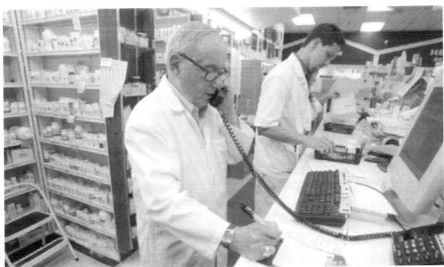

15

Mistakes when nurses and receptionists phone prescriptions to the pharmacy

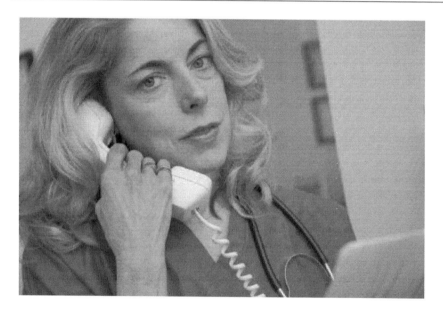

A not uncommon source of error is when a nurse or reception-ist phones the pharmacy with a prescription. Young pharmacists are surprised that doctors so often allow inexperienced staff with very little knowledge of drug names to phone prescriptions to the pharmacist. It's as if the nurse or receptionist is doing nothing more critical than phoning the local sub shop with a lunch order.

When the nurse or receptionist calls the pharmacist, it is not uncommon for us to hear her ask for help in deciphering a drug name. Pharmacists commonly hear her say: "You'll have to help me with this one" or "This one looks like" or "I'll need to spell this one for you." Pharmacists are not only amazed that doctors allow such inexperienced people to relay prescriptions to the pharmacy, but we are often worried that we can be blamed if an error occurs.

The nurse or receptionist can misread the doctor's prescription but, if an error occurs, that nurse or receptionist can claim "I phoned in the right medication! The pharmacist must have written it down wrong!" Obviously, we as pharmacists don't have proof (a handwritten prescription in our files) that the nurse or receptionist made a mistake.

I was filling in at a pharmacy in Durham, North Carolina, for a week for a pharmacist's vacation. One day I came to work and the other pharmacist said to me that I had taken a phoned-in prescription from a doctor's office in which I wrote down Prilosec (which was then a prescription-only drug), when, in fact, the prescription was for Prozac. Apparently the patient had questioned the medication received, called the doctor's office, asked the nurse or receptionist what had happened, and then, apparently, that same nurse or receptionist claimed to have called in the right medication.

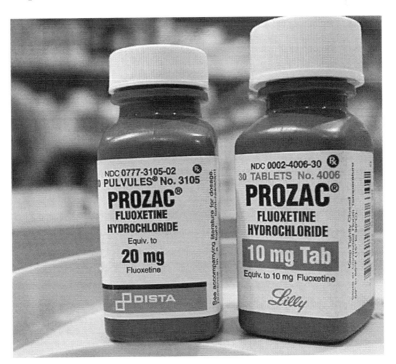

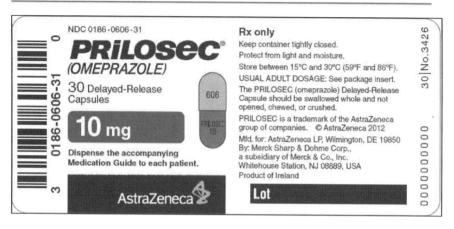

Of course, it is very possible that I did indeed write down the wrong drug. Both Prilosec and Prozac can sound very similar on the phone, especially when there's background noise in the pharmacy: another phone ringing, technicians jabbering, customers talking and complaining, etc.

So, I could have made the error, or the nurse or receptionist may have misread the doctor's prescription. It's possible that I misunderstood the drug name. Perhaps I had just filled a prescription for Prilosec and consequently I had that drug on my mind.

When the other pharmacist informed me that the nurse or receptionist claimed I simply wrote down the wrong drug, I had no way of proving otherwise. The nurse or receptionist may have misread the doctor's handwriting and she may have been covering up for her own error.

On another occasion, a different nurse or receptionist phoned me with a prescription for Inderal LA 40 mg. Inderal is used for conditions like hypertension, angina, or migraine. I didn't recall that this sounded like a strength that was available so I asked the nurse or receptionist to repeat the drug name and strength. She said again, "Inderal LA 40mg." I said, "Could you hold on just a second?" I wanted to take a quick look at our shelves to see whether we had such a strength. We didn't but this doesn't necessarily mean that it is not on the market. We were extremely busy at that time, so I didn't have the opportunity to check the appropriate reference material to see whether it was indeed on the market. So I returned to the phone and repeated again, "Inderal LA 40 mg." The nurse or receptionist again said "Yes." When I finally had time to look it up, I discovered what I suspected. The drug is not available in that strength. The long-acting form of Inderal (known as Inderal LA) is available only in the following strengths: 60 mg, 80 mg, 120 mg, and 160 mg. I called back and asked to speak with the same nurse or receptionist with whom I had spoken previously. I said to her, "Inderal LA 40 mg is not listed." She said, "Hold on and let me check." She returned a few minutes later and said, "It's supposed to be Inderal LA 160 mg." I told my partner about this incident and she commented, "If people only knew how many mistakes are made in doctors' offices!" The bottom line is that this nurse or receptionist called in a dose that was one-fourth of the intended dose. Under other circumstances, this could have been a dangerous mistake.

Here is an example of a nurse calling a pharmacy about a commonly prescribed drug. In this case, the nurse was apparently inadequately familiar with the drug to be able to prevent an obvious misinterpretation of a doctor's directions. Examples like this happen all the time in pharmacies across America. This example involves the anti-diarrheal drug Imodium which is available as 2 mg capsules. A fancy term for "diarrhea" is "unformed stools." Hospital pharmacist Steve Timmerman writes in *Drug Topics* ("Strange Rx Stories: Now That's a Smart Stool," July 1, 2002, p. 42):

It's not unusual to receive orders for Imodium as "two capsules now and then one after each loose stool." One evening, a nurse called and told me she needed Imodium 4 mg for an initial dose and then 2 mg for every time there was an "informed stool." I repeated this order back to her and questioned the "informed" part. She was confident the order read "informed stool." I brought the initial dose to the patient care area and picked up the copy of the order. The physician had actually written for 2 mg to be given after each "unformed" stool.

The point is that the system is absolutely fraught with the potential for errors from the time a doctor decides to prescribe a drug until that medication is picked up at the drugstore.

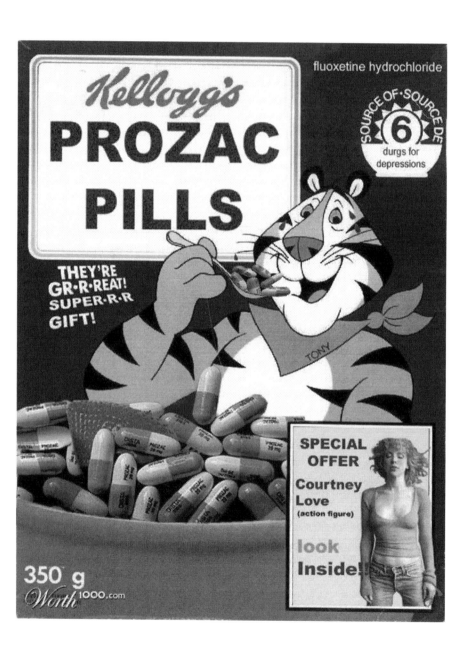

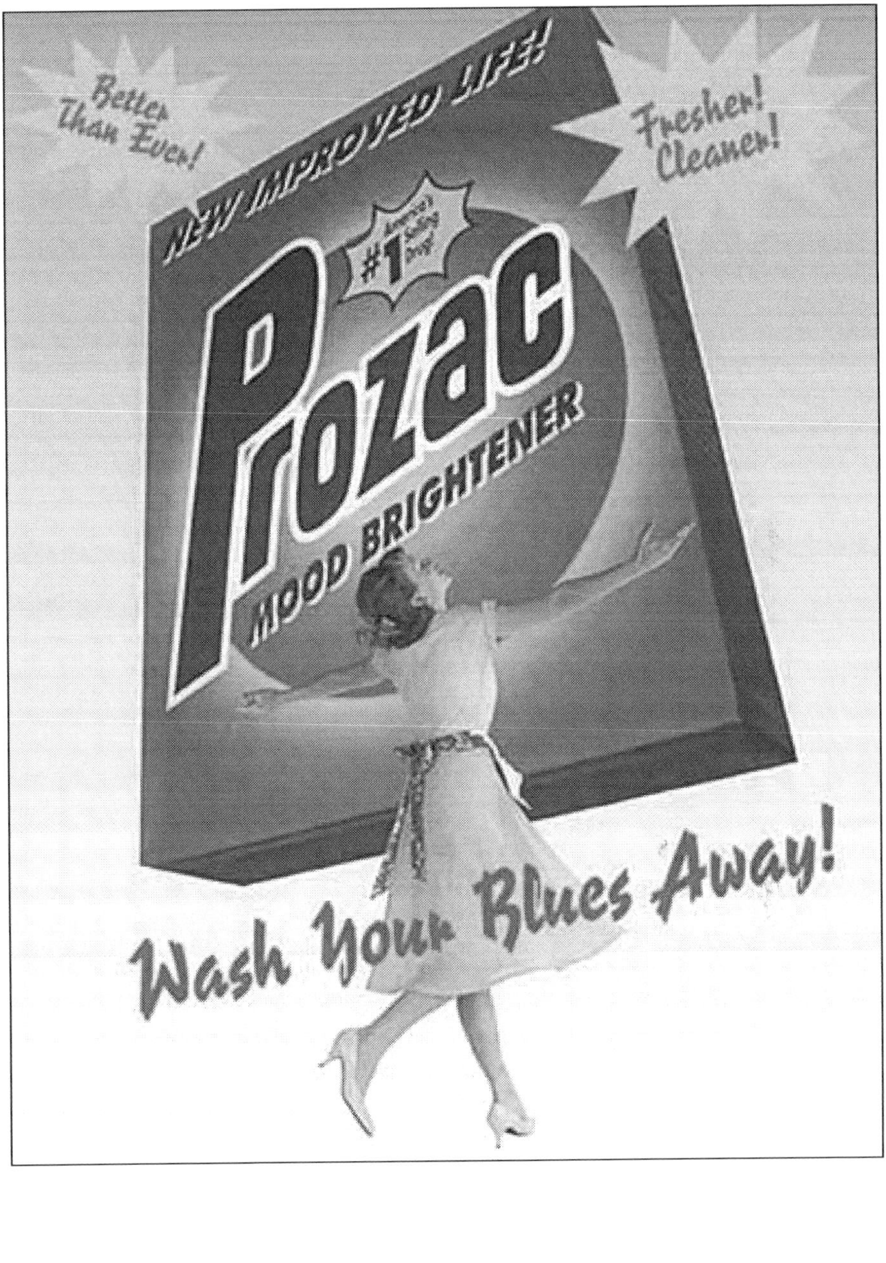
Better Than Ever!
NEW IMPROVED LIFE!
Fresher! Cleaner!
America's #1 Selling Drug!
Prozac
MOOD BRIGHTENER
Wash Your Blues Away!

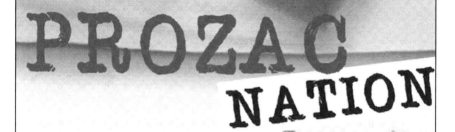

CHRISTINA **RICCI**   JASON **BIGGS**   ANNE **HECHE**   MICHELLE **WILLIAMS**   JESSICA **LANGE**   JONATHAN **RHYS-MEYERS**

PROZAC
NATION

**BASADA EN EL BEST-SELLER
AUTOBIOGRÁFICO DE ELIZABETH WURTZEL**

   manga films

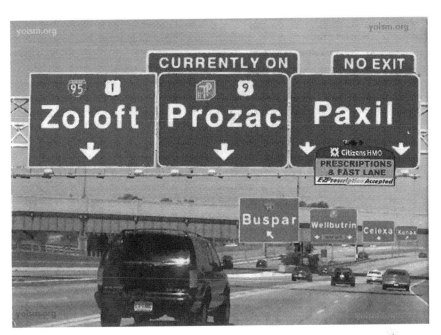

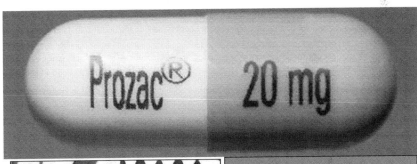

ST CHUR

JESUS IS MY PROZAC

God made us neighbors and Prozac made us Friends

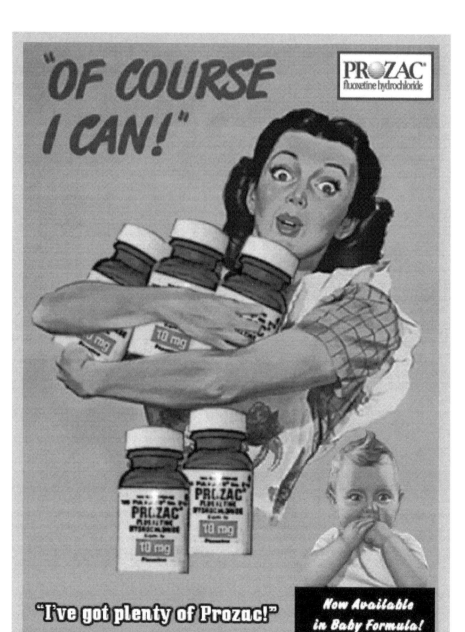

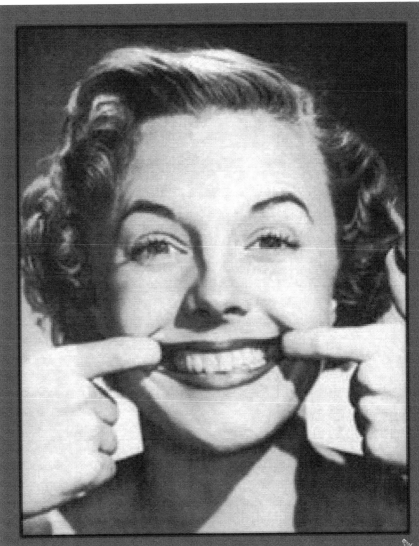

I took my
Prozac today

PLATO
NOT PROZAC!

APPLYING ETERNAL WISDOM
TO EVERYDAY PROBLEMS

"You don't need a prescription for this mind-opening, possibly life-altering, book. . . . The thinking person's guide to understanding yourself."
—*Cleveland Plain Dealer*

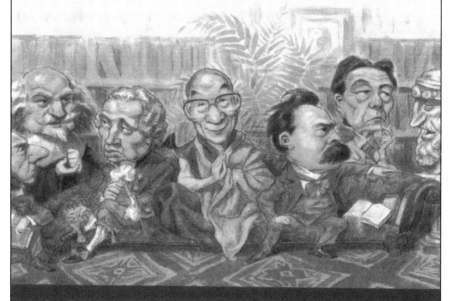

LOU MARINOFF, PH.D.

IF YOU'VE BEEN
LISTENING TO PROZAC,
YOU HAVEN'T HEARD
THE REAL STORY...

AS SEEN BY
MILLIONS ON
OPRAH!

TALKING
BACK
TO
PROZAC

WHAT
DOCTORS AREN'T
TELLING YOU ABOUT TODAY'S
MOST CONTROVERSIAL DRUG

PETER R. BREGGIN, M.D.
BESTSELLING AUTHOR OF *TOXIC PSYCHIATRY*
AND GINGER ROSS BREGGIN

"THERE IS UNQUESTIONABLY A GREAT DEAL OF TRUTH IN WHAT BREGGIN
WRITES. LET THE PILL-SWALLOWER BEWARE."—Los Angeles Times

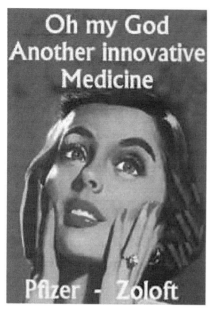

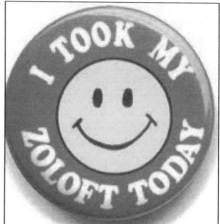

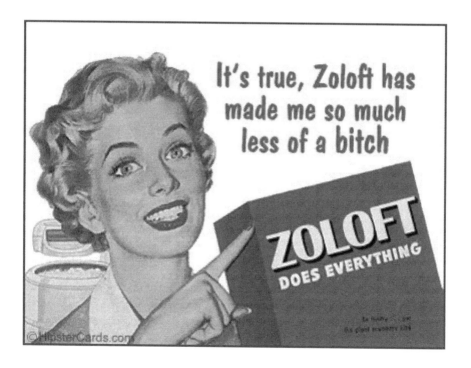

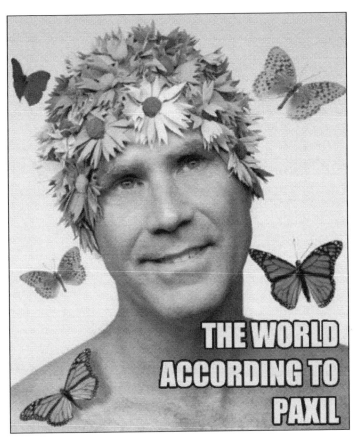

THE WORLD
ACCORDING TO
PAXIL

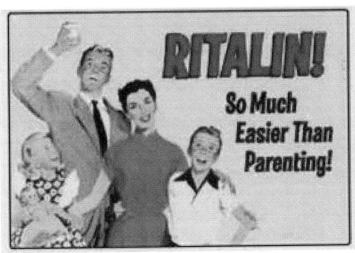

RITALIN!
So Much
Easier Than
Parenting!

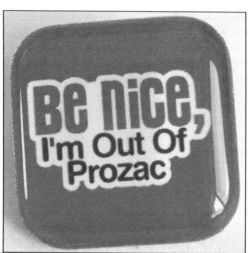

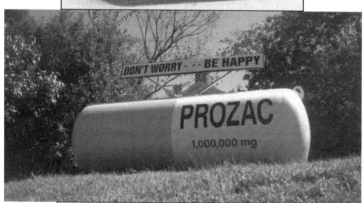

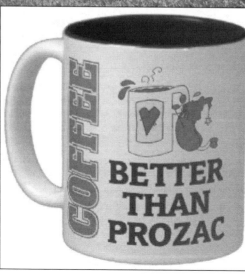

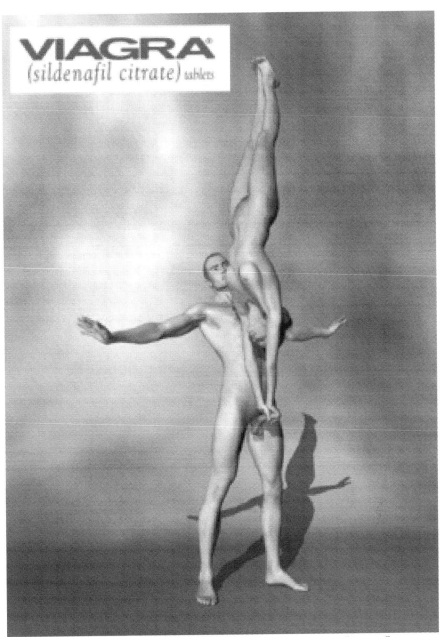

Viagra is used to treat erectile dysfunction. The drug name "Viagra" conjures up the immense power of Niagara Falls. If you replace the letter "r" in Viagra with an "n" and rearrange some letters, Viagra becomes "Vagina."

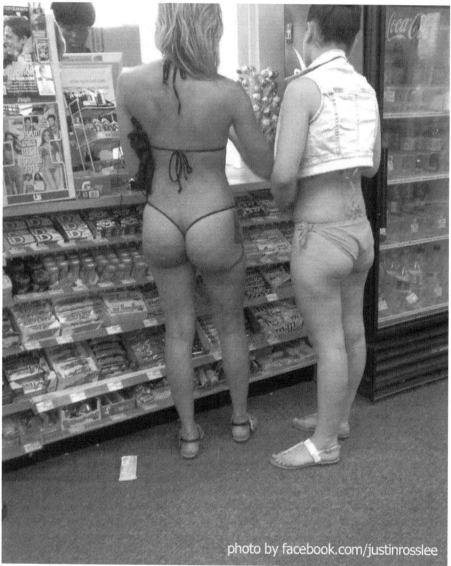

Not typical CVS customers but a welcome diversion from a tightly regimented workplace.

16

Mistakes when prescriptions are faxed from doctors' offices

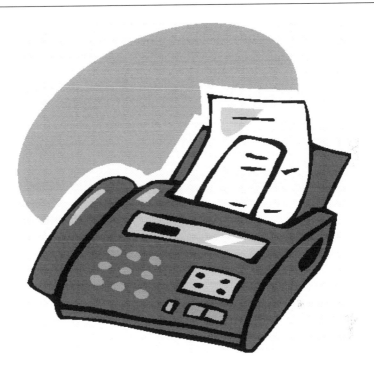

Prescriptions faxed from doctors' offices can be another significant source of errors. Here are three separate incidents involving prescriptions faxed to pharmacies. The first incident involved Neurontin, the second incident involved Monopril, and the third incident involved lisinopril/hctz. (Kate Kelly, PharmD, and Allen J. Vaida, PharmD, "'Fax Noise' Can Result in Medication Errors," *Pharmacy Times*, July 2004, p. 28)

Most health care practitioners would agree that facsimile (fax) machines have facilitated communication of prescriptions. There are, however, inherent problems associated with this technology. In fact, a recent article in the *Journal of Managed Care Pharmacy* found that prescriptions received by fax required a greater number of clarification calls than those received by other methods of communication.

We received a report from a longterm care facility about a patient who had been receiving Neurontin (gabapentin) 600 mg tid [three times a day]. An order had been faxed to the pharmacy that the pharmacist thought read to change the Neurontin dose to "300 mg 1 tab qid [four times a day]." The change was made, and the new dose was sent to the facility.

Later, when the pharmacist received the original order and compared it with the faxed order, he realized that the physician had actually requested a change to "800 mg 1 tab qid." The left side of the order had been cut off during the fax transmission, making the "8" look like a "3." Fortunately, because the pharmacist had been sent the original order for comparison, he quickly realized the mistake. Unfortunately, not all outpatient pharmacies receive the original prescription for comparison.

In another report, a faxed prescription was received at a pharmacy for what appeared to be for Monopril (fosinopril) "10 mg #90 one tablet daily." Despite the fact that the fax machine created a definite vertical streak that ran between the drug name and the strength, the pharmacist felt confident in her interpretation of the prescription. Unfortunately, the prescription was actually for "40 mg." The streak had run through the "4" in "40 mg," making it look like "10 mg" instead.

A prescription was faxed to a mail-order pharmacy... for "lisinopril/hctz." (Note: Institute for Safe Medication Practices does not condone the use of the abbreviation "hctz.") The pharmacist interpreted this order as "20/25 mg." What the prescriber had actually written, however, was "20/12.5 mg." A subtle vertical gap in the faxed copy (which also can be seen "breaking" the circles around "3 months supply") had obliterated the "1" in "12.5." In addition, the pharmacist reading the order had misinterpreted the decimal point as one of many stray marks.

17
Mistakes with e-prescriptions

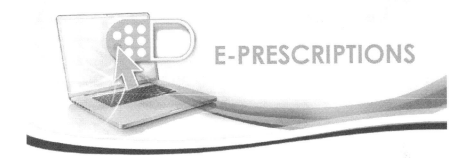

Much has been written lately about how transmitting prescriptions electronically to pharmacies can drastically cut down on errors. Many articles imply that this technology can virtually eliminate errors caused by doctors' illegible handwriting. But few of these articles explain that electronic prescriptions (e-prescribing) can introduce a new set of problems. Pharmacists have many stories about problems that can result from the use of this technology. For example, here is a post from the Internet discussion group sci.med.pharmacy by a pharmacist who goes by rxempress (rxempress@mmchsi.com) (Subject: What do you think about medication errors? Newsgroups: sci.med.pharmacy, Sept. 16, 2004)

I have caught quite a few errors on electronic prescriptions. Our local doctors are using palm pilots which involve a touch sensitive screen. I have seen a couple cases where they selected the wrong drug (touched the wrong one). Last week one was sent to me with the directions "one tablet 4 times daily". This was 4 times the regular dose. Dr keyed in QID (4 times daily) and meant QD (once daily). This is exactly the type of error that these systems are supposed to prevent. (It is very easy to misread a handwritten QID and a QD). The mistakes are still being made... it's just easier to read the mistake. It's catching the mistake that's the tough part and in this case contacting the doctor and explaining the mistake took about a week to do.

There are advantages and disadvantages to having doctors transmit prescriptions electronically to the pharmacy. One pharmacist sent me an e-mail in which he stated one advantage:

Electronic prescriptions seem to be increasing all the time. Depending on the store I think they are about 10% of the total. One positive way to look at these prescriptions is that in the past each one would have been the phone ringing. The telephone ringing in my ear has a Pavlov's dog reaction in me. I am sure the sound raises my pressure a bit each time. The phone is such an intrusion on what you are doing at the moment.

Here is a disadvantage of electronic prescriptions. This is a case from the Institute for Safe Medication Practices in which a hospitalized patient died from respiratory arrest after a physician entered drug orders electronically under the name of the wrong patient. ("Oops, Sorry, Wrong Patient!: A Patient Verification Process is Needed Everywhere, Not Just at the Bedside," Institute for Safe Medication Practices—ISMP Medication Safety Alert! Acute Care Edition, posted May 17, 2011, http://www.medscape.com/viewarticle/742372?src=mp&spon=30)

A dehydrated lung cancer patient was admitted to the emergency department for IV hydration. Another patient from a motor vehicle accident (MVA) was awaiting intubation and transfer to a local trauma center. The same physician was caring for both patients. The physician gave verbal orders for vecuronium and midazolam for the MVA patient, but he inadvertently entered the medication orders electronically into the cancer patient's record. The nurse caring for the cancer patient went on break, and a covering nurse administered the paralytic and sedative to the cancer patient even though he was not intubated. The patient experienced a respiratory arrest and died.

Here is another case from the Institute for Safe Medication Practices. In this case a doctor's error on an electronic prescription was made worse when a pharmacist edited the prescription in an attempt to correct that doctor's error. The patient suffered respiratory arrest as a consequence of the pharmacist's error in the process of correcting the doctor's error. The patient was fortunately resuscitated. ("Keeping patients safe from iatrogenic methadone overdoses," Institute for Safe Medication Practices—ISMP Medication Safety Alert! Acute Care Edition, Feb. 14, 2008 http://www.ismp.org/newsletters/acutecare/articles/20080214.asp)

ISMP received a report about a 17-year-old patient with a traumatic brain injury who received 25 mg of methadone BID [twice a day] instead of methylphenidate. Using the hospital's computerized prescriber order entry system, the physician had increased the patient's methylphenidate dose from 20 to 25 mg, but he accidentally selected a 2.5 mg tablet strength, which was available in the hospital (1/2 tablets of the 5 mg strength were routinely packaged by the pharmacy). During the order verification process, the pharmacist edited the order to indicate that 10 mg strength tablets should be used, but he accidentally changed the order from methylphenidate to methadone. The mnemonics for these drugs were almost identical: methadone 10 mg = METH10, and methylphenidate 10 mg = METH10T. The computer system did not alert the pharmacist that he had inadvertently changed the ordered medication, rather than the strength of tablets used to prepare the dose. The patient suffered a respiratory arrest after taking two doses of methadone; fortunately, he was resuscitated.

When pharmacist **Joe Laborsky** was the publisher at *Drug Topics*, he maintained a "Publisher's Blog" in which he invited feedback from pharmacists. During one period in the latter part of 2007, Laborsky's blog dealt with electronic prescribing. Several pharmacists posted comments questioning the accuracy of e-prescribing. ("Publisher's Blog: E-prescribing—Pharmacy Pays To Play," *Drug Topics*, Sept. 13, 2007). Here is a sample:

Kelly / Pflugerville, Texas / Posted Oct 31, 2007 It has been my experience thus far that the chance of errors in prescribing is much greater with electronic prescribing than traditional methods. Those who tout e-prescribing as safer obviously haven't worked much in a pharmacy to observe the system in actual practice. Their interests are self-serving in trying to sell technology for the sake of technology and their profits, without any practical advantages whatsoever. It is so much easier to erroneously click on the wrong button than to write out the wrong drug. I have spent much more time contacting doctors in the past several months to clarify electronic prescriptions (wrong drug, strength, directions) than I have in the last several years with traditional prescriptions.

Ken / Mendham, New Jersey / Posted Oct 16, 2007 Accuracy? I have found more errors by e-prescribers than with written Rxs. The difference is that when the error is made, the e-script makes it look appropriate. ...As for improved accuracy "studies", who's paying for these studies?

Frustrated R.Ph. / Iowa / Posted Oct 17, 2007 I agree with others. I have seen horrible errors with electronic generated prescriptions.

Drug Topics **publisher Joe Laborsky, R.Ph. comments / Nov. 7, 2007:** Thanks to all of you who took the time to respond to my e-prescribing blog. ...I have to tell you that I was surprised to hear from many of you about mistakes M.D.s have made using this technology. This alarms me even more in that one of the primary advantages of this technology is that it should be a more accurate and reliable means of communicating the prescriber's choice of medication(s) to the pharmacy.

   Harold E. Cohen, R.Ph, Editor-in-Chief at *U.S. Pharmacist,* **offers his perspective on electronic prescriptions** ("The e-ffective Pharmacist," *U.S. Pharmacist*, Feb. 2008, p. 2):

   There is much discussion lately about how e-prescribing is the answer to all of pharmacy's woes, particularly drug errors. In fact, a spokesperson for General Motors was quoted in the *Detroit News* as saying, "The benefits of ePrescribing are overwhelming in terms of reducing medication errors." I'm not so sure. There is little doubt that e-prescribing will certainly all but eliminate prescription errors caused by sloppy physician handwriting, but it does nothing for prescriptions that are written incorrectly in the first place, and that seems to be a far bigger issue than illegible handwriting. One New York pharmacist recently wrote me that she has personally witnessed several errors with prescriptions that were electronically transmitted. She recalled one instance in which a very legible electronically transmitted prescription had the wrong drug prescribed on it. The pharmacist caught the mistake because the prescription was not consistent with her patient's medical and drug history. Other problems she's encountered are prescriptions containing "strengths which do not exist, directions which are terminated before the prescription was sent electronically [she thinks the directions may have been too long and didn't entirely fit into that data field], and no indication of whether the physician prescribed a generic or brand." She has also received prescriptions for patients who normally do not get their prescriptions filled in her store. She said that several times patients have arrived to pick up an electronically transmitted prescription that was not yet transmitted. In such cases, she must then call the doctor and get the prescription over the phone. The electronic prescription generally arrives after the patient has already left the store with the filled prescription in hand. That wouldn't be so bad if it weren't for the fact that she is paying a transmission fee for every e-prescription she receives. She concludes: "I haven't found electronic transmissions to have decreased mistakes or saved time; it just changed the nature of mistakes being committed and causes me to call the physician for a different reason. Adding insult to injury, my pharmacy is paying for these mistakes to be transmitted."

Estimates vary regarding the precise frequency at which prescriptions are transmitted electronically from doctors to pharmacies. Eighteen percent of prescriptions were being sent electronically in 2010, up from six percent in 2008, according to a National Progress Report on e-prescribing released by SureScripts, which operates an e-prescription network. SureScripts says that e-prescribing was used by one in four prescribers in 2010. SureScripts also says that the federal government's leadership and incentive structures are part of the reason for this increase. ("E-Prescribing Nearly Tripled in 2009: Report," *U.S. Pharmacist*, September 2010, p. 59)

Why have doctors been slow in embracing computer-based prescribing? Perhaps a big reason is the cost and complexity of computerizing a medical practice. Perhaps doctors fear what happens when their system crashes in the middle of a very hectic day. Of course, one of the biggest reasons for doctors continuing to embrace handwritten prescriptions is that they're so handy.

Perhaps computers make the doctor feel that the computer is in charge, not the doctor. That's certainly how I feel in the drugstore. The computer is the nerve center of the pharmacy nowadays. Pharmacy has become largely a data entry enterprise in which the ability to type fast is a major asset for technicians and pharmacists. But computers are very humbling and egalitarian.

I'm speculating but perhaps doctors don't want to become servants to computers wherein their large egos are subsumed by the strict dictates of this technology. Perhaps doctors see the computer as a threatening cultural shift in medicine that moves the emphasis toward technology and away from the view that the doctor is the center of the universe. Perhaps doctors would like their patients to believe that the prescription is too magical and mysterious for something as pedestrian as a computer. Perhaps doctors view computers as appropriate for data-entry, bookkeeping, billing, and scheduling, but inadequate for perpetuating the belief that doctors are gods.

According to a study supported by the federal Agency for Healthcare Research and Quality and the Harvard Risk Management Foundation, e-prescriptions are just as error-prone as paper scripts. (Robert Lowes, "E-Prescriptions Just as Error-Prone as Paper Scripts," *Medscape Medical News*, July 1, 2011. *J Am Med Inf Assn*. Published online June 29, 2011 www.medscape.com)

Government and the healthcare industry have placed big bets on digital technology, and electronic prescribing in particular, for the sake of patient safety, but a new study reports that the error rate with computer-generated prescriptions in physician offices roughly matches that for paper scripts: about 1 in 10.

However, results from the study, published online June 29 in the *Journal of the American Medical Informatics Association*, are not as damning as they may initially appear. Error rates varied widely depending on the type of e-prescribing software used, with some programs outperforming pen and paper. In addition, software improvements could eliminate more than 80% of the mistakes, most of them involving omitted information.

In 2010, an estimated 190,000 physicians were electronically prescribing, the technical term for transmitting scripts directly to a pharmacy computer, according to a pharmacy industry group called Surescripts. That number does not include physicians who create a prescription with computer software and then either fax it to the pharmacy or give patients a printout.

Since 2009, the federal government has been paying hundreds of millions of dollars in Medicare bonuses to physicians and other clinicians who electronically prescribe. The government operates an even pricier incentive program for electronic health records, and e-prescribing is one of the prerequisites for earning a 6-figure bonus.

The new study study examined nearly 3900 computer-generated prescriptions received by a pharmacy chain in 2008 in Florida, Massachusetts, and Arizona, regardless of whether they were faxed or electronically transmitted to pharmacies or were printed out. Of those prescriptions, 11.7% contained at least 1 error. Researchers did not ascertain whether errors were corrected by the pharmacy chain or whether they led to an actual adverse drug event. Lead author Karen Nanji, MD, MPH, writes that the 11.7% figure is "consistent with the literature on manual handwritten prescription error rates."

Roughly one third of the errors represented potential adverse drug events, none of them life-threatening.

Software Improvements Must Be Physician-Friendly

Omitted information such as drug dose, duration, and frequency accounted for almost 61% of the errors detected by the authors. The rest of the errors stemmed from unclear, conflicting, or clinically incorrect information.

Software improvements, Dr. Nanji and coauthors write, could eliminate the vast majority of these mistakes. E-prescribing programs can incorporate so-called forcing functions that would prevent physicians from completing a prescription unless they enter required information, including complete drug names and proper abbreviations. Likewise, decision-support tools can issue alerts about a wrong drug dose or frequency. However, the authors note, physicians may rebel against e-prescribing software if antierror safeguards make it too slow or annoying to use.

Some e-prescribing programs included in the study appeared to give users a technological edge. The error rate associated with one such program was only 5.1% compared with a whopping 37.5% for another. However, the study did not assess whether the root cause was system design or how well or poorly the systems were implemented in physician offices. Training physicians and staff on new software systems, the authors note, is often given short shrift.

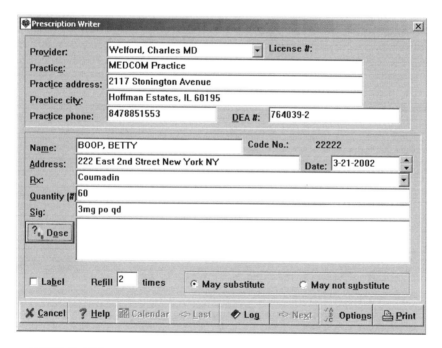

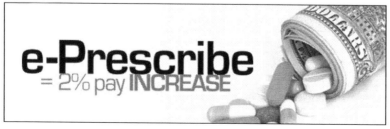

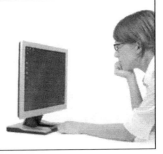

Prescribe medicine electronically.

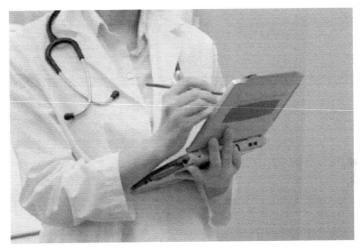

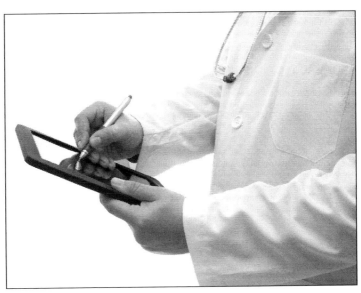

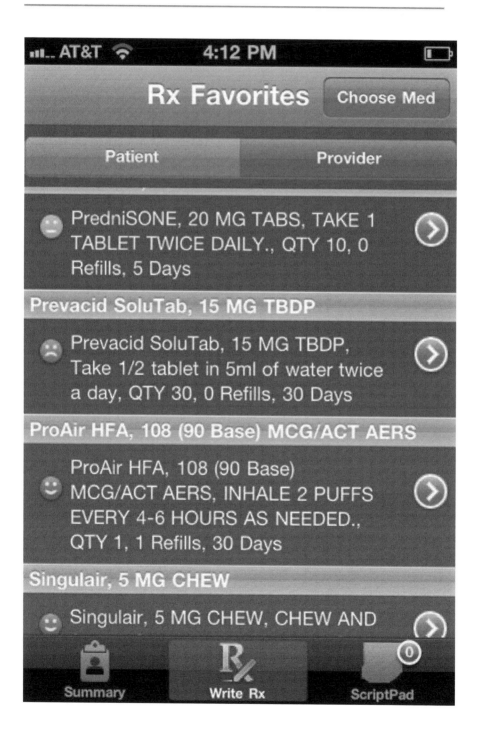

18

Getting prompt answers from doctors is difficult

The process of trying to resolve questions about wrong doses or potential interactions is a source of tremendous frustration for pharmacists. In my experience, what usually happens is something like this. The pharmacist calls the doctor's office and says something like, "I have a prescription here that Dr. Smith wrote today for [Drug X] for Mary Jones. Our computer has flagged a "most significant interaction" between [Drug X and Drug Y]. Could you check with Dr. Smith to make sure we should go ahead and fill the prescription?"

What I'm really saying is that I'm not eager to fill the prescription since our computer flags the interaction as "most significant." I'm trying to put the ball completely in the doctor's court (and give the doctor full notice) so if the patient suffers harm, the doctor is to blame. Of course, it's not that simple because pharmacists have a right and duty to refuse to fill any prescription that the pharmacist feels is not in the patient's best interest. Pharmacists can be liable if the patient suffers harm from the interaction even though the doctor confirmed in a phone call that we should go ahead and fill the prescription as written.

The nurse-receptionist who takes the pharmacist's phone call does one of the following things.

Phone Scenario #1 (Least likely): The doctor is not busy and is standing nearby so the nurse-receptionist immediately says to the doctor, "CVS is calling about a prescription for Mary Jones. The pharmacist says there's a drug interaction."

Then the doctor either tells the nurse-receptionist to tell the pharmacist to go ahead and fill the prescription as written or the doctor tells the nurse-receptionist to tell the pharmacist to change the offending drug (to drug Z) to avoid the potential interaction.

Some doctors do indeed get on the phone and read the pharmacist the riot act for calling about what the doctor considers to be an insignificant interaction. That has happened to me a few times. It has the effect of dampening pharmacists' enthusiasm for calling that doctor in the future about potential interactions (and, indeed, for calling doctors about anything).

When I worked at one drugstore in North Carolina, a local doctor phoned one day and said that we were calling his office too often about potential interactions. That particular store is very busy with many different pharmacists rotating in and out on different days. These relief pharmacists understandably haven't worked in that store long enough to have learned the personal preferences of local doctors. These relief pharmacists have no idea that this particular doctor doesn't like to be phoned about potential interactions. I mentioned this to another pharmacist who worked there occasionally. This pharmacist suggested to me in disgust that the doctor needed to mail us a letter relieving us of any liability in the event that one of his patients suffered harm resulting from an interaction between drugs he prescribed. Obviously we never requested such a letter from that doctor. And obviously that would not relieve the pharmacist of responsibility for filling a prescription for drugs that interact adversely.

In my opinion, modern medicine is primarily about power, ego, status, and wealth. Health is further down the line. I suspect that it looks bad in the nurse-receptionist's eyes when a pharmacist phones and says that the doctor made an error in dosage or with regard to a potential interaction. So the doctor occasionally feels he needs to protect his ego and reputation in front of the nurse-receptionist by calling the pharmacist and reading him the riot act.

Phone Scenario #2 (Much more likely): The nurse-receptionist tells the pharmacist, "I'll check with Dr. Smith and get back to you." I would say that, on average, it may take forty-five minutes for us to get a call back from the nurse-receptionist. Most likely fifteen minutes to an hour, but it can easily be two or three hours before the pharmacist gets a return call from the nurse-receptionist. Many nurse-receptionists do not call back until the end of the day (5 PM or 6 PM). Some doctors do not address pharmacy calls until they have seen ALL their patients. (Likewise, when patients themselves call their doctors about some question, many doctors do not call the patient back until after the doctor has seen all his patients for that day.)

It is unrealistic for a patient to assume that the pharmacist can immediately resolve a dose or interaction question with a quick phone call to the doctor's office. Nurse-receptionists usually wait for an opportunity to ask the doctor about the dose or interaction. A few nurse-receptionists immediately call the doctor on the office phone system and the doctor gives an instantaneous answer. But that's doesn't seem to be particularly common in my experience.

If a customer brings a prescription to the drugstore after the doctor's regular office hours or on a weekend or holiday, getting in touch with the doctor is even more difficult. Yes most doctors pay an answering service for these situations. But, too often, when we do call the answering service, the doctor who calls us back is actually the on-call partner who knows nothing of the situation but, thankfully, he is usually willing to make the necessary changes in the prescriptions if warranted.

So patients should never expect that dose or interaction or illegible handwriting questions can be resolved quickly. Having a patient wait at the pharmacy for the matter to be resolved with the doctor is something that most pharmacists have learned is not a good idea.

Of course, many customers get very upset at having to wait. In addition, telling the customer what we're doing can be tricky. It doesn't instill much confidence in patients when we tell them "Your doctor just prescribed a dose that's far too high for a child" or "Your doctor prescribed a drug for you that may interact with another drug you're taking." If we say this to the customer, we are essentially saying that their doctor doesn't know what proper dosages are for the drugs he prescribes or their doctor doesn't know about interactions among the drugs he prescribes. So the pharmacist might say, "I need to phone your doctor to clear up something." Then the customer is in a complete fog as to what's going on. Many pharmacists are indeed quite forthright and do indeed tell the customer that the doctor prescribed a questionable dose or a drug that may interact with other drugs the patient is taking. Some pharmacists are indeed very direct in explaining what's going on. Other pharmacists try hard to protect the reputation of local doctors from whom we get lots of prescriptions. (Doctors can easily steer patients to competitors.) Some pharmacists don't care whether the explanation to the customer makes the doctor look bad.

There is tremendous variation in the threshold that different pharmacists use when deciding when to phone the doctor about a questionable dose or potential interaction. Many young pharmacists just out of pharmacy school call doctors' offices very often, whereas many veteran pharmacists call doctors only in cases of the most blatant or serious dosage or interaction questions. Young pharmacists working in busy chain drugstores soon learn that they don't have time to call doctors' offices as often as they were instructed to do in pharmacy school. In the real world, chain pharmacy is about quantity, not quality.

Physicians almost never call the pharmacist back promptly. Doctors seem to give priority to the patients being seen rather than drop everything and address the pharmacist's concerns. I think this contrasts with what doctors do when other doctors are on the phone. Short anecdote: When my father was visiting several doctors before being diagnosed with lymphoma, I accompanied him on several of these visits. One time my father mentioned to one of these doctors that he had recently been to another local doctor for an evaluation. Immediately, the doctor phoned that other doctor and got thru to him right away. My impression is that doctors give much greater priority when other doctors phone, in contrast to when pharmacists phone.

Sometimes we never hear back from the doctor's office. Sometimes the doctor is out of town, or on vacation, or not on call that weekend, etc. Not hearing back from doctors' offices is not unusual. Pharmacists often have to make an additional call to doctors' offices to remind the nurse-receptionists that we never received an answer to the dosage or interaction question. Consequently, many customers go home in limbo, without the prescription. We tell the customer we can't fill the prescription until the nurse-receptionist or the doctor calls us back. Some customers get angry. Other customers are accustomed to these difficulties in dealing with very busy doctors or their disorganized/incompetent staffs.

In general, I would say that doctors view pharmacists' calls as nuisance calls. The hierarchy in modern medicine is very rigid. Doctors are at the top of the pyramid and pharmacists learn very quickly we are not viewed by doctors as professional equals. Way too many doctors view themselves as gods. How dare the pharmacist phone and claim that there is a potential drug interaction or wrong dose!!!!! Very few doctors seem to view the pharmacist's call as one health professional (the pharmacist) consulting with another health professional (the doctor) on equal terms for the best interests of the patient.

Over my career of 25 years, I spoke with hundreds (perhaps thousands) of doctors. My view (and, I suspect, that of many pharmacists) is that issues of power and hierarchy are, at the very least, as important to doctors as is the health of their patients.

My pharmacy school was in the same medical center complex as the medical school. Pharmacy students see what types of students go into medicine. The competitiveness that is required to gain admission to medical school is often precisely the opposite personality trait that is needed to be a truly compassionate physician. It is my opinion that many pharmacists, as a result of years of talking to doctors on the phone, have a skeptical view of the humanitarianism of many doctors.

Let me emphasize that some pharmacists do indeed call doctors too much. Some pharmacists call about interactions that are unlikely to cause a significant problem. But, of course, an interaction can be much more serious in one person than another. Pharmacy computers seem to be programmed to flag every potential problem, rather than only the most serious problems. Some pharmacy computers grade the seriousness of the interaction as "Level 1," "Level 2," or "Level 3." Many times I have seen pharmacists call doctors about interactions that I would not have called about. So, from the perspective of doctors, it is fair to say that some pharmacists are making calls of marginal significance. Some pharmacists seem to like to parade their drug knowledge in front of doctors, as if the pharmacist is saying "Gotcha!"

I would say that half of the students in my pharmacy school class were serious students and serious people. The other half seemed to be interested in learning the least they could to graduate. I guess my point is that I don't really have much respect for perhaps half the pharmacists I know and I suspect that many doctors have come to the same conclusion as a result of some of the phone calls they (doctors) get from pharmacists.

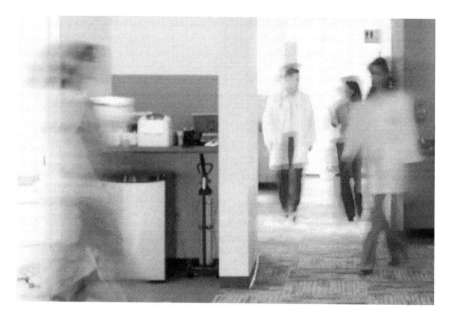

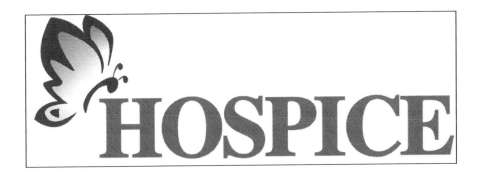

HOSPICE

19

A Florida hospice couldn't reach my mother's oncologist for morphine continuation when she was transferred from a local hospital

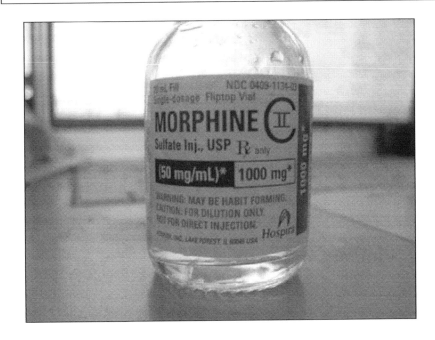

Here's a disturbing incident that occurred when my mother was in a hospice in Florida. It illustrates many things about our health care system, including the fact that it can often be difficult to get prompt answers from doctors, even in emergencies.

I was fortunate to be able to be with my mother for the last several days before she died from colon cancer that spread to her liver. At our nearby community hospital, she was given a continuous drip of morphine for her intense pain. Her oncologist had given orders that the nurse on duty could supplement that morphine drip with a direct injection from a syringe as needed in the event of any breakthrough pain (i.e., anytime my mother experienced especially severe pain that exceeded the ability of the continuous drip of morphine).

For example, I vividly remember one occasion when my mother began moaning terribly in pain. I ran out to find her nurse who happened to be with a patient in a room a couple of doors down. I told the nurse that my mother was moaning in pain. The nurse immediately accompanied me to my mother's room and administered maybe half of a syringe containing morphine. This seemed to help my mother quite quickly.

After a few days in the community hospital, my mother was transferred to the local hospice. I rode in the medical transport vehicle with my mother from the hospital to the hospice, a distance of about ten miles. While sitting in my mother's hospice room, I noticed that something wasn't right. Where is the morphine? In the hospital, a bag or bottle of morphine was her constant companion, hung near the head of her bed.

I went to the nurse's station and asked my mother's hospice nurse (a very professional and caring person), "Where is the morphine?" Suddenly, one of the other workers at the nurses' station piped up and said, "We have a call out to her oncologist."

So I went back to the room and waited. And waited. And waited. No morphine. I knew that my mother would soon be in excruciating pain without the morphine. She still had some morphine in her system from the hospital but I knew her pain would return when the effects of the hospital morphine wore off. So I went back to the nurses' station and asked about the status of the morphine.

That same worker (I don't think she was a nurse) told me again, rudely, "We have a call out to her oncologist." I asked her (almost pleading for anything at this point), "Can't you just call the hospital where we just came from and get a confirmation of the morphine order she had there?" This MEAN WOMAN again rudely told me that they were awaiting a return call from my mother's oncologist.

I was getting very nervous because my mother had been without the morphine drip for over an hour (possibly approaching two hours) and I was afraid that at any moment she would be in excruciating pain. So I told this MEAN WOMAN who was speaking to me as if I had no understanding of the medical system, "I'm a pharmacist. I know you have to stay on 'em [doctors] when they don't return calls." This MEAN WOMAN at the nurses' station suddenly shut up.

Even though I try very hard to avoid confrontations with people, this MEAN WOMAN could see I was very tired of her attitude. My mother's nurse was standing nearby and heard my entire conversation with this MEAN WOMAN at the nurse's station. But the nurse did not say anything.

Several minutes later when my mother's oncologist finally called the hospice, the nice nurse came in my mother's room with the morphine. She told me "You were absolutely right" [to confront that MEAN WOMAN at the nurse's station]. I had the impression that the nice nurse had had other bad experiences with that MEAN WOMAN. The nice nurse told me that my mother's oncologist requested that she relay to me his very sincere apologies for failing to arrange the morphine order prior to my mother's arrival at the hospice.

A few weeks later, I received what looked like a standard questionnaire from the hospice, asking me to answer a few multiple choice questions as a way to assess my experience during my mother's brief stay at that hospice. There was also a space to add any additional comments. I had wanted so badly to tell the hospice administrator personally about this entire incident, but I was afraid that the administrator would think it was the nice nurse who was the person who rude to me, rather than the MEAN WOMAN at the nurses' station. So I didn't make any comments.

My mother died less than 36 hours after arriving at the hospice. I stayed with her the entire time, sleeping on a cot that was in the room. I think each nurse's shift lasted 12 hours. My mother had a different nurse assigned to her for each of the three shifts. The first nurse was absolutely spectacular. The overnight nurse was horrendous. And the nurse the next morning was average. But I'll never forget that MEAN WOMAN at the nurses' station who was handling the call to my mother's oncologist for the morphine order. During this time of profound sadness as I stayed with my mother before she died at the hospice, the situation was made worse by that MEAN WOMAN at the nurses' station who was a first class asshole.

I think this incident illustrates the following: (1) Patients in hospitals and hospices need a friend or family member present (preferably around the clock) to try to assure that the patient is getting reasonable attention. (2) Don't assume that your doctor will arrange pain relief medication orders ahead of time when a patient is transferred from a hospital to a hospice. (3) Don't assume that the physician can be contacted immediately in the case of an emergency. (4) Don't assume that all hospice workers will be helpful.

Both of my parents died from cancer and they both had different oncologists. (My father died from lymphoma). My father's oncologist was arrogant, aloof, and, in my opinion, a real jerk. In contrast, I really liked my mother's oncologist. He was much younger than my father's oncologist and a really down-to-earth person who didn't seem to have a big ego.

The day that my mother was transferred from the hospital to the hospice, my mother's oncologist told me (at the hospital) that he made rounds through the hospice in the mornings so I would probably see him there if I were in the room with my mother. It turns out that I was indeed there the next day and the oncologist never showed up. I don't know what the reason was but I suspect it may have been because he was so embarrassed for having failed to authorize the morphine prior to my mother's arrival at the hospice.

My mother's oncologist seemed to have a British sense of humor even though I could not detect a British accent. When the nice nurse informed me that he sincerely apologized on the phone for not having made arrangements for the morphine prior to my mother's arrival at the hospice, the nurse said that he said he was "aghast" to be informed that my mother was at the hospice without morphine. That sounded precisely like a word he would have used.

I never saw that oncologist after this event so I was never able to discuss it with him. I could certainly have visited his office and told him about my displeasure, but I realize that things like this happen all the time in our health care system where patients routinely fall through the cracks. He was a decent enough person up to this event so I saw no reason to stop in to see him.

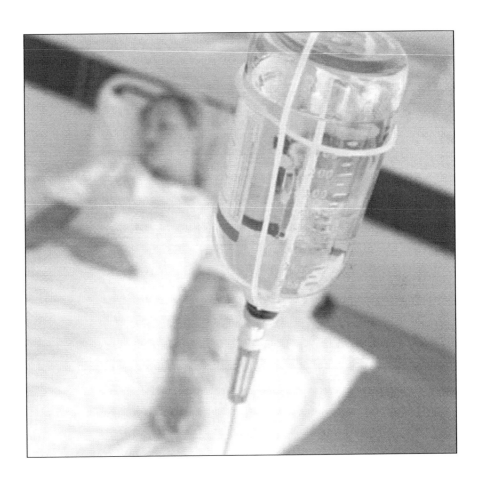

20

When doctors prescribe the wrong dose

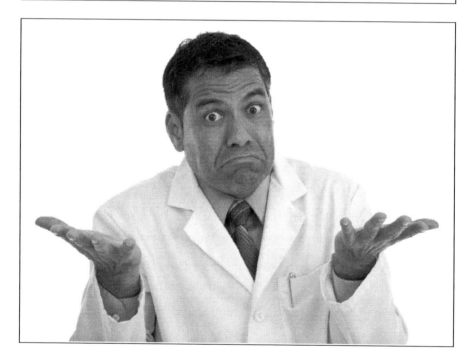

---

1. Doctor prescribed wrong dose of Compazine

One Saturday I received a prescription for a child aged 2 years 9 months. The prescription was for Compazine 12.5 mg suppositories, a drug used to treat severe nausea and vomiting. The doctor's directions were "Insert 1 suppository rectally every 6 to 8 hours." If these suppositories were inserted every 6 hours (four times a day), the child would receive 50 mg of Compazine per day. However, the recommended dose for severe nausea and vomiting for a child weighing 30 to 39 pounds (my estimate of the weight of a child at this age) is "not to exceed 10 mg per day." (2003 *PDR*, p. 1491) If the child were given 4 suppositories per day, he could well have gotten five times the recommended dose.

The *PDR* (2003 ed., p. 1491) lists the following symptoms of overdosage, among others: "Symptoms of central nervous system depression to the point of somnolence or coma. Agitation and restlessness may also occur. Other possible manifestations include convulsions, EKG changes and cardiac arrhythmias...."

It so happened that I did not catch the doctor's error until after the child's father already picked up the finished prescription. We were very busy at that time and I was working as fast as my hands would allow me. About a half hour later, I got an uneasy feeling that the doctor had overdosed the child. So I looked up the recommended dose and discovered that the doctor had indeed made a big error.

The prescription had been written at the local hospital emergency room so I called there hoping the doctor was still on duty. Luckily, he was. I said to him, "I just filled a prescription for Compazine suppositories for [child's name]. You probably know more about pediatric dosing than I do, but isn't the dose you prescribed a little high?" I said "a little high" in an attempt to be nice. Actually, it was dangerously high. He said, "Okay, let's make it twice a day." I said, "That's still a daily dose of 25 mg which is still more than double the recommended dose for a child who weighs 30 to 39 pounds." Incredibly, he asked, "What's the recommended dose?"

I told him that the *PDR* says the recommended dose for nausea and vomiting in a child 30 to 39 pounds is "not more than 10 mg per day." He seemed to be quite concerned at this point. Then I told him that I had already dispensed the prescription and that the child's father had already left the store. Then he made a statement that irritated me. He said, "You went ahead and dispensed the prescription?" I said "It wasn't 'til after the child's father left that I got worried." I had the impression he was trying to shift some of the blame to me even though he was the one who had written the prescription. He was, however, essentially quite decent during our exchange. But he seemed to become even more worried. I told him, "I've got the father's home phone number and I'll give him a call if you like." He said, "Please do."

Luckily, the child's mother answered the phone when I called and luckily she hadn't given the child a suppository yet. I told her that the doctor and I decided that the child would be better off with a lower dose. I did not tell her that the doctor had made a potentially serious mistake and that I had failed to catch it before dispensing the drug. The mother didn't seem to be upset. She said that she would have her husband return the suppositories as I requested.

I called the doctor back and said that I had reached the child's mother and that she hadn't given the child a suppository yet. The doctor was audibly relieved. He then told me to change the prescription to 2.5 mg every 6 to 8 hours (a total daily dose one-fifth of his original order). Then he said "I really appreciate what you did a whole lot."

My comment: The doctor sounded very young and very hurried. I'm probably not as young but equally hurried. When customers demand that prescriptions be filled with lightning speed, errors like this are inevitable.

2. Doctor prescribed wrong dose of albuterol

One day I received a prescription from another doctor for Albuterol inhalation solution for asthma. This medication is put in a special breathing machine.   It comes two ways: as a concentrated solution and as a pre-diluted solution. The user or caregiver is to mix, usually, half a cc of the Albuterol with 2.5 cc of a diluting solution before administration. This prescription was for a child.

When I received this prescription, it had a few numbers on it that made no sense. The child's mother told me that she was in a hurry. But I still had to call the doctor who wrote the prescription to clear up the confusion. The child's mother only seemed to be interested in getting the medication. She did not seem to understand or appreciate my efforts to clear up this doctor's confusing prescription.

The customer had just received the prescription from the local hospital emergency room. I called the doctor there and asked him what, in particular, two numbers were supposed to indicate. He told me that he had never prescribed that particular product before so he was not very familiar with it. He said that he had prescribed it as a result of the child's mother's request. He apologized for the resulting confusion. He said that he had started to prescribe the concentrated solution but the child's mother had asked for the dilute solution because she had used the dilute solution before. He said that he had never prescribed the pre-diluted solution before and asked me to describe the form in which it was available.

The doctor was very nice and apologetic. Yet the fact remains that he prescribed a product with which he was not familiar. This hospital emergency room is usually quite busy so I am not surprised that he did not have time to investigate the product before he prescribed it. I sympathize with him as regards his workload.

Yet the fact remains that this child could have ended up receiving six times the intended dose if this prescription had not been clarified. The child's mother did not seem to appreciate my efforts. She just seemed to resent that she had to wait while I cleared up the confusion.

I was recently told of another incident at another drugstore involving these same two products. A pharmacist who had been licensed less than four months told another child's mother that the concentrated solution could be given without being diluted. Somehow the child's mother found out that this was incorrect and returned to the pharmacy crying over the potential harm that could have resulted. Another pharmacist was on duty at that time and apologized for the error.

---

3. Doctor prescribed wrong dose of Tussionex

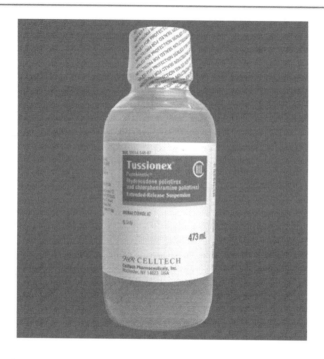

Another doctor prescribed the cough syrup Tussionex for a 14-year-old girl, with the directions: "Take 1 to 2 teaspoonsful every 8 hours." The official prescribing information for Tussionex reads as follows (2003 *PDR*, p. 1174): "Adults: 1 teaspoonful every 12 hours; do not exceed 2 teaspoonsful in 24 hours. Children 6-12: one-half teaspoonful every 12 hours; **do not exceed 1 teaspoonful in 24 hours.**" The bold-faced print appears in the *PDR*.

This was a refill bottle that another pharmacist had originally filled. The customer's request for the refill took place on a weekend. The directions were so evidently an excessive dose that I re-typed the directions on the label with the manufacturer's recommended dose. In my experience, Tussionex is one of the drugs most frequently prescribed with the wrong directions. Most doctors forget—or never knew—that Tussionex is unusual in that it is long-acting and it is used in small doses.

I didn't even notify the doctor's office that I changed the directions. It was so clearly an error that it was pointless to notify the doctor and risk appearing to "rub it in" that he made an error.

What usually happens is that we call the doctor's office and tell the person who answers the phone (usually the receptionist) that there appears to be an error in the doctor's directions. Then the receptionist tells the doctor or a nurse. I suspect that it is embarrassing for the doctor to be told by his receptionist or nurse that the drugstore is calling with what appears to be an error. Then (assuming it is indeed an error), one of two things can happen:

1. The doctor is honest with himself and agrees with the pharmacist that an error has been made. The doctor tells his nurse or receptionist to tell the pharmacist to correct the directions.

2. The doctor's ego and his desire to appear faultless in front of his staff cause him to tell his nurse or receptionist to relay to the pharmacist that the doctor wants it kept as he wrote it on the prescription. The doctor knows that he is clearly in error but refuses to acknowledge that fact.

In this case with the Tussionex, I felt there was no reason to notify the doctor's office, even if this incident had occurred during the doctor's normal business hours. (As I said, this was a weekend.) We get lots of prescriptions from this doctor, so why risk upsetting him? I know that he has a very busy practice and that mistakes like this are inevitable. Having spoken with him many times over the years as he relays prescriptions to us, he seems to be the type of doctor who would prefer that we just make the correction in the dose without making a big fuss about it.

The difficult part was telling the child's father that the directions we had typed on the label originally were what the doctor had written but that it was best to use a lower dose. I implied that the doctor knew better but must have been in a hurry. Whether or not the doctor actually knows the maximum recommended dose for Tussionex is something I don't know.

As I said, the doctor wrote on the prescription, "Take 1 to 2 teaspoonful every 8 hours." Every eight hours means three times per day. So the doctor's directions could have led the child to take up to six teaspoonful per day. This is three times the recommended adult dose. Sometimes doctors prescribe a somewhat higher dose when the patient is large. However, this 14-year-old girl appeared to be of average weight for her age. It is even stretching it somewhat to put her in the adult category because, at 14, she's only two years past the child category according to the manufacturer's recommended dose. So it is not stretching things a lot to say that six teaspoonsful per day could be six times the recommended dose. I asked the girl how often she was taking it and she said she was taking one teaspoonful in the morning and two teaspoonsful at night (three teaspoonsful per day).

So I acted as if the doctor knew the correct dose but just must have been in a hurry when he wrote the directions. Whether or not this is the case I'll never know, but at least it got me out of a fix. I didn't want to refill the Tussionex with the original directions that the previous pharmacist had typed on the label. I was legally liable for dispensing a drug with incorrect directions. My employer was also liable. I just acted as if it was no big deal and re-typed the directions on the label with the manufacturer's recommended directions. I implied that the doctor knew the correct dose but must have been in a hurry. I was protecting myself and my employer against a lawsuit. The doctor had clearly made an error.

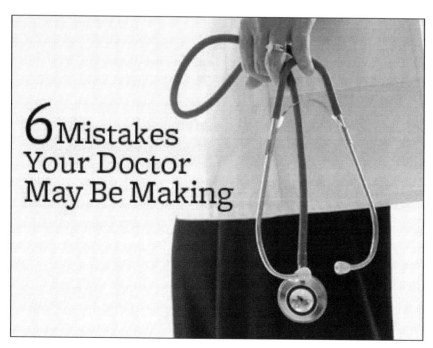

21

Many doctors don't welcome pharmacists' calls about drug interactions

In my experience, most doctors don't seem too happy to hear that a pharmacist is calling to point out a drug interaction. They too often interpret this as a turf battle or an implication that they are not sufficiently knowledgeable about interactions among the drugs they prescribe.

Pharmacists are overwhelmed with prescriptions, yet some doctors think we have nothing better to do than call about interactions. One doctor told my partner we were calling his office too often. I told this to another pharmacist who suggested we request written permission from the doctor never to call him again about drug interactions. But I doubt that would relieve us of liability in the event of a lawsuit.

One Saturday I called a doctor about his prescribing erythromycin for a customer who was on carbamazepine from a different doctor. This is a "Level 1," or "most significant," interaction. When the doctor finally called back, he said rudely, "I'm making a long distance phone call for this? The interaction is extremely mild!" He finally said (as if only to please me), "All right! Change the erythromycin to Duricef!" I told the patient her doctor had changed her antibiotic, but not about the potentially serious nature of the interaction or how angry the doctor was that I called him.

Here is what the *United States Pharmacopoeia* says about the interaction between erythromycin and carbamazepine (*USP-DI*, 1997, p. 1351): "Erythromycins may inhibit carbamazepine metabolism, resulting in increased anticonvulsant plasma concentrations and toxicity; it is recommended that erythromycin be used with caution if at all in patients receiving carbamazepine."

On a different occasion, I called another doctor's office about another Level 1 interaction. I wanted to make sure I should dispense the drugs as written. When the receptionist called me back, she said, "I checked with the doctor, AND HE SAID IT'S OKAY!" Her attitude implied that I was an idiot for calling. I assume that is because the doctor was irritated that a pharmacist had called about yet another drug interaction and took out his anger on her.

Pharmacists are put in the impossible position of having to decide which patients will experience clinically significant effects from drug interactions. In any large statistical sample, some people will end up with adverse consequences from a drug interaction. Others will not.

I believe the doctor should be the one to weigh the statistical probability, not the pharmacist. The doctor should have ultimate responsibility for screening for drug interactions. He/she should have a duty to review all current meds a patient is taking (including the ones prescribed by other doctors) before prescribing another drug. Liability for detecting drug interactions resulting from doctors' carelessness should not fall on the shoulders of pharmacists. (Of course, if we had adequate staff in the pharmacy, I would more willingly accept part of the burden of screening for drug interactions.)

In understaffed pharmacies, we simply don't have enough time to call doctors as often as we should. Customers are in a hurry, and they don't seem to recognize the significance of our phone calls. Yet these same customers will not hesitate to sue us if they suffer harm from an interaction. When we do call, the doctor's response to the interaction often seems arbitrary or based on inadequate knowledge. Or the doctor simply uses the occasion to display his ego.

Because of doctors' attitudes, we may tell customers something like this: "Our computer flagged a potential interaction between your medications. I called your doctor and he feels there will be no problem." Essentially, we're telling customers that we, as pharmacists, are concerned about an interaction but their doctor is not, so if they develop a problem, BLAME THE DOCTOR!

Patients would probably be surprised to learn that considerations such as a doctor's ego factor into whether their pharmacist calls about a potential drug interaction. Customers likely assume that health professionals are collegial and that everyone works together for the benefit of patients. In reality, some doctors' attitudes and egos are a serious impediment to ensuring safety in the dispensing of medications.

I'm sure a few pharmacists enjoy parading their drug knowledge in front of doctors. And I'm sure many pharmacists call doctors about potential interactions that indeed have a low probability of causing a problem. But the longer a pharmacist has worked in a busy store, the quicker he realizes there simply is not enough time to devote to potential drug interactions.

Pharmacists: Do you have adequate time to call doctors about drug interactions? Are you worried that your pharmacy technicians are overriding significant drug interactions?

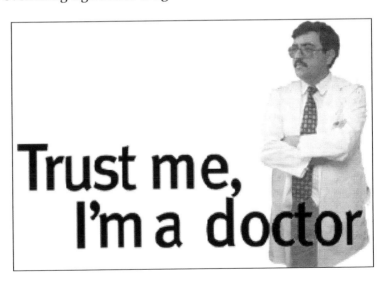

INCLUDES SHOCKING NEW INFORMATION
ON HAZARDOUS INTERACTIONS

PROTECT YOURSELF FROM HARMFUL DRUG,
FOOD, AND VITAMIN COMBINATIONS

DANGEROUS DRUG INTERACTIONS

The People's Pharmacy® Guide

Joe Graedon and Teresa Graedon, Ph.D.

22

Many doctors don't keep up with the latest drug warnings

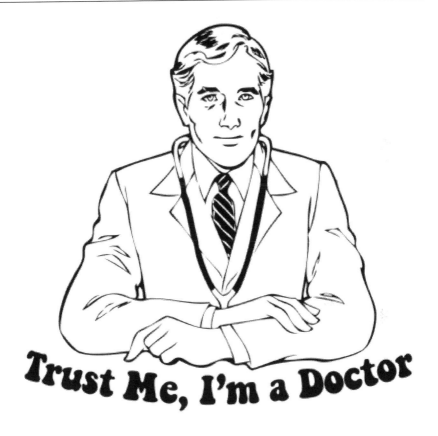

Trust Me, I'm a Doctor

In his excellent book on the FDA, Philip J. Hilts discusses how doctors often ignore FDA warnings in the official prescribing information, known as the label. Hilts quotes one FDA staffer, "Doctors aren't often paying attention. We may put crucial information in a label and have it end up as a dead letter." Hilts says, "Studies confirm it: the labels are largely unheeded and often completely unread." (Philip J. Hilts, *Protecting America's Health: The FDA, Business, and One Hundred Years of Regulation,* New York: Knopf, 2003, pp. 234-5)

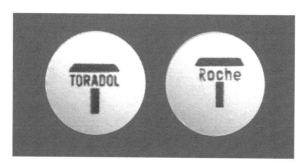

I wrote the following in May 1995: A local doctor continues to prescribe the pain killer Toradol for an excessive duration of time. He often prescribes it to be taken for ten days with four refills. This is a potentially 50-day supply. However, the medical literature says that Toradol should not be taken for more than five days because of the possibility of serious gastrointestinal bleeding and other problems.

The recommendation for short duration therapy with Toradol was a big story in 1995. How could this doctor have missed it?

One day I said to my partner, "There's a local doctor who's using a drug for much longer than is recommended." To my great surprise, my partner immediately said, "Yeah. It's Dr. Smith and it's Toradol." I was surprised that my partner had the same concern that I had.

I told my partner that one of us needed to call this doctor and wake him up because he's jeopardizing the health of his patients and exposing us and Revco to liability. Every time we enter "days supply" into the computer when filling one of his prescriptions for Toradol, the computer flags this as an excessive duration of therapy.

But Dr. Smith is such a know-it-all that we both decided that neither of us wanted to call him. We get a lot of prescriptions from

Dr. Smith, so we fear that he'll direct his patients elsewhere if we tell him he's greatly exceeding the recommended total duration of therapy for Toradol. Hopefully some other drugstore in town will make him aware of this fact.

June 1995: The daughter of the customer my partner and I were concerned about brought in another prescription for Toradol. Against my better judgment, I went ahead and dispensed thirty more tablets. Later on that afternoon, I called the customer herself and asked her how long she had been on the Toradol. I could have looked it up in our computer records, but I wanted her to actually tell me how long she had been on the Toradol. She told me that she had been taking Toradol for a little over a year for her headaches.

The revised prescribing information (December 1994) for Toradol specifically states that patients should not take this drug for more than five days and that it should not be used for chronic conditions. There have been many reports of serious gastrointestinal bleeding and even death from this drug. It turns out that this customer has had ulcers in the past even though she told me she doesn't currently have an ulcer. (How can she be so sure that some ulceration is not occurring without her realizing it?) Toradol should be used even more cautiously in patients with a history of ulcers.

Sidney Wolfe, M.D., and his Public Citizen Health Research Group, advised against use of this drug as early as August 1993. ("Health Letter," August 1993, p. 5:)

A widely-used painkiller, especially used in patients after surgery, has been temporarily suspended from sales in Germany and the German government gave Syntex, the drug's U. S.-based manufacturer, three weeks to provide evidence that it should not be permanently removed from the market. The drug, which is in the same family of non-steroidal anti-inflammatory drugs (NSAIDs) as Feldene, Naprosyn and aspirin has been associated with a large number of cases of serious gastrointestinal bleeding, including dozens of deaths as well as life-threatening allergic reactions similar to Zomax, another NSAID which is no longer on the market.

...For now, we urge patients not to use ketorolac [generic name for Toradol].

The official prescribing information sounds equally scary. From the package insert, revised December 1994:

Toradol, a nonsteroidal anti-inflammatory drug (NSAID), is indicated for the short-term (up to 5 days) management of moderately severe, acute pain, that requires analgesia at the opioid level. It is NOT indicated for minor or chronic painful conditions. Toradol is a potent NSAID analgesic, and its administration carries many risks. The resulting NSAID related adverse events can be serious in certain patients for whom Toradol is indicated, especially when the drug is used inappropriately. ...

Toradol can cause peptic ulcers, gastrointestinal bleeding, and/or perforation. Therefore, Toradol is contraindicated in patients with active peptic ulcer disease, in patients with recent gastrointestinal bleeding or perforation, and in patients with a history of peptic ulcer disease or gastrointestinal bleeding. ...

The combined use of [intravenous, intramuscular, and oral forms of Toradol] is not to exceed 5 days. ...

Serious gastrointestinal toxicity, such as bleeding, ulceration, and perforation, can occur at any time, with or without warning symptoms, in patients treated with Toradol. Studies to date with NSAIDs have not identified any subset of patients not at risk of developing peptic ulceration and bleeding. ...

The incidence and severity of gastrointestinal complications increases with increasing dose of, and duration of treatment with, Toradol. ...

Toradol is a potent NSAID and may cause serious side effects such as gastrointestinal bleeding or kidney failure, which may result in hospitalization and even fatal outcome.

Physicians, when prescribing Toradol should inform their patients of the potential risks of Toradol treatment. ...

Remember that the total duration of Toradol therapy is not to exceed 5 (five) days.

I told our customer that the recommendation for a decreased duration in the use of Toradol was very recent. I told her that I was going to call her doctor to see whether he had heard about it. The fact is that her doctor had plenty of time to hear about it but I needed a way to make it sound like her doctor was a good doctor, even though there are many people in this community who hold a very low opinion of this doctor.

That evening, I called my partner at home and said that we needed to do something about this situation NOW!!! He agreed, particularly after I read him the warnings from the official prescribing information and after I read him from Sidney Wolfe's "Health Letter."

My partner has worked at this store for nearly fifteen years. I work in this particular store only on a part-time basis, yet I happened to fill a few prescriptions for Toradol for this customer. We agreed that it was best that he call the doctor and act like this was very new information that the doctor possibly had not heard about, even though, as I said, it's been in the medical literature for several months.

My partner has spoken on the phone with this doctor countless times in these nearly fifteen years, usually for routine questions like permission to refill various drugs for our customers, and, significantly, for help in deciphering his handwriting. This doctor has some of the worst handwriting I've seen in the twenty years since I graduated from pharmacy school.

We concluded that if we were to make this doctor mad (a not unlikely possibility), my partner should be the one to handle the situation since my partner was the one who needed to maintain ongoing relationships with the doctors in this town.

My partner called this doctor on a Monday morning. It turns out that the doctor didn't get mad but his reaction to the situation was quite inadequate and quite disappointing. For the recommendation that Toradol not be taken for more than five days, the doctor said that he had told the patient to always skip a day after five days (what a joke!) and that he had told her not to take more than twelve tablets a week, even though he allowed her to take it every week for over a year.

Then the doctor made an absolutely incredible statement. He said that it was his experience that warnings in the prescribing literature come and go and that it was his experience that one's own judgment should guide the physician's prescribing practices.

I guess this doctor has no use for the FDA. Why worry about official FDA warnings? Since he had not personally run into problems with his patients on Toradol, that fact apparently superseded data gathered from around the country and around the world.

In discussing this situation with me, my partner said that we should document all our concerns and conversations (with the patient and doctor) on the prescription and in the computer. I told my partner that I still was not satisfied. I said that we are still liable for dispensing a drug that we have reason to believe is not in the patient's best interest. As pharmacists seek a greater role in drug therapy decisions, lawyers are not exempting pharmacists from lawsuits when something goes wrong. In the past, it was usually only the doctor and the drug manufacturer that were found liable.

I told my partner that I plan to refuse to dispense any more Toradol to this customer and that he should do the same. I also said that I pray that she doesn't have any gastrointestinal bleeding in the meantime. I told him that we should possibly contact the Revco legal department for further guidance.

This customer gets all her prescriptions at Revco, so it would probably cause a problem in our relationship with this doctor if we told the customer that we would fill all her other prescriptions but refuse to dispense any more Toradol.

I transferred to a different city shortly after this episode, so, unfortunately, I never found out whether this customer continued to take excessive quantities of Toradol.

DON'T BE A STATISTIC

TOP SCREWUPS DOCTORS MAKE AND HOW TO AVOID THEM

- Top 10 Doctor Errors • Top 10 Pharmacist Errors
- Diagnostic Disasters • Prevent Hospital Screwups

JOE GRAEDON, M.S., AND TERESA GRAEDON, PH.D.

Bestselling authors of *The People's Pharmacy*

23

Doctors and placebos

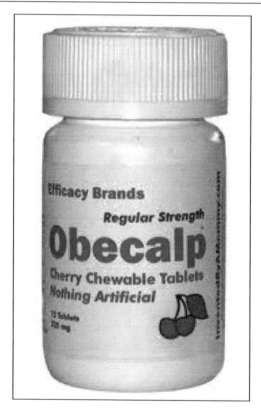

In the early 1990s I worked at several drugstores in North Carolina, including one in a town called Henderson. Henderson is a forty minute drive on the Interstate from Durham, the city in which Duke University is located. Drugstores in a wide radius from Durham receive lots of prescriptions from the Duke University Medical Center. One day a customer handed me a prescription for her son from a Duke doctor. The customer decided to hang around in the drugstore and wait for the prescription to be filled—rather than return later to pick it up.

When I began filling the prescription a few minutes later, I noticed that the Duke doc had prescribed a drug with which I was not familiar. The Duke doc had prescribed Obecalp. I called the customer over and told her that I would have to phone her doctor at Duke because I wasn't familiar with Obecalp and I couldn't find it listed in any of our order books. The customer said that would be fine. She remained nearby as I called the Duke doc. Luckily, I got through to the Duke doc quickly. I said, "I have a prescription here for Obecalp for [patient's name], but I can't find it listed anywhere." He said, "Oh. That's placebo spelled backwards."

The doctor proceeded to explain the situation to me. He was considering prescribing Ritalin for this child (for attention deficit-hyperactivity disorder, I presume). He wanted to see whether the mother could actually tell a difference in her child's behavior on days that he took Ritalin and on days that he took the placebo. The plan was to alternate the Ritalin and the Obecalp (placebo) in some way—I can't recall the precise plan. Perhaps the placebo was to be taken every other day, or every other week, or every other month.

I told the Duke doc that, even though I was well aware of the placebo effect, I could not recall ever having actually dispensed placebo pills (commonly known as sugar pills or inert pills). He said, "Why don't you just dispense, say, a low dose of Vitamin C tablets if you don't have any placebo pills." (Placebo pills—containing no active ingredients—were indeed available from our suppliers under "Placebo," but not, at that time, under the name "Obecalp.")

This doctor was extremely nice during the entire conversation, but I was left worrying that I had blown the cover on his experiment. The child's mother was standing nearby during this entire conversation and she must have heard almost everything I said to her child's doctor. I think I went ahead and dispensed Vitamin C tablets, as the doctor suggested, rather than actual placebo pills since we didn't have any placebo pills on hand. I did not tell the Duke doc that I may have ruined his experiment since the child's mother was standing nearby and had overheard most of my conversation. The mother now seemed to be highly curious about what was going on.

I greatly admire this Duke doc for considering the possibility that the child may not need the Ritalin. And I greatly admire his attempt to see whether the child's mother could tell any difference in her child's behavior on the days he took the Ritalin versus the days he took the placebo (actually Vitamin C tablets in this case). But I just wish the doctor had handled the situation a little differently by, perhaps, calling me before the child's mother arrived with the prescription for Obecalp. He could have called beforehand to explain to me what he was planning to do with this unconventional prescription for Obecalp.

Of course, I was equally guilty for handling this situation poorly, since the child's mother had heard almost all of my conversation with the doctor before I concluded that the doctor probably didn't want her to know that the Obecalp pills are indeed placebo pills (i.e., a dummy or inactive pill). I don't know how much of this experiment the mother was aware of before she walked into the drugstore, but she certainly understood much more after my bumbled conversation with the doctor.

Too many doctors seem to prescribe Ritalin reflexively, so I admire the way this Duke doc was trying to determine whether the child really needed the drug. But the way he and I handled the situation was not good at all.

Here's an unrelated but (perhaps) funny anecdote about placebos. This is a letter-to-the-editor published in *Drug Topics*, written by a New Jersey pharmacist. This pharmacist, in cooperation with a physician, dispensed placebo pills to one of that physician's patients. (Letters, "Score 1 for placebo ... make that 2," *Drug Topics*, December 2010, p. 10)

In 1957, I was a brand-new pharmacist in a New York hospital. An elderly female patient of the arthritis clinic adjacent to my pharmacy had no clinical disease in reality but constantly sought treatment. The rheumatologist, the director, and I conferred and decided to give her a 2-month supply of saccharin tablets with ad lib refills [refillable as needed] to be taken 1 tid [one tablet three times a day]."

This went well for several months, with the patient reporting good results, until she came to my window one day, shouting, and accused us of giving her substandard medication. The previous night she had tried to commit suicide by taking the entire supply — "And look at me: I'm standing right here in front of you, and I'm alive!"

We sent her for a psych consult. I didn't know whether to laugh or to cry. *—Irving Gerber, RPh,* Fair Lawn, N.J.

There has been a great deal of discussion about whether it is ethical to prescribe placebos to patients without those patients knowing it. How would you feel if your doctor—without informing you—decided to put you on a dummy or inert pill to see, for example, whether your symptoms of depression or anxiety responded as well to the placebo pill as to, say, Prozac or Xanax? Would you feel that your doctor thinks you're nuts?

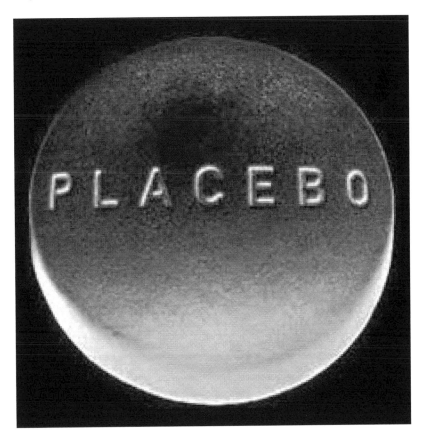

PART IV

PHARMACY TECHNICIANS

24

Some pharmacy technicians are a threat to the public safety

Pharmacy technicians are those people you see in the pharmacy who wear white coats but are not pharmacists. They do things like accept prescriptions from customers, count pills, answer phones, stock pharmacy shelves, and operate the pharmacy computer.

For example, if you are allergic to penicillin, the person entering this fact into your computer record may be no more than a high school student. This critical information allows the computer to flag any subsequent prescription for penicillin or penicillin-like drugs. If the person entering this information does so incorrectly, your notifying the pharmacy of your penicillin allergy has been a waste of time.

Pharmacies are turning over more duties to techs. Techs decipher your doctor's oftentimes poorly legible handwriting to determine which drug you doctor prescribed. Commonly, it is the technician—not the pharmacist—who inputs the drug name, strength, quantity, number of refills, and directions (once a day, twice a day, every 4 hours, etc.). Techs attach those colorful little stickers to your prescription bottle like: "Take with food" or "Avoid prolonged exposure to sunlight" or "Take this medication one hour before or two-three hours after a meal."

Techs are allowed to do almost everything that the pharmacist does, under the pharmacist's supervision. The pharmacist is always responsible for checking the tech's work. There are a few things that techs are not allowed to do. For example, techs are not allowed to release a prescription without a pharmacist's approval.

The chains love techs. Techs usually make around $10.00 to $15.00 per hour. Pharmacists make $90,000 to $110,000 or more per year. The chains say that with profit margins squeezed by managed care, pharmacy technicians are essential to ensure a profit in the pharmacy. The chains say that techs hold down the cost of your medication.

There are several hundred thousand pharmacy techs in the United States. An increasing number of techs are becoming certified, allowing them to place the initials CPhT (Certified Pharmacy Technician) after their name. In addition, many of the nation's pharmacy technicians are attending technical schools or getting associate's degrees. Many techs favor licensure or certification, seeing it as a way to increase their wages. Some employers oppose the licensing of techs, figuring it will increase their labor costs.

Facts from the Pharmacy Technician Certification Board website (https://www.ptcb.org/AM/Template.cfm?Section=Regulations&Template=/CM/HTMLDisplay.cfm&ContentID=4108, accessed Aug. 23, 2011):

• Since 1995, the Pharmacy Technician Certification Board has certified 413, 447 pharmacy technicians through the examination and transfer process.
• The following states require certification of pharmacy technicians: Arizona, Idaho, Illinois, Iowa, Louisiana, Maryland, Massachusetts, Montana, New Mexico, Oregon, South Carolina, Texas, Utah, Virginia, Washington State, Wyoming.
• The following states do not require registration, licensure, or certification of pharmacy technicians: Colorado, the District of Columbia, Georgia, Hawaii, Michigan, New York, Pennsylvania, and Wisconsin.

Is licensure or certification of techs the answer to safety concerns? Or is lack of adequate staffing in the pharmacy the real problem? Can licensed or certified techs make up for dangerous understaffing in the pharmacy? Many pharmacists say that understaffing is the most serious problem in the pharmacy, causing a dangerous dispensing environment.

Many chains define a tech as anyone who helps out in the pharmacy, regardless of her level of experience. As soon as she walks into the pharmacy from the street, some chains define her as a tech. This is absurd and dangerous.

Auburn University School of Pharmacy conducted a study of pharmacy errors, concluding that "51.5 million errors occur during the filling of 3 billion prescriptions each year." (Eliz. Flynn, et.al., "National Observational Study of Prescription Dispensing Accuracy and Safety in 50 Pharmacies," *Journal of the American Pharmacist's Assoc.*, March/April 2003, pp. 191-200) Can pharmacists be expected to catch all the mistakes made by techs in high pressure pharmacies in which hundreds of prescriptions are filled daily? I have worked in pharmacies that fill up to 50 prescriptions per hour during the busiest times of the day.

A pharmacist can safely check the work of how many technicians? Tech-to-pharmacist ratios are hotly debated. Some observers say that with more than two techs per pharmacist, the pharmacist is unable to safely check all the prescriptions techs churn out. Common sense says that the faster people work and the less training they have, the more likely it is that errors will occur. The question is whether your pharmacist can catch all the inevitable errors in this fast-food environment.

Do techs increase the likelihood of errors in the pharmacy? In some cases, they undoubtedly do. Having a good tech, however, is almost like having another pharmacist present. It all depends on the quality of the techs. I know many techs who make fewer errors than pharmacists. I know many techs who I trust more than pharmacists to accurately type your doctor's directions on your label. It's not that these techs know more than pharmacists. It's just that some techs are inherently more careful than many of the pharmacists I know. Techs and pharmacists span the entire spectrum as regards accuracy. Some techs and pharmacists rarely make errors. Other techs and pharmacists are an accident waiting to happen. You have no way of knowing whether the pharmacists and techs at your pharmacy are in the former category or the latter.

I worked in one very busy store in which the best tech could churn out as many prescriptions as the three or four worst techs combined. I know many techs who can churn out far more prescriptions than pharmacists. Given the choice between working alongside a great tech or a slow pharmacist, I would choose to work with the great tech every time.

With so many look-alike or sound-alike drug names like Prilosec and Prozac or Xanax and Zantac, should you trust a person with little or no formal training in drugs to decipher your doctor's handwriting? Is the tech sophisticated enough to investigate a poorly legible prescription to determine that acid reflux is your problem, implying that your doctor wants you to have Prilosec; or that depression is your problem, implying that your doctor is prescribing Prozac? If pharmacists often have difficulty reading doctor's handwriting, does it make you comfortable to know that the person attempting to decipher your doctor's handwriting may have just begun working in the pharmacy?

Upon becoming a pharmacist, I was surprised that many of the big chains would allow high school students and inexperienced techs to have such a critical role in filling prescriptions. I was surprised that on-the-job training has been accepted practice with something as critical as prescription drugs. Prescriptions are often filled so quickly that they are just a blur as they pass by technicians and pharmacists. Pharmacists frequently say to themselves, "Mrs. Smith was in today but I don't even remember filling or checking her prescriptions."

25

Should technicians run the pharmacy computer?

The pharmacy computer is the heart of the pharmacy and the repository for all the data about your prescriptions. If data is entered into the computer incorrectly, the current prescription and each subsequent refill will reflect that erroneous information. Unless there is some obvious reason to go back and change the data that's entered, a serious error can be perpetuated for months or longer. That means the customer can receive the wrong drug, the wrong strength, the wrong directions, etc., for the current prescription and subsequent refills.

Pharmacy software providers pride themselves on the number of warning flags they can raise as pharmacists and techs enter prescriptions into the pharmacy computer. This gives technicians the impossible task of separating critical warnings from those that are unlikely to result in significant harm. Pharmacists, themselves, are frequently uncertain about which warnings justify taking action such as notifying the doctor who wrote the prescription(s). Most pharmacists agree that expecting pharmacy technicians to evaluate these oftentimes complex warnings is absurd. Yet most of the big drug chains expect pharmacy technicians to input most of America's prescriptions and to evaluate the huge numbers of warnings that pop up as technicians speed through a large number of computer screens in the filling of millions of prescriptions across America every day. Granted, pharmacy computers usually grade the severity of each warning. But many techs seem to have a very relaxed attitude toward these warnings, regardless of the severity level assigned by the computer software. It is true that their level of concern often reflects the attitude of the pharmacists with whom the techs work.

U. S. News & World Report conducted a large-scale undercover investigation of pharmacists' ability to catch drug interactions. ("Danger at the Drugstore," August 26, 1996, pp. 46-53) The investigation revealed that pharmacy staff did not do a good job of catching potential drug interactions. Even though this investigation was conducted in the 1990s, I would be willing to bet that similar results would be obtained today, since the problem of pharmacy understaffing is probably more acute today than it was in 1996. Understaffing translates into prescriptions filled at incredible speed. Does it make any sense to have technicians screen your record for drug interactions that even pharmacists overlook? Some computer programs do not even require that the tech call the pharmacist over to view the most serious interactions and enter his secret password or authorization before proceeding.

Statistically, overriding a drug interaction warning is unlikely to harm the customer since most of the warnings that pop up on the computer screen do not require a change in the drugs the doctor has prescribed. Yet the chains seem to be gambling on statistics. Drug interactions vary tremendously in their potential to cause harm. In my experience, most interactions that the pharmacy computer flags have been of theoretical concern and do not require notifying the doctor who prescribed the drugs. For several years, I have been collecting articles that describe lawsuits against pharmacists. I see that "overlooking a drug interaction" is not one of the more common reasons for a lawsuit against pharmacists. The most common reason that pharmacists are sued is for dispensing the wrong drug (for example, dispensing Coumadin instead of Cardura). Another common reason for being sued is typing wrong directions on a child's liquid prescription medication (for example, "Give 1.5 teaspoonsful" instead of "Give 1.5 milliliters."

Employers say that technicians free up the pharmacist from mundane tasks like counting pills and operating the pharmacy computer. Supposedly this allows the pharmacist time to advise customers about the proper use of medications. It is a fact that employers greatly prefer to hire techs when business increases, thus making the pharmacist responsible for checking, for example, the work of three techs rather than two. The addition of techs does not necessarily give the pharmacist more time to advise customers, because chain staffing is usually kept at the bare bones level to increase profitability.

Pharmacy technicians are the workhorses of pharmacy. Busy drugstores often have one or two pharmacists supervise techs who prepare several hundred prescriptions per day. The onerous workload of this nation's increasing prescription volume is being placed on pharmacy techs. It's a high-pressure assembly line with the pharmacist responsible for verifying the end product.

I once had a conversation with the head of a state board of pharmacy. He compared the modern drugstore to one famous episode of *I Love Lucy* in which Lucille Ball places chocolates in boxes at the end of an assembly line. The actress has a hard time keeping up as the speed of the assembly line increases so she begins stuffing the chocolates in her mouth and pockets. The head of this state board of pharmacy told me that he worries that we may be heading in a similar direction in pharmacy.

Here's another food production analogy: The filling of prescriptions in America is much like the making of sausage: You don't want to watch the process. With some understanding of what's involved in the filling of prescriptions, if you were to step behind the pharmacy counter in a busy drugstore for a few hours and watch how prescriptions are processed, you might never again assume that:

• the right pills are in your bottle,

• the directions on the label are correct,

• your medications have been properly screened for drug interactions, or

• your pharmacist has had enough time to carefully check each prescription technicians have filled.

You might also see that time constraints sometimes force pharmacists and technicians to take educated guesses about doctors' poorly legible handwriting or questionable doses, and to sometimes override potentially risky drug interactions.

When pharmacists fill in at other stores for pharmacists who are sick or on vacation, we are at the mercy of those stores to have competent techs on duty. Most pharmacists are very familiar with the extremely unpleasant experience of working in an unfamiliar pharmacy with techs who make lots of errors, or working with no tech at all. Some pharmacists insist on proper tech staffing before agreeing to work in an unfamiliar pharmacy. Sometimes this gives the pharmacist a reputation for being uncooperative, too demanding, not a team player, etc.

As pharmacy customers become more impatient and expect instant service, many of the large chains have responded with drive-thru windows. This reinforces in the minds of our customers the perception that prescriptions are a commodity like hamburgers. It is very dangerous to add oftentimes untrained technicians to an already hyper-stressed environment. Do you want—in some cases—a high school student preparing your medication order as if she were preparing a burger order? Do high school students have the maturity required for the pharmacy? Are ongoing conversations about their boyfriends and social activities conducive to the accurate filling of prescriptions? Are you comfortable with people of widely varying experience levels having an increasing role with today's potent prescription drugs?

The practice of having techs run the pharmacy computer seems to be a corporate decision at most of the big chain drugstores. Yet some pharmacists refuse to let techs run the computer. These pharmacists feel that running the pharmacy computer is the most critical job in the drugstore and that only the pharmacist should be trusted to read all the warnings that pop up on the screen as we enter prescriptions. So the question is: *Should techs indeed be allowed to run the pharmacy computer even though doing so is routine in most pharmacies today?*

In my opinion, the corporate attitude of the big chain drugstores toward the doctorate in pharmacy degree (Pharm.D.) illustrates the same corporate attitude that endorses techs running the pharmacy computer. It is clear to me that the bean counters at the big chains believe Pharm.D.'s are overeducated for work in drug-stores. The best indication of this is that many of the big chains want technicians to run the pharmacy computer, not the pharmacist. The most often stated reason is that this allows the pharmacist to be free to answer customers' questions, speak on the phone with doctors' offices, check prescriptions that have been completed by technicians, make recommendations to customers for non-prescription products for coughs and colds, etc.

Apparently many of the big chains do not attach much significance to the endless number of warnings (Drug Utilization Review or DUR alerts) that pop up on the computer screen. If you have any doubts whether the big chains think Pharm.D's are overeducated for retail pharmacy, consider the fact that the big chains don't think it is necessary for a pharmacist (B.S. *or* Pharm.D.) to review the warnings, contraindications, precautions, high/low dose alerts, drug interactions, etc.

Pharmacists: Can you name a task in the pharmacy that requires more education than responding to drug therapy questions or evaluating DUR alerts? Supposedly technicians are not allowed to screen for drug therapy problems but isn't that exactly what they're doing when they routinely zip past a blizzard of DUR alerts of varying levels of importance?

The pharmacy computer software generates a remarkable number of these DUR alerts. Pharmacists assumed that the evaluation of these DUR alerts is precisely the reason we were required to graduate from pharmacy school. Some of these warnings are highly complex and they leave the pharmacist scratching his head and wondering what is indeed the practical significance of these warnings. Some pharmacists choose to ignore the vast majority of warnings as simply "noise." Other pharmacists consult reference books in the pharmacy in order to understand more fully the implications of the DUR alerts.

The big chains design their computer systems as they see fit, with "filling and billing" functions given top priority. The fact that most of the big chains encourage the pharmacy technicians to run the pharmacy computer demonstrates to me that the big chains view the pharmacy computer as mainly a data-entry tool for the processing of prescriptions, rather than a medical tool for assuring that all prescriptions are screened for possible drug therapy problems.

Are pharmacists and techs like airline ticket agents? Airline ticket agents spend a large part of their day on the computer: checking fares, flights, the availability of seats, and entering the customer's name, address and phone number, etc. But airline ticket agents don't also need to examine the plane's maintenance records to determine the safety of the planes on which the customers fly. In contrast, the pharmacy staff must screen each prescription to be sure that there are no pertinent warnings, contraindications, drug interactions, etc. that can affect the customer's safety.

What conclusion can one reach other than that the big pharmacy chains do not place a lot of importance on the warnings? If the big chains took seriously the endless number of warnings, only pharmacists would be allowed to run the pharmacy computer. The big chains seem to view the operation of the pharmacy computer as simply a clerical job, not a job that requires substantial knowledge of drug therapy.

I bet that most pharmacists have often wondered what warnings the technicians are ignoring. In my experience, only a small percent of the warnings require changing anything about the prescriptions, so, statistically, the pharmacy staff finds little danger in having a relaxed attitude toward the endless number of warnings that pop up. But surely we are overriding a few very important warnings. In that huge sea of warnings generated by the pharmacy computer software, surely we are overlooking a few very important ones.

If the big chains are sued, they can claim that the pharmacist was negligent in overlooking the warnings that do indeed pop up on our computer screen. Thus the big chains can blame the pharmacist, rather than admit that staffing levels determined by the corporation don't allow the pharmacist enough "warm bodies" in the pharmacy to assure that all prescriptions are filled with maximum care.

I occasionally worked in one store with a tech who would call me over—in what seemed to be a random fashion—to look at various warning messages. She seemed to be proud of herself for being conscientious enough to call me over. Yet she seemed to have no idea which warnings were the most serious and which were unlikely to result in significant harm. I suspect that she, like many techs, overrode the vast majority of warnings, but, feeling guilty, wanted to assuage her guilt by randomly calling me over. She was more likely to call me over during times of the day when the pharmacy was less busy. She seemed to be much less likely to call me over when everyone in the pharmacy was stressed to the max as a result of our running far behind in the filling of prescriptions.

I am at least partly guilty in this situation. I should have stressed to her the importance of closely monitoring the grading system that the computer software uses to warn us about the severity level of each warning. But there just never seemed to be enough time. I felt that, since I was only filling in at that store occasionally, it was the duty of the regular pharmacists to teach her.

Because of all the things that can go wrong when techs run the pharmacy computer, some pharmacists insist on running the pharmacy computer themselves. However, in very busy pharmacies with several computer terminals, it is almost impossible to prohibit the technicians from running the pharmacy computer. High prescription volume often requires substantial use of the pharmacy computers by technicians.

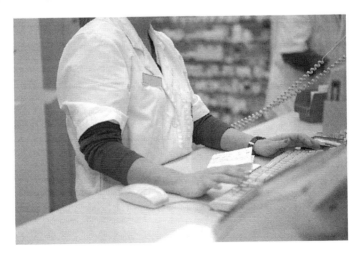

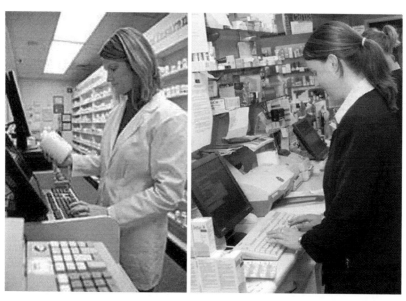

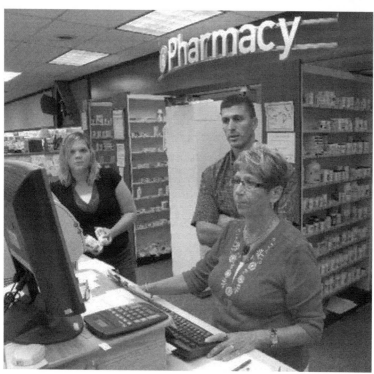

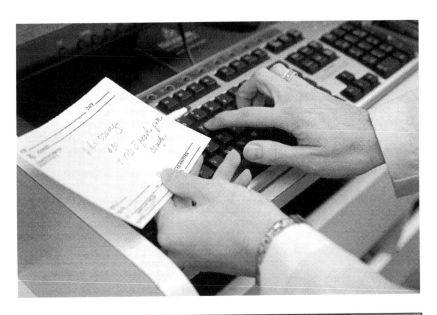

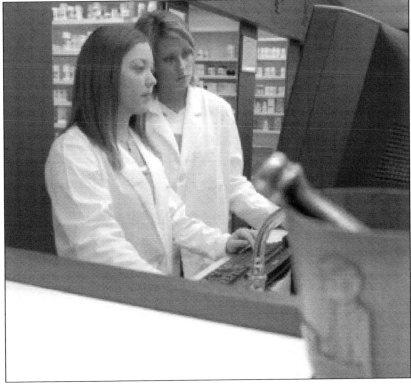

26

Should technicians override computer warnings on their own?

I used to work for a large national chain that required the pharmacist to review drug interactions by typing his secret password in the computer before proceeding. The computer screen would lock until a valid pharmacist's password was entered. This meant that the technician had to interrupt the pharmacist from whatever he was doing (like answering a customer's question or talking on the phone with a doctor's office). The technician would say something like "I need you to look at this drug interaction." The pharmacist had to walk over to the computer, examine the potential drug interaction, and then enter his secret password if the pharmacist determined that the drug interaction was unlikely to result in significant harm.

When our chain was sold to another large chain, all pharmacists at our chain began using the computer program used by the chain that bought our chain. Our new employer's pharmacy computer system does not require the pharmacist's secret password to proceed. Many pharmacists told me that they are scared to death that a technician will proceed past critical drug interaction warnings without notifying the pharmacist. Pharmacists worry about the real potential that a customer can be harmed, resulting in a lawsuit.

Our new employer held a meeting for the fifty or so pharmacists in our district. The purpose of the meeting was to familiarize us with the new computer system. There was a loud groan among many pharmacists in attendance when we were informed that the computer system we would be adopting (with transition to the new employer) did not require the pharmacist's secret password to proceed. The trainer told us, "It's a training issue!! Train your technicians to call you over whenever a drug interaction pops up on the computer screen!!" Pharmacists in attendance mostly said, "Yeah, right!!"

With dangerously inadequate staffing in too many pharmacies, pharmacists don't welcome frequent interruptions from technicians (or customers, for that matter). In many such cases, technicians become reluctant to interrupt the pharmacist and simply proceed past drug interaction warnings with the new computer system that doesn't require the pharmacist's secret password to proceed. Since, in my experience, most drug interactions are indeed overridden by the pharmacists themselves, technicians see that the course of least resistance is to override the interaction without interrupting the pharmacist.

Overriding potential drug interactions doesn't often result in harm to the customer, since most of the drug interaction warnings that pop up on our computer screen seem to be more of a theoretical concern than a real world concern. But the fact remains that this attitude toward drug interactions by techs and pharmacists occasionally results in overriding potentially serious interactions. Can anyone seriously deny that?

The big chains seem to feel that slowing down the prescription filling process by having pharmacists and technicians obsess over each potential drug interaction is not worth the time. It is as if the big chains prefer to pay customers who suffer harm from drug interactions rather than slow down the prescription filling process across the entire chain. The big chains seem to base their operations on how often they get sued for something, rather than basing it on assuring that prescriptions are filled with extreme care. Filling prescriptions with extreme care does not seem to be profitable under managed care. It is more profitable to herd customers and then pay that small fraction of customers who are inevitably harmed.

Many pharmacists were very unhappy with the fact that our new employer's computer system does not require the pharmacist's secret password to proceed past potential drug interactions. But the common attitude among the pharmacists I know seems to be: *This is just one more example of the ease with which the big chains place our license (and the corporation itself) at risk in order to fill prescriptions quickly.* One of the biggest surprises for me in pharmacy has been the ease with which big chains seem to expose themselves to tremendous liability (for both their pharmacists and the corporation itself). Many pharmacists feel that the big chains will continue in this reckless manner until the cost of settlements from lawsuits exceeds the cost of adequate staffing in the pharmacy.

Let me be perfectly clear that I do not mean to denigrate technicians. Some technicians are absolutely fantastic. There are many technicians with whom I would rather work than pharmacists. I know many technicians who are more accurate and faster than pharmacists. My concern is simply whether technicians are capable of determining the significance of oftentimes highly complex warnings when pharmacists themselves are often uncertain of their practical significance.

There is as much variation in the quality of technicians as there is in the quality of pharmacists. The public thinks that surely one pharmacist is as good as the next. Not so. Same with techs. Great techs are an absolute delight to work with. I've seen pharmacy managers who schedule the best techs to work the pharmacy manager's shift and leave the worst techs to work with the other pharmacists.

Some chains seem to feel that once we've got a warm body in the pharmacy, that's the equivalent of having a seasoned tech. When we have an opening for a tech, many pharmacists hire the first person who walks in the door and asks for a job. Pharmacists should, in my opinion, go back through their employment applications on file to find the most promising candidate. Hiring a good tech is one of the most important of the pharmacist's duties. Many pharmacists put a tremendous amount of thought into whom they hire as a tech. Other pharmacists hire the first person who asks for a job.

Hiring a tech is more difficult than I first assumed. I used to think that I was a good judge of people, that I could size them up after a short conversation and predict how well they would do as a tech. In one store, the store manager transferred one of his clerks to the pharmacy when we needed a tech. At the time, I assumed the store manager was dumping his worst clerk on us, and I guess I shouldn't be surprised that a store manager would not want to part with one of his top employees. I worked with her for a few weeks and was very disappointed in her performance. I had heard her tell another tech, "The more you learn, the more they'll expect you to do." So I assumed she was pretty much hopeless. Apparently something caused her to change her attitude, because she gradually became a super tech. To my amazement, she turned out to be one of the best techs I ever worked with. She was quiet but turned out to be fast as lightening.

Even though predicting who will be a good tech is very difficult, I wish more pharmacists would put a much greater effort into screening whom they hire. When I fill in at other stores, I find techs who are absolutely terrific, and others who are horrendous, a threat to the public safety. It seems that young pharmacists are more likely to hire the first person who asks for a job as a tech. Perhaps more experienced pharmacists realize how important it is to hire promising applicants.

Techs can definitely make the difference between a day that's tolerable and a day that's an absolute nightmare. I worked in one busy pharmacy in which we had three or four techs on duty at one time (plus two pharmacists), and a total of seven or eight techs on the payroll. I am not exaggerating in saying that the output of the top two techs was equal to the combined output of the other five or six techs.

I enjoy working with fast, accurate, and friendly techs and hate working with techs who are slow and immature. I'd rather work with a fast tech who makes a few errors than a slow tech who is extremely accurate. In the real world, many pharmacists would consider the slow tech to be a greater danger to the public. That is because the chaos caused by being covered with prescriptions is much worse than the usually straight-forward task of catching and correcting tech errors. I'd rather work with a tech who is extremely fast but makes a few mistakes during her shift, than I would to work with a tech who makes no errors but is painfully slow. Slow techs cause confusion in the pharmacy because prescriptions back up, customers start complaining, and tempers flare. Some techs can absolutely make the computer keyboard sing. Other techs seem to stare at the computer screen endlessly when they are stumped—rather than ask a pharmacist or another tech for assistance. Perhaps the tech doesn't want anyone to know that she doesn't understand something in the computer.

Error-prone techs are a particular hazard when working with floater pharmacists or pharmacists who fill in for sick days or vacation days. Many floater or fill-in pharmacists assume the techs they work with are accurate. That is a dangerous assumption. It is wise to be extra-vigilant when working with techs we are not familiar with.

Technicians often fight among themselves over whose turn it is to answer the phone or wait on a customer at the drive thru window. Understandably, techs don't like interrupting their work on the pharmacy computer to ring up a customer or accept a prescription from a customer who has just approached the pharmacy. I occasionally worked in a pharmacy in which the drive thru window is an incredibly long distance from the dispensing area. One day a pharmacist commented that the architect who designed the layout for that pharmacy should be hung from one of the rafters in the ceiling. Techs routinely became upset with each other over whose turn it was to walk the long distance to wait on a customer at that drive-thru.

Working with a tech who's a mature and interesting person can sometimes make my day almost tolerable. Pharmacy can be an intellectually deadening job even though pharmacists can't allow our brain to become less than fully alert in viewing drug interactions, contraindications, drug allergies, and in making sure the right pills are in the right bottle. In my opinion, the activity of filling prescriptions is inherently unfulfilling (profoundly so) because it is like a hamburger assembly line. (I have lots of adjectives to describe my dislike for my job: piece work, production work, intellectually unsatisfying, vacuous, monotonous, repetitive, robotic, physically ex-hausting grunt work in a factory.) Working with a fast tech who's also an interesting person can sometimes turn a nightmarish day into one that's tolerable. If she's cute, that's an added bonus.

I try hard to be a likeable person. Despite my best efforts, some techs and I just don't hit it off, probably due to us having totally different personalities.

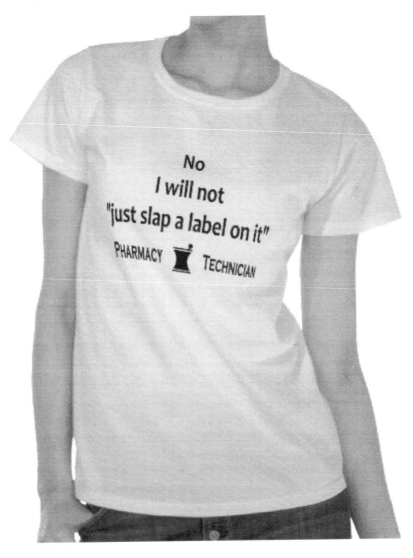

27

Is it possible to have too many technicians on duty?

Some state boards of pharmacy have maximum "tech-to-pharmacist ratios." In states that have such a regulation, what this means, for example, is that no more than two (or sometimes three) techs can be on duty for each pharmacist on duty. I've never heard of a maximum ratio of four techs to one pharmacist. State boards of pharmacy pass regulations mandating such maximum ratios in an attempt to force employers to hire a second pharmacist, i.e., when the prescription volume exceeds the capabilities of a single pharmacist to adequately check every prescription filled by that pharmacist and the techs. It is obviously cheaper for the corporation to keep hiring techs as prescription volume increases, rather than pay the salaries of two pharmacists working simultaneously.

Unfortunately, I've only seen such "tech-to-pharmacist ratios" actually enforced after-the-fact. In other words, when the board of pharmacy investigates a particular pharmacy or pharmacist for an infraction of some type (a pharmacy mistake reported by a customer, a pharmacist found to be distributing drugs to dealers, a pharmacist found to be abusing drugs or alcohol, etc.), the investigator may notice that the tech-to-pharmacist ratio in that pharmacy is being exceeded. That infraction will be added to the other infraction(s) in the board of pharmacy citation.

In my opinion, if the state boards of pharmacy imposed severe penalties for exceeding these maximum tech-to-pharmacist ratios, it might have some effect. However, in the cases I've read about, the penalties for exceeding the maximum ratio amount to a slap on the wrist. As I state in my chapter on boards of pharmacy, I feel this is because the state boards of pharmacy are afraid of the immense legal and political clout of the big chains. And the state boards don't want to appear to be anti-business in the eyes of state legislatures that are strongly pro-business.

I would, in fact, love to work in a pharmacy that had an excess number of techs. Yes, after perhaps three techs per pharmacist, the techs can churn out more prescriptions than one pharmacist can safely check. But I don't recall ever having the luxury of working with too many techs. The usual problem is having too few techs on duty.

During my entire 25 year career, I've only worked in one store which had two pharmacists on duty simultaneously. That pharmacy averaged over 300 prescriptions per day, a nightmare for a single pharmacist. But even at this store, there were days when one pharmacist was forced to work as the only pharmacist on duty, usually due to the illness or vacation of another pharmacist and due to the fact that no other pharmacists in the district were available to work that day.

I think the state boards are naïve if they think that their loose, after-the-fact enforcement of tech-to-pharmacist ratios will force the big chains to have, say, two pharmacists on duty at the same time. The big chains only have two pharmacists on duty at the same time when the volume for one pharmacist becomes extremely burdensome. Most chains have strict internal guidelines on the level of prescription volume required before two pharmacists are allowed to work at the same time. These guidelines are usually far above what pharmacists feel is realistic or safe.

28

Should technicians be allowed to give advice to customers?

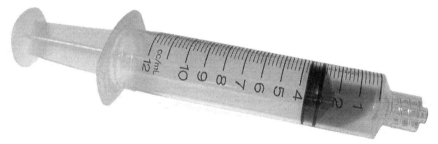

Some technicians have a habit of advising customers or answering customers' questions in a manner that exceeds the tech's level of knowledge. Sometimes this occurs because the tech is overzealous or over-confident, but sometimes the problem is that the tech knows that the pharmacist she's working with doesn't like to be bothered or interrupted with questions. Some pharmacists are simply arrogant and technicians understandably avoid speaking with these pharmacists. Working with pharmacists who don't like to be disturbed, the tech is placed in the uncomfortable position of feeling compelled to try to give advice to customers or answer customers' questions when the tech knows that the pharmacist is the person who should be answering those questions from customers.

Here is an example from the Institute of Safe Medication Practices (www.ismp.org) in which a technician gave a wrong syringe and wrong instructions to a customer. There is, of course, no way of knowing whether the pharmacist didn't have the time or desire to advise the customer. Some pharmacists love to talk with customers. Other pharmacists try hard to avoid speaking with customers because of shyness or because they're so far behind with a huge backlog of prescriptions.

Whenever you get a prescription filled or refilled, be sure that the pharmacist talks with you about your medications. This means more than just telling you the name of the medication. If the medication needs to be measured, ask the pharmacist to show you how to measure it. A mother gave her 7-week-old baby 5 mL of Tagamet (cimetidine) instead of 0.5 mL for acid reflux because a pharmacy technician gave her the wrong syringe. The technician told the mother that the "5" on the syringe meant 0.5 mL. After four doses, the baby was very drowsy, vomited and had loose stools. The mother took the baby to the emergency room for observation, but, fortunately, the baby did not have to be treated. When prescriptions are dispensed, no one but a pharmacist should be giving you advice about the medication. If a pharmacist does not offer to counsel you, insist on it.

A similar incident occurred involving the dispensing of the acid reducer Axid to an infant. In this case the medicine dropper was incorrectly marked by a technician. This incident, which occurred in 2008, resulted in a disciplinary action by the North Carolina Board of Pharmacy against pharmacist A. P.
(http://www.ncbop.org/Disciplinary%20Actions%20%20-PHAR-MACISTS/PickensAsa05790.pdf#search="error")

On August 25, 2008, [Pharmacist A. P.] dispensed a prescription for Axid to an infant patient with a medicine dropper that was incorrectly marked, so that the patient received approximately four and one-half times the prescribed dose of the medication. A technician had hand-marked the medicine dropper, and requested that [Pharmacist A. P.] confirm the marking. Without visually inspecting the medicine dropper, [Pharmacist A. P.] approved the marking. [Pharmacist A. P.] accordingly failed to physically review the dispensed product and the medicine dropper before they were delivered to the patient. Furthermore, when [Pharmacist A. P.] dispensed the drug, he failed to counsel the patient, instead improperly allowing the technician to counsel the patient.

The drug was administered to the patient, and the patient twice ingested the drug at the incorrect dose. As a result, the patient suffered from diarrhea for over a week while the large dose passed through her system.

29

Potentially serious consequences when pharmacists, technicians, and patients don't "Shake Well"

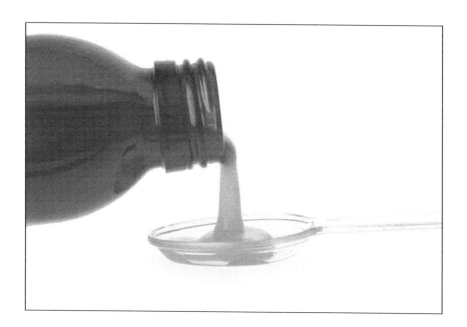

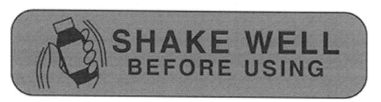

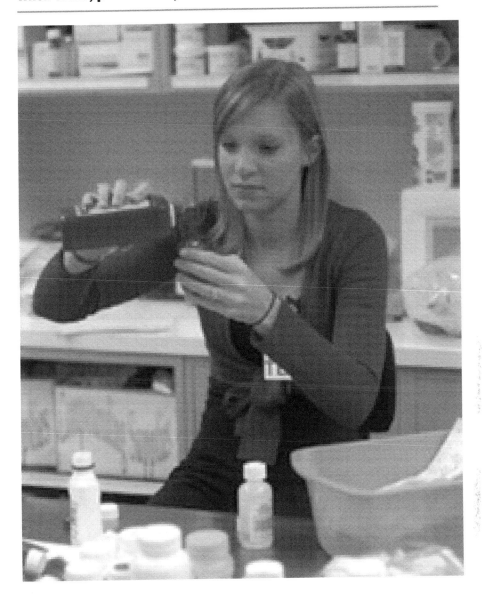

Here's an example of a problem that can occur because of poorly trained or inadequately supervised technicians. I fear that this problem is more common than most pharmacists realize. First, some background on the critical difference between liquid medications that are solutions and those that are suspensions.

Most of the drugs in the pharmacy are tablets and capsules but a large number are liquids. Liquids are used primarily for children since children often have a hard time swallowing tablets or capsules. An exception to this generalization is that products for cough are usually in the liquid form for both children and adults.

Many of the products in the pharmacy need to be shaken by pharmacy staff before being dispensed to the customer. Then the customer (or parent) must shake the product again at home before it is swallowed. Drug products available in the liquid form are usually in one of two categories: solutions and suspensions. A solution is a product that does not normally need to be shaken. A non-pharmacy example of a solution is any of the soft drinks you buy in a supermarket such as Coke, Pepsi, Mountain Dew, Dr. Pepper, etc. These products obviously aren't supposed to be shaken before you drink 'em.

On the other hand, think of a suspension as a product like a salad dressing. When a salad dressing has been sitting on a shelf for a period of time, we see that a significant portion of the contents has settled to the bottom of the bottle. For example, we shake Italian dressing before pouring it over our salad. Very few people who know anything about salad dressings would ever consider pouring it over their salad without first shaking the bottle. A very similar situation exists in the pharmacy, i.e., there are several products that are analogous to salad dressings. These products must be shaken well before being dispensed. The trouble is that many pharmacy technicians are not fully aware of the importance of shaking these products when pouring them from our stock containers when filling a prescription. I have seen many instances in which techs shake the bottles in the most cursory and superficial fashion. Would you be contented with shaking your salad dressing, perhaps, once up and once down? I've seen techs do that with pharmacy products that need to be shaken before being transferred to the customer's bottle.

Among the products that sit on the pharmacy shelves as suspensions (and thus need to be shaken before being dispensed to the customer) are Septra (trimethoprim/sulfamethoxazole) suspension and Tegretol (carbamazepine) suspension. These prescription products must be shaken before they are dispensed to the public because a heavy concentration of active ingredient settles to the bottom of these bottles while sitting on our shelves. These products must also be shaken well at home before *each* dose is taken.

Many technicians do not fully comprehend the importance of shaking these suspensions in our (typically) 16-ounce stock bottles before pouring out a smaller quantity to fill a waiting prescription. If the bottle is not shaken well, most of the active ingredient may be sitting at the bottom of the bottle so the first prescriptions filled from our stock bottle would tend to be subpotent, whereas the last prescriptions would tend to be superpotent. Notice that the little sticker we apply to your Rx bottle says "SHAKE WELL." It does not say "SHAKE LIGHTLY."

Many children's' antibiotics arrive at the pharmacy in the form of a dry powder, to which pharmacists or technicians add a specified quantity of water before dispensing the product. It is important that parents shake these products thoroughly before each dose is given to a child. Otherwise, most of the active ingredient is sitting at the bottom of the container.

Here is a real world example of the consequences of the pharmacy staff not adequately shaking a child's anti-seizure medication before dispensing it. (Kate Kelly, Pharm. D., "Shake Well Before Dispensing," *Pharmacy Times*, October 2005 http://www.pharmacytimes.com/article.cfm?ID=2652)

Obviously, it is important to ensure that the active ingredient(s) in a suspension is (are) properly dispersed throughout the vehicle before administration. "Shake well before use" is a common reminder (in the form of directions typed on the pharmacy label, an auxiliary label, or verbal instructions) given by pharmacists to patients who receive oral suspensions. Yet, how often is this important reminder forgotten by pharmacy staff members when preparing a smaller quantity of a suspension from a large stock bottle? What happens if the stock bottle is not shaken or is inadequately shaken?

One mother knows all too well. In a report to the Institute for Safe Medication Practices, she explained that her son had been diagnosed with epilepsy, and his seizures were well controlled with carbamazepine (Tegretol) oral suspension. His prescription called for 8 oz of carbamazepine to be dispensed with each refill. Because the medication is available in a 16-oz stock bottle, smaller bottles were prepared for each refill.

Several days after starting a new bottle, the son had a recurrence of seizures that lasted about a week. During this time, his mother noticed that the suspension had a different appearance from the previous prescription. She mentioned this difference to the prescribing physician, who recommended getting a new refill. She was subsequently more aware of the appearance of the suspension whenever she had the medication refilled. Whenever the suspension looked different from what was expected, she would ask the pharmacist for a replacement, dispensed from an unopened manufacturer's bottle and shaken in her presence.

After a few of these occurrences, however, she insisted that the pediatrician write prescriptions instructing pharmacists to dispense the medication only in the 16-oz unopened manufacturer's stock bottle. She saved several of the more suspicious-looking suspensions dispensed in 8-oz bottles and sent them to the manufacturer. Assays performed by the manufacturer's Quality Control Division revealed that three of the bottles contained suspensions that were significantly less concentrated than the expected 100-mg/5-mL concentration, and one bottle of suspension was three times more concentrated than was expected!

The problem appears to have stemmed from pharmacy staff members not shaking or inadequately shaking the stock bottle of carbamazepine suspension before preparing the smaller bottle. If an unopened stock bottle of a suspension was inadequately shaken before preparing a smaller bottle, the suspension that was poured out could potentially be less concentrated than expected. The remainder of the stock suspension would then be more highly concentrated. Both situations could potentially lead to significant variability in doses, which could affect disease control (i.e., recurrence of seizures resulting from the less-concentrated carbamazepine suspension dispensed). This variability is particularly significant for drugs with a narrow therapeutic index. Even if the suspension is adequately shaken prior to dispensing, if patients do not shake the medication properly, similar variability in doses can occur.

In order to prevent such problems, pharmacy staff members should be sure to adequately shake all suspensions. Education may be required for pharmacy technicians and students, who may not be aware of the difference between a solution and a suspension. Visually check that the suspension is uniformly dispersed before it is transferred from its original container. Pharmacists involved in the final check of a suspension should verify with the individual who prepared it that this important step was performed before allowing the suspension to be dispensed.

Consider making auxiliary labels as reminders for pharmacy staff members that read "Shake well before dispensing," and add them to appropriate pharmacy stock bottles. In addition, attention could be drawn to suspensions by highlighting or circling the word "suspension" on product labels. Make sure that patients receiving suspension preparations are counseled so that they fully understand the need to shake the medication well before each use. The "Shake Well" auxiliary label, which commonly accompanies the pharmacy label on suspension preparations being dispensed, could easily be overlooked. It should not be used as the only means of communicating this important information, but rather it should serve as a reminder for patients.

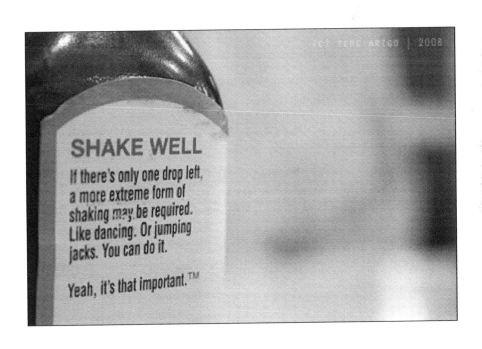

SHAKE WELL

If there's only one drop left, a more extreme form of shaking may be required. Like dancing. Or jumping jacks. You can do it.

Yeah, it's that important.™

30

Two technicians and their supervising pharmacist missed this error involving two drugs with similar generic names

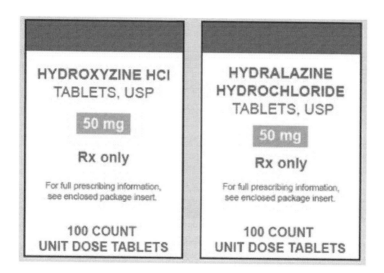

HYDROXYZINE HCl TABLETS, USP	HYDRALAZINE HYDROCHLORIDE TABLETS, USP
50 mg	50 mg
Rx only	Rx only
For full prescribing information, see enclosed package insert.	For full prescribing information, see enclosed package insert.
100 COUNT UNIT DOSE TABLETS	100 COUNT UNIT DOSE TABLETS

This example illustrates the dilemma with techs. In one store in which I worked, one evening a customer came in with a swollen face. She approached me and asked, "Has my doctor called in a prescription for this?" She then pointed to her swollen face and said that that happens to her occasionally because she reacts to some (as yet undetermined) substance. I was startled by the swelling but she assured me that she had had it more than once before and that medication helps to clear it up. I went to the bin where we keep prescriptions that are ready to be picked up. I noticed that the computer label on the bag indicated that the contents was hydralazine, a blood pressure medication. I said to the customer, "What we have ready for you is a blood pressure medication." She was startled and said that that made no sense. I asked, "Have you not been on this drug before?" She said, "I don't even have hypertension."

I had that sinking feeling in my stomach as I sensed that all-too-common scenario: another prescription error. I went over to our pile of new prescriptions that had been filled that day and retrieved her doctor's phoned-in prescription. To my dismay, the prescription called for hydroxyzine (a drug that treats allergies or allergic reactions), rather than the blood pressure drug hydalazine. Without explaining to the customer that we had made an error, I changed the prescription to the proper medication. I did my best to act as if nothing had happened, even though she left with a very quizzical expression on her face, wondering what had indeed happened.

I was working the evening shift that day. It turns out that the pharmacist who had filled that prescription in the morning had not caught the tech's error. How do I know a tech had made the error? Let me explain: There were two techs working during the day, but only one remained with me to work the slower evening shift. After the customer left, I asked the remaining tech if she had any idea how this could have happened. As it turns out, the tech who was there with me has a lot less experience than the other tech. The evening tech told me, "I asked Mary if this was the right drug. She said it was." Mary is the more-experienced tech, by far.

So it turns out that the less experienced tech asked the more-experienced tech to verify the drug the doctor wanted. The less experienced tech picked the wrong drug. The more experienced tech did not catch the error when asked for verification by the less-experienced tech. And the pharmacist, who has ultimate responsibility for detecting errors, also did not catch the error. Two techs and a pharmacist missed this error. I remember the other pharmacist commenting to me, as she left for the day, "It's been a very busy day today."

Here is an example of an actual lawsuit in which Walgreen's was sued after a mix-up involving these same two drugs (hydroxyzine and hydralazine) contributed to a patient's death. Any involvement by pharmacy technicians is not described. (Kansas City Injury Lawyer Blog: "Pharmacy Sued Over Fatal Drug Error," March 19, 2012, by The Horn Law Firm, Doug Horn, Lead Attorney http://www.kansascityinjurylawyerblog.com/2012/03/pharmacy-sued-over-fatal-drug.html)

The family of an elderly Kentucky woman has filed suit against Walgreens pharmacy after an alleged mix-up of her prescription medication led to her death. Mary Moore, a Louisville resident, had just left the hospital after receiving treatment for high blood pressure, kidney failure, and congestive heart failure on November 10, 2010. Her doctor had written her a prescription for the high blood pressure medication hydralazine. The pharmacy allegedly gave her the antihistamine hydroxyzine by mistake.

Because of the medication error, Moore's high blood pressure went entirely untreated for about two weeks. The pharmacy reportedly noticed the error and provided Moore with the correct medication, but by then "it was too late," according to the lawsuit. Moore could not tolerate the dosage of the blood pressure medication. Her blood pressure reportedly continued to increase, putting additional strain on her heart. This caused "decompensation" of both her congestive heart failure and her kidney disease. She was hospitalized again, and died on December 6, 2010.

Hydralazine, according to the National Institutes of Health, is a muscle relaxant used to treat high blood pressure. It allows blood to flow more easily by relaxing the muscles in the blood vessels. Hydroxyzine is an antihistamine used to treat allergic reactions such as itching, and to control symptoms of motion sickness. It can also treat anxiety and alcohol withdrawal symptoms. The NIH specifically cautions people over the age of 65 to not use hydroxyzine, as other medications that treat the same conditions are considered safer for older patients.

Moore's family filed a lawsuit in Jefferson Circuit Court in Louisville on February 15, 2012 against Walgreens and the pharmacist in charge at that particular location. The lawsuit claims negligence and wrongful death, as well as strict liability, negligent failure to warn, and breach of warranty. The pharmacy's error in dispensing the wrong medication, according to the lawsuit, was a "substantial factor" in Moore's injuries, in enhancing her existing injuries, and in causing her death. The suit also alleges that, by not counseling Moore about the drug at the time she filled the prescription, the pharmacy violated state law. Had the pharmacist spoken to Moore at that time, the pharmacist likely would have noticed that the medication was incorrect, the lawsuit says.

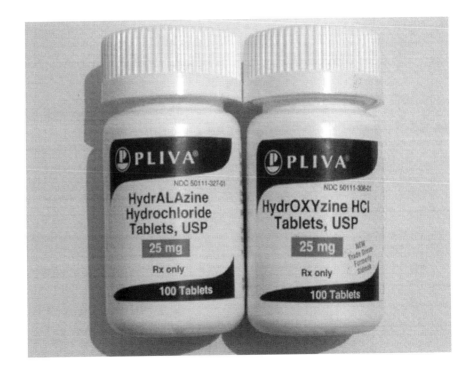

31

More examples of
typical technician mistakes

Technician errors span the entire spectrum from those that are trivial to those that are potentially catastrophic. Here are a few routine tech errors that I recall:

PCE 500 and Entex PSE

A tech filled two prescriptions as follows. One was for the antibiotic PCE 500 mg (erythromycin), taken twice a day. The other was for Entex PSE, a drug used for colds, also taken twice a day. The tech filled both prescriptions correctly in every detail except one. She put the PCE 500 in the Entex PSE bottle. And she put the Entex PSE in the PCE 500 bottle. So the medications that the patient would have received were correct but they were in the wrong bottles. In this case, it would likely have resulted in no harm since both tablets are taken twice a day. Under other circumstances in which the label directions were different, the results could have been disastrous. Even in this case, if the patient had decided to take the decongestant only as needed and the antibiotic for the full course, he would likely have ended up taking the antibiotic for a few days and the decongestant for the full course, i.e., exactly opposite of what's usually recommended.

Ibuprofen 600 and Ibuprofen 800

There are lots of garden variety errors that occur in pharmacies. For example, a technician recently put Ibuprofen 600 mg (a drug that treats pain, inflammation, and fever) in a bottle that was supposed to be Ibuprofen 800 mg. This error was discovered before the customer received the wrong strength. This is a minor error but it is still an error.

Coumadin 4 mg confused with Cardura 4 mg

One technician put Coumadin 4 mg in a refill bottle that was supposed to be Cardura 4 mg. I told her that Coumadin is probably the most dangerous drug in the pharmacy and that I just prevented her from killing someone. I made a joke out of it because I didn't want her to lose confidence in her abilities or dislike working with me. Yet she needed to know that she made a potentially very serious mistake. Coumadin is a blood thinner. It is very similar to the substance that is used in d-Con rat killer. Rats eat the d-Con and then hemorrhage internally. Cardura is used for blood pressure. I was not kidding when I told her that Coumadin is the most dangerous drug in the pharmacy. In lawsuits against pharmacists and pharmacies, Coumadin is one of the drugs most frequently involved. This was, indeed, a potentially very dangerous mistake.

Expiration dates and refrigeration

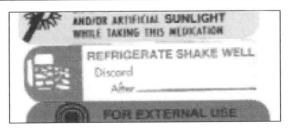

Technicians frequently put wrong expiration dates on children's antibiotics. Most children's antibiotics arrive in the pharmacy as a dry powder. The pharmacist or technician adds water to the powder immediately before dispensing. Once the water is added, the antibiotic is good only for ten or fourteen days, depending on the particular antibiotic. The majority of these antibiotics (amoxicillin and Keflex, for example) are good for fourteen days. So, techs get in the habit of putting a fourteen day expiration date on the label of all these antibiotics, even the ones that are good only for ten days. Most of these antibiotics are supposed to be kept in the refrigerator during these ten or fourteen days. However, there are a few that are supposed to be kept at room temperature. As is the case with expiration dates, the techs often seem to be so accustomed to attaching labels instructing the patient to refrigerate these liquids that they do so even for the ones that are not supposed to be refrigerated.

After I discovered a mistake that one tech made and pointed it out to her, she said to me that she needed to slow down. I said, "No. You need to continue at the same speed. If you slow down, we'll get completely covered with prescriptions. It's my job to catch your mistakes."

Some more examples of tech errors:
• A tech filled a prescription for Levlen birth control pills with TriLevlen.
• A tech filled a prescription for Septra DS (a drug used frequently to treat urinary tract infection in women) with ten tablets rather than twenty specified by the doctor.
• A tech typed a label for Motrin suspension (a drug used for pain and fever in kids), "Take three-fourths teaspoonful" rather than what the doctor specified, "Take one and three-fourths teaspoonsful."
• A tech typed the directions for Naprelan (an analgesic and anti-inflammatory drug) as "Take 1 daily" rather than what the doctor specified, "Take 2 daily."
• A tech put a "Keep in refrigerator" sticker on two bottles containing tablets. These tablets are not supposed to be refrigerated. This clerk does everything with lightning speed and never looks back to see if she has made an error.
• A tech filled a prescription with Rondec DM Drops rather than plain Rondec Drops specified by the doctor. These are medications

for colds in infants. One contains dextromethorphan (DM), a cough suppressant. The other does not.

• A tech filled a prescription with Cefzil rather than what the doctor specified, Ceftin. These are both antibiotics. I caught myself making the same mistake on a separate occasion.

• A tech gave a customer the correct pills in his two refill containers but switched the contents of both containers. In one container labeled glyburide (a drug used to treat type II diabetes), she placed methotrexate (a powerful drug used to treat cancer, rheumatoid arthritis, and psoriasis). In the container labeled methotrexate, she placed the glyburide.

This last example is a potentially very dangerous mistake. Of course, there's a good chance that if this customer had been on these drugs for awhile, he would have caught such an error and no harm would have occurred. Customers catch a lot of our errors. So an error that we make doesn't necessarily mean that harm will occur, even with potentially dangerous drugs. An ever-vigilant patient is a requirement in today's "speed is all that matters" environment.

These are, as I said, just a few of the errors that I recall catching in the last few months. If I were to list all the errors that I've caught techs making in the twenty-five years since I graduated from pharmacy school, the list would fill a book. Catching errors of varying levels of seriousness is a routine part of the pharmacist's job. The errors I've seen and caught are no different (in terms of seriousness) than those seen by every pharmacist in America.

PART V

STORE MANAGERS

32

Store managers are too often clueless about pharmacists

I think that many of the big chains need to go back to the drawing board and figure out a better management structure for their stores. In almost every store I've worked in, there is a constant battle between the pharmacists and the non-pharmacist store manager. In the best-run stores, the pharmacists and the non-pharmacist store manager get along well and enjoy working with each other. But, in my experience, that is the exception.

The fundamental nature of the conflict between managers and pharmacists hasn't changed since I graduated in 1975. This conflict is truly Topic A in many of the stores in which I've worked. Many pharmacists talk about this situation constantly and passionately. Too often, the relationship between the pharmacists and the non-pharmacist store manager is like a bad marriage where both partners desperately need a divorce. We see each other so much that we get under each other's skin.

Pharmacists resent the fact that someone with so little appreciation for the problems in the pharmacy has so much power in the store. Pharmacists feel that our years of schooling entitle us to more respect than we receive from the non-pharmacy management. Pharmacists resent that someone who often has little or no college education is (or acts like he is) our boss. Many pharmacists feel that district managers too often hire low caliber management trainees.

Whether the non-pharmacist store manager does indeed have authority over the pharmacy is a question that's often avoided by chain management. Pharmacy supervisors tell pharmacists that the non-pharmacist store manager isn't really our boss. But the non-pharmacy supervisors seem to tell the non-pharmacist store manager the opposite.

In many stores, the pharmacy accounts for over half of the total sales. Pharmacists at these stores feel they should be given more respect for this fact. In contrast, the non-pharmacist store manager prefers to look at the situation in terms of square footage. The non-pharmacist store manager takes pride in the fact that he commands much more square footage than the pharmacists.

Pharmacists understandably don't want any more responsibility than we already have. Pharmacists don't have time to be in charge of the entire store. The solution that most pharmacists would like is for the non-pharmacy supervisors to tell the manager to keep out of the pharmacy's business. Many companies have a separate chain of command for the pharmacy but this doesn't prevent the non-pharmacy supervisors from getting involved in pharmacy affairs. In my ideal world, the non-pharmacy people would have absolutely no authority over the pharmacy and this fact would be made clear to all store employees.

The non-pharmacist store manager thinks we should be able to sling out prescriptions as quickly as McDonald's slings out burgers. I don't know any non-pharmacist store managers who seem to genuinely comprehend that each prescription we fill is a potential lawsuit—an event that can have devastating consequences for our customers and ourselves. Pharmacists view the non-pharmacist store manager's single-minded emphasis on speed as cavalier and ignorant of the realities of a litigious society.

As long as the non-pharmacist store manager views prescription drugs as a commodity similar to hamburgers, he will never truly understand pharmacists' concerns. Perhaps it is unrealistic to think that the non-pharmacist store manager would understand what worries pharmacists since our customers don't seem to understand either. The only thing that customers seem to care about is how long they will have to wait for their prescriptions to be filled and how much it will cost. Customers seem to have absolutely no idea how easy it is to make an error in the pharmacy. Many customers are even surprised (or shocked) to learn that drugstores do indeed make errors.

Even many pharmacy technicians don't seem to truly under-stand how high the stakes are in the pharmacy. Some techs ask the pharmacist to take a quick look at a prescription because a customer is in a hurry. These techs don't seem to understand that if it's OK to look at one prescription quickly, then it's OK to look at every prescription quickly.

An outside observer would probably think that all store employees routinely take up for each other in our daily battles with rude and arrogant customers. But, too often, the tension between pharmacists and non-pharmacist store managers leads to backstabbing incidents. I got into a dispute with a rude customer one day. The non-pharmacist store manager, who knew nothing about the situation, stepped in, taking the customer's side. The customer mailed a complaint card to corporate headquarters, at the manager's suggestion. When a customer complains to the non-pharmacist store manager about something in the pharmacy, the manager often seems to enjoy giving customers complaint cards that are mailed to corporate headquarters.

The non-pharmacist store manager has a leisurely lunch and dinner each day in his office and can't understand why pharmacists don't have time for the same. Nor does he understand why we don't have time to go to the bathroom or sit down for a break. Too often, he seems to be jealous of our wages. He acts as though he's the boss of our pharmacy technicians.

The non-pharmacist store manager takes every opportunity to criticize pharmacists (behind our back) and he tells his supervisors that he would have a good store if he had better pharmacists. The pharmacy is always the source of all the problems in the store in the eyes of the non-pharmacist store manager.

When a floater pharmacist fills in for us, the non-pharmacist store manager has only one assessment of the floater the next day: "He (or she) was too slow!!" The non-pharmacist store manager does not seem to understand that pharmacists are slower in unfamiliar pharmacies. The non-pharmacist store manager's favorite subject is the speed of pharmacists. He tells our supervisor we're slow. "Slow" becomes our middle name.

The company encourages the non-pharmacist store manager to help out in the pharmacy and allow other non-pharmacy employees to do likewise during extremely busy times. In the best stores, non-pharmacy staff help out in the pharmacy frequently. I agree with the non-pharmacist store manager that this puts an extra burden on him because he doesn't get enough staffing to complete his own work on the sales floor so allowing the non-pharmacy staff to help out in the pharmacy puts him even further behind. Understandably he resents it when the pharmacist wants to pull a clerk off the sales floor to help out in the pharmacy.

The professional model stressed in pharmacy school (a professional pharmacist with highly trained colleagues and co-workers) is at wide variance from daily reality in the drugstore. Personality conflicts simmer for months—until, by chance, the pharmacist or non-pharmacist store manager transfers to a different store. Too often, even with new pharmacists or non-pharmacist store managers, the patterns of tension and resentment soon re-emerge. I don't deny that the pharmacist is sometimes to blame. Some pharmacists are indeed very immature.

The hyperstressful working conditions bring out the worst in all of us. Best friends become bitter enemies. Employees blame each other for being too slow, for spending too much time talking to customers, for taking too much time filling each prescription. In the extreme stress of understaffed drugstores, employees blame each other rather than pull together as a team.

The following e-mail was forwarded to me in 2006. It is written by a former K-Mart pharmacist who describes a very unpleasant interaction with the non-pharmacist store manager at K-Mart.

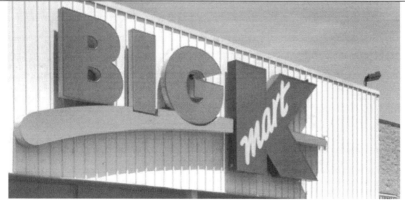

Here is how I handled my problem with the chains. It was unprofessional but it did make me feel better.

I used to work for K-Mart and life there was miserable. High volume, high pressure. I grew to hate it. I had a store manager who was a jerk. No other word for it. He was tough to work for. It was a chain pharmacy and I was chained to the counter.

Every day at noon, he (store manager) would pull my clerk to cover a register up front while one of the cashiers up there was on lunch hour break. My tech/clerk would come back at 1 PM only to go on her lunch. I had no lunch break. He would leave me all alone in the pharmacy putting extra pressure on me. One day I complained about the lack of help, the disservice to customers and the problems involved. He said "Get used to it."

My other pharmacist was on vacation so I was doing 12 hour days. One day, since it was a high volume store and it was busy, I told every customer during the morning that the computer was down and things would be all okay at 2 PM and that their Rx would be ready at 2 PM. I took in plenty of Rx's. I had them lined up and down the counter. I told customers who called in that their Rx's would be ready at 2 PM. During my two hour "lunch break" I did nothing. Absolutely nothing. I stopped, I ate, I had a cup of coffee, I read a magazine. I ignored the phone—all three lines. There were about 50 people waiting in the store.

At 1:55 PM I closed the pharmacy, locked the door, went to the main office and put the key in the wrong safe knowing it would be found only hours later. There were plenty of customers waiting for the 2 PM pick up. I told them the pharmacy was closed, their Rx's were not ready and to complain to the store manager about the lack of service. I waited while the customers lined up at the service desk and yelled at the store manager, and yell they did. Loud and clear. The customers were upset and vented complaints at the manager. I felt sorry for the customers but not the manager. He was under pressure and the customers threatened to call K-Mart (Troy, Michigan) headquarters. This would bring hell down on the manager.

I then told the store manager, "I quit." He got very upset and was visibly angry. Explosive would be more appropriate. He said, "What about all the unhappy, yelling customers waiting for their

Rx's?" I said "That is your problem. Get used to it." I left and never went back to work for any chain ever again.

Life is good! I work where I am appreciated, from owner above and customers below. **—[Pharmacist B. K.]**

Here are two e-mails I received from pharmacists as a result of my editorial in *Drug Topics* titled "Pharmacists versus non-R.Ph. store managers." (Sept. 15, 2003, pp. 18, 21)

Subj: Drug Topics Viewpoint article
Date: 9/23/03
From: [Pharmacist G. P.]
To: dmiller1952@aol.com

Dennis,

I truly enjoyed your article on pharmacists vs. store managers. I am one of the few lucky ones. I work for a supermarket chain, and my store manager does not interfere with pharmacy, but rather supports and assists me to the best of his ability. Yet I hear the horror stories from my colleagues. Your points are very true. Community pharmacy has quite a ways to go. We are trained professionals in health care, yet many times we are simply viewed as another department, pill pushers, and treated with little respect. I recently had a customer call corporate because I asked him to wait 15 minutes and he insisted that I was "touching the pills". Just to retaliate.

I graduated from pharmacy school in 1999 at age 46 (my second career) and enjoy my job immensely. Yet my biggest gripe is how patients view us versus their physicians. On a day-to-day basis, I receive incorrect prescriptions from doctors, e.g. Levaquin 500 qid [four times a day] rather than qd [daily]; a refill with a higher strength than the one patient was originally on; Augmentin for children with a PCN [penicillin] allergy; Zocor 20 mg tid [three times a day]. The list goes on and on. Yet the patients are quick to "forgive," if you will, their physicians for the mistakes. Yet, they become furious when we make a mistake in filling; no mercy; it is as if they hold us to a higher standard, or yet, they forgive their physicians because they are "so busy." Well, so are we. They will wait 2 hours for the physician but expect us to fill their script in 10 minutes!!!

I work in community pharmacy by choice. I enjoy the interaction and 90% of my customers are appreciative and understanding. Yet that 10% have no respect for our profession and they would never speak to their physician the way they speak to us.

Getting back to your topic, one of my pet peeves is when a customer wants to register a complaint with the "store manager." I quickly approach them and explain that I am the pharmacy manager, but no, they want to speak to the store manager (who obviously has no concept as to what we do).

I feel that we as pharmacists must work diligently to promote our profession as one that is to be respected; in fact, we should be treated in the same category as physicians. Sometimes when I am counseling a patient, I will be interrupted by a patient who asks me to hurry up their script. It is downright insulting. Being of Hispanic descent, I marvel at the way Hispanics respect their pharmacists—a different respect, just like those from European culture.

Good luck to you.

[Pharmacist G. P.]

Subj: Pharmacist vs. non-R.Ph. store manager (Feedback)
Date: 10/9/03
From: [Pharmacist Z. M.]
To: dmiller1952@aol.com

Hello Mr. Miller,

I enjoyed reading your article in *Drug Topics* in the September 15th 2003 issue and it was like you were reading my mind. I don't know of any other health professional who is treated in the same manner that pharmacists are treated. It's like they think that we are machines and not human beings. We are not allowed to get sick, have family emergencies, take vacations, or leave the pharmacy on time. The same managers who want you to hurry up and fill prescriptions are the same individuals who want to leave at posted store hours although we have a backlog of customers waiting on their prescriptions and they would not approve the necessary help to service these customers. And, of course, they were supposed to help out in the pharmacy but they hate coming to the pharmacy to help out so they hide or wait thirty minutes to show up.

I feel the major problem that we have in our profession is that we don't have strong lobbying associations. Everyone looks at us as well-paid servants and part of the problem is that we don't speak up enough. Our profession needs more unity. The boards of pharmacy in each state only look out for the best interests of the consumers and they are a watch dog for them. But, as for us, we have no such organization. I really don't know how we are able to do our jobs as well as we do with store managers and the state boards breathing down our backs. We need to form a reliable organization that is going to look out for us. I don't know how much more our profession can handle with the managed care companies forcing their clients to utilize mail order and the poor reimbursement which insurance companies give us. It makes you wonder what I was thinking when I chose this as a profession. And pharmacy school does not even give you a clue of what to expect in the real world. All they tell you is that you are a professional and you must conduct yourself accordingly. But they never tell you that you will be the only person who understands that you are a professional. This is why we don't understand how someone who may not even have finished high school—let alone completed one year of college—can be our supervisor.

We need a change. I don't know how or when it's going to happen but if something doesn't happen soon, the baby boomers won't have anyone to fill their meds. I can't tell you how many pharmacists I know of trying to pursue a new career because they are so burned out and broken-hearted by the current plight of our profession.

Sincerely yours,

[Pharmacist Z. M.]

PART VI

DISTRICT SUPERVISORS

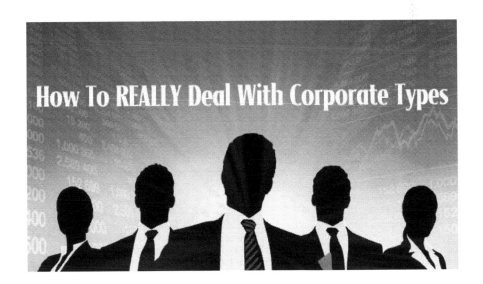

33

District supervisors drink the corporate Kool Aid

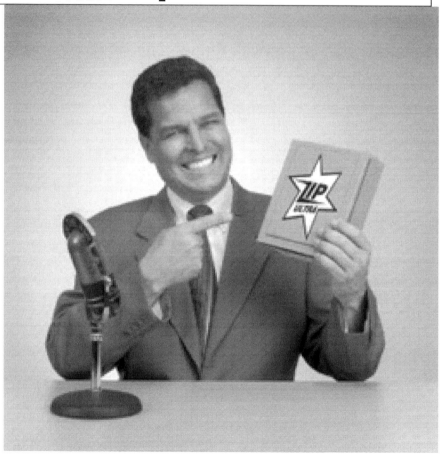

District pharmacy supervisors are usually pharmacists who are in charge of somewhere around 10 to 20 pharmacies and 20 to 40 pharmacists, assuming an average of two pharmacists per pharmacy. District supervisors don't usually fill prescriptions themselves except in cases of a severe shortage of pharmacists. They

usually travel between stores in carrying out their management duties, which include hiring pharmacists. Pharmacists might see their
district supervisor once every two or three weeks. The district supervisor might stay in the store for an average of an hour or two
with each visit. I've had more than a dozen district supervisors in
my career.

Some of my district supervisors stress that no food is allowed in
the refrigerator. Apparently, food in the refrigerator is unprofessional, causes a cluttered appearance, and poses a problem of cross-
contamination with the drugs. (A moldy sandwich might contami-
nate the drugs in the refrigerator.) The prohibition against food in
the refrigerator has always struck me as heartless. Would the supervisor be so cavalier if his own lunch or dinner were prohibited
from being kept in the refrigerator? Food is one of the last pleasur-
able things at work for a pharmacist who's absolutely exhausted. If
there were another refrigerator in the store (like in the break
room), I wouldn't have a problem with the prohibition against food
in the pharmacy refrigerator. As regards the possibility of moldy
sandwiches contaminating drugs, the supervisors should simply
stress that we need to be extra careful to make sure that the refrigerator is routinely checked for old food. Eating is a requirement for
Homo sapiens. Somehow, many supervisors seem to view food as a
luxury, not a necessity.

Some chains require pharmacists to wear a tie. I have always
found a tie (and tight collar) to be uncomfortable, but many district
supervisors get agitated when pharmacists don't wear ties. Is this
gender discrimination against men? I am not aware of any dress
code for female pharmacists.

One day my district supervisor told me, "You think too much
about what you're doing." I was shocked by his comment because I
felt I did a pretty good job of hiding my personal feelings about my
job. Perhaps my body language revealed more about me than I assumed. Certainly my boss had no understanding of my profound
disillusionment with a health care system based on pills rather than
on prevention. Nevertheless, I extrapolated his comment to its
logical conclusion: I need to work my shift each day on automatic
pilot rather than ruminate endlessly about the absurdity of it all.

One of my district supervisors was always disappointed to see that we were sitting on a stool when he visited our store—even for a short break. He actually made a big speech one day (on voice mail) about stools. He said that they should be kept off to the side somewhere and used at a minimum. We are forbidden to use stools when entering data into the computer because this creates the impression that we are lazy. Incredibly, the district supervisor hinted that stools would be banned from the pharmacy if he found them to be used excessively.

In pharmacy school, there is no dress code, class attendance is optional, and the professors let students be individuals. Chain pharmacy is nearly the opposite. Pharmacists must wear the company smock and name tag. When I graduated, tennis shoes were prohibited. This rule seems to have been relaxed, possibly because management finally (amazingly!) realized that pharmacists are more productive when they wear comfortable shoes.

District supervisors are adamant that we do everything to avoid confrontations with customers. What this means is that we cannot say even one word to incredibly rude and arrogant customers. We are required to swallow any personal attacks against us without any anger. For example, one of my district supervisors put out a voice mail: "Swallow your pride. Swallow your gum. But don't have a confrontation with the customer!" In my experience, when a pharmacist gets into an argument with a customer, and his or her supervisor finds out about it, chances are the supervisor will support the customer's side. That's because supervisors want to end the argument at the store level rather than have the angry customer contact people higher up the corporate ladder. Pharmacists shouldn't be surprised if their supervisor appears to inexplicably support the customer's side, even when that customer richly deserves to be forcibly removed from the store.

One day I overheard my district supervisor's phone conversation with another pharmacist. Apparently the pharmacist on the other end of the phone had gotten into a big argument with a customer. My district supervisor told the pharmacist on the phone, "Don't argue with him. Take his money." The implication was: *You can't get the customer's respect so get his money!* Presumably, making a sale and making someone poorer by the cost of his prescription should be satisfaction enough.

I once had a supervisor who directed all pharmacists, techs, and clerks in his district to answer the phone "Thank you for calling Revco. This is (employee's name). How can I help you?" During one period when this supervisor was tightly enforcing this policy, he listened closely to see how employees answered the phone when he called. The net result was that store employees became afraid to answer the phone, afraid that it was him calling. So all customers who phoned the store experienced long wait times before any employee in the store found the courage to answer the phone.

A prominent characteristic of chain pharmacy is the rigid hierarchy that closely resembles military hierarchy. I once had a district supervisor mention to me that one of the pharmacists in his district was guilty of "insubordination" for going over the supervisor's head and speaking directly with the division manager. The chain hierarchy usually consists of (starting from the bottom): staff pharmacist, chief pharmacist, district supervisor, division manager, regional vice-president, president.

Many pharmacists fear visits by their district supervisor, feeling that he comes to criticize us, not to help us. One of my former partners decided to make a career change by getting a Ph. D. in public health. I ran into her one day and asked her why she decided to leave pharmacy. She said, "The district supervisors would only tell you when you did something wrong. They would never tell you when you did something well."

We fear our bosses because they have the power to fire us if we don't fill prescriptions fast enough. The blood pressure of pharmacists often goes up when our supervisor visits our store. Our bosses' main concern is whether prescription volume (number of prescriptions filled per week) is up compared to the same period the previous year.

District supervisors routinely speak disparagingly of pharmacists in their districts who are slow. In twenty-five years as a pharmacist, I can recall only one instance in which a pharmacist was terminated because of an excessive number of dispensing errors. I am not saying that completely reckless pharmacists are retained forever. In my experience, inadequate speed and rudeness toward customers are much more likely to give pharmacists a bad name with district supervisors than dispensing errors.

The most serious confrontation I have ever seen between another pharmacist and a district supervisor involved the pharmacist's supposed inadequate speed in filling prescriptions. I happened to be in the pharmacy as my shift had just ended. I was tying up some loose ends. Even though I ended my shift fully caught up, a lot of customers came in at the same time with new prescriptions and my partner was covered up with prescriptions when our district supervisor walked in. The district supervisor almost immediately began criticizing my partner for being so far behind. My partner was very agitated by our supervisor's single-minded focus on speed, given the fact that corporate policy set staffing levels ridiculously low.

Our district supervisors often speak about other pharmacists in the district. It is highly unusual for a supervisor to say something like "Bill is very knowledgeable about drugs." It is much more likely for a supervisor to say something like "Bob can really crank 'em out!" (i.e., fill prescriptions quickly). Supervisors praise fast pharmacists to let it be known that speed is a very important criterion in our job evaluation.

District supervisors say that more errors are made when things are slow than when we're very busy. We complain to our district supervisor that the overwhelming workload increases the opportunity for misfills. Our district supervisor recites his favorite self-serving mantra: "More errors occur when things are slow because you're not focused." I'd like to ask him, "Does that mean we should regularly exceed the speed limit on the highway because speeding causes us to be more focused on our driving?"

It may just be the district supervisors I know, but when they're forced to work in a pharmacy themselves because of a severe shortage of pharmacists, they seem to make an inordinate number of errors in filling prescriptions. District supervisors place a high value on speed and it shows when they fill prescriptions. They are correct in believing that they are nearly immune to criticism from the company for dispensing errors (after all, they *are* the company). But they are certainly not immune to a lawsuit filed by a customer.

In my experience, it is not the best pharmacy students who become district supervisors. In my experience, the district supervisor personality is more extroverted, outgoing, and more likely to have been a party animal in school than a serious student. In pharmacy school, the serious students did not respect the party animals, but in the real world, the party animals are now our bosses. In my experience, the party animal personality is less concerned with accuracy than the serious student personality. In pharmacy school, the party animals seemed to be in college mainly to have a good time.

How well do our district supervisors really know the pharmacists under their control? I've seen many pharmacists put on a good act when our district supervisor is present. As soon as the district supervisor leaves, that pharmacist resumes his or her rudeness toward customers and techs. Sometimes the supervisors gradually learn what the pharmacist is really like. But I've seen many instances in which supervisors never figure out what the pharmacist's true personality is and how that pharmacist is, in reality, very bad for business.

I once worked with a pharmacist who was extremely professional and quite knowledgeable about drugs. She was very thorough and precise with paperwork. She took great care in learning the proper procedures for submitting claims to various insurance companies. Pharmacists would often call her for advice in solving some paperwork question or some quirk in insurance procedures. Yet this pharmacist had a very negative attitude toward customers. When the large chain we were working for bought a small local chain, my district supervisor asked her to transfer for a few weeks to one very high volume store that was just purchased. My district supervisor viewed her as one of his best pharmacists and he felt she would be of great assistance in transitioning that high volume store since this pharmacist was an expert in the policy and procedures for our chain. One day I visited her at that pharmacy. I asked her how things were going. I was not surprised when she said that the prescription volume was overwhelming. She commented to me that things would improve "when we get the volume down to a manageable level." In other words, she was saying that that store *has too many customers!* This statement would have been viewed as absolute blasphemy in the eyes of our district supervisor. My supervisor had no idea that that pharmacist's solution for the overwhelming workload in that pharmacy was to *shed customers.* Chain supervisors have one overarching obsession, i.e., that Rx volume grows, not shrinks.

I once had a district supervisor (in charge of, say, fifteen stores) tell me about an incident in which a local pharmacist had gone over the head of this district supervisor and complained about something to the division manager (in charge of, say, a hundred stores). My district supervisor was very unhappy with this pharmacist and referred to it as "insubordination." In pharmacy school, I never thought I'd hear the term "insubordination" coming from one of my bosses in the world of community pharmacy. If I were a pharmacist in the military, I could understand it. As a chain pharmacist, it was surprising.

The hierarchy in chain drugstores is, indeed, as rigid as that in the military. It looks something like this: staff pharmacist, pharmacist-in-charge (PIC), district supervisor, division manager, regional vice president, director of operations, and president. With thousands of stores, the big chains have a clearly defined chain of command. My district supervisor didn't look kindly on the pharmacist who did not seem to understand the power hierarchy.

Store level employees often referred to these people above the store level as "the suits." That's because they visited us in the stores wearing a suit or sports jacket, in contrast to store employees who wore smocks or pharmacy jackets. The suits enjoyed displaying their power over store-level employees by constant use of the telephone when visiting stores under their command. This was meant to show store level employees that "the suits" were important people.

The number of stores under the command of the various bosses was not set in stone. I think I recall my district supervisor having as few as a dozen stores, and as many as two dozen when he had to take temporary control over the adjacent district when that supervisor was transferred or quit. During this period when my district supervisor had two dozen stores, he mentioned to me that all he had time to do was "go around and put out fires." In other words he didn't have time to work with individual managers in any significant way. All he had time to do was things like intervene in a store in which the pharmacist-in-charge and the non-pharmacist store manager were close to killing each other (not a rare situation by the way).

A pharmacist once told me a story about a division manager (in charge of perhaps one hundred stores) or regional vice president (in charge of perhaps five hundred stores) who visited one of the local stores and awarded a pharmacist, on the spot, somewhere around three thousand dollars for suggesting something that almost anyone could have suggested. Have you ever been in a grocery store and noticed those little advertisements that are about the size of a license plate attached to your shopping cart with a little plastic frame that is similar in shape to a license plate frame? This incident occurred a couple of decades ago and apparently this "suit" had not been in too many grocery stores. It is true that the use of such advertisements on shopping carts was not yet commonplace, but it was not rare. So this suit, in what I would describe as a display of power, awarded this pharmacist around three thousand dollars for suggesting that our drugstore chain begin using similar advertising attached to all of our shopping carts. I don't recall discussing this incident with anyone besides the pharmacist with whom I worked at that time. Both he and I agreed that the cash award seemed excessive, bordering on reckless. But that's the way power often shows itself.

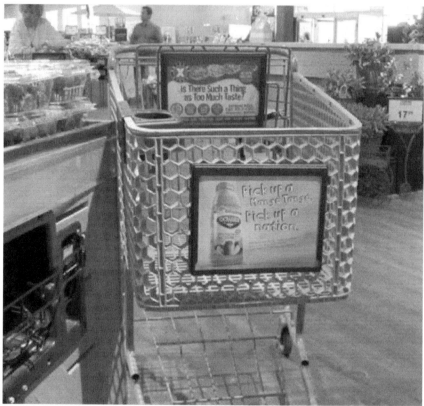

One of the "suits" from corporate paid a pharmacist a hefty sum for pointing out what was then relatively new—the placement of advertisements on store shopping carts. Most people I spoke with had already seen advertisements placed on shopping carts. Apparently this corporate "suit" didn't shop at large grocery chains very often.

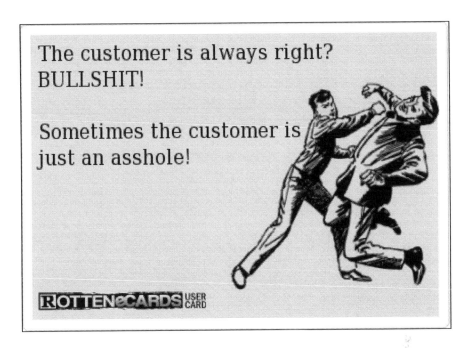

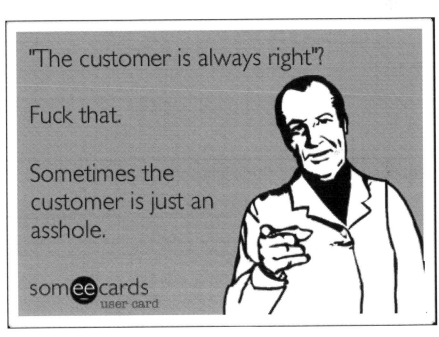

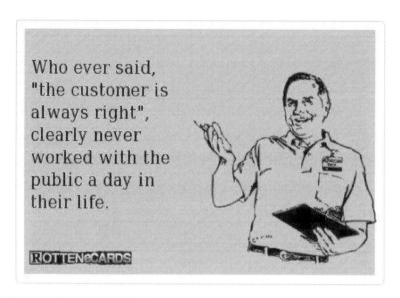

Who ever said, "the customer is always right", clearly never worked with the public a day in their life.

ROTTENECARDS

PART VI

PHARMACY CUSTOMERS

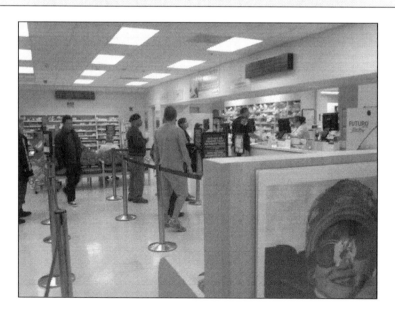

34

How customers really irritate pharmacists

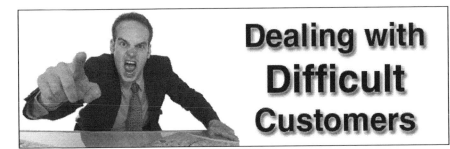

My pet peeves with pharmacy customers

1. Most customers don't seem to realize that pharmacists can and do make mistakes. Some customers are so confident in their pharmacist's abilities that they don't even question when the color or shape of their pills suddenly looks completely different. These customers have been led to believe that a change in the appearance of the pills always means they received a generic. A change in the appearance of your pills most often means that the pharmacist gave you a generic. But sometimes a change in appearance means the pharmacist has made a mistake. There are some customers who have very little trust in pharmacists. These customers immediately go home and count their pills to verify that we gave them the correct quantity. Not a bad idea.

2. Most customers evaluate pharmacists based solely on how fast we fill prescriptions. Customers do not realize that some pharmacists are much more thorough in calling doctors about illegible handwriting, questionable doses, and drug interactions. Customers do not realize that some pharmacists make many more

errors than others. Customers do not realize that "speed" is not the most important criterion in judging a pharmacist.

3. Many customers think that clearing their throat or clanking their keys on the counter or staring at us will cause us to fill their prescriptions faster. They ask "Why does it take more than a few minutes to put a few pills in a bottle?" or "Why does it take so long to fill my birth control pills? The pills are already in the pack." or "Why does it take so long to fill a prescription for a skin cream? The cream is already in the tube." Customers do not realize that, even though there may be only one or two other people nearby, we have a backlog of maybe fifty prescriptions, including those for customers shopping elsewhere in the store. Customers seem to think that the pharmacist should be able to fill prescriptions as quickly as McDonald's fills burger orders. They have no idea that rushing their pharmacist increases the likelihood of an error.

4. Many customers expect vitamins to cure any and every problem. Customers ask us to recommend a vitamin for "nerves" or "lack of energy." Customers seem to interpret their anxiety, depression or angst as a sign that their nerves are "acting up." Customers don't seem to realize that vitamins are not the best way to address "lack of energy." Customers don't seem to be interested in advice that they should consider getting more sleep at night, eating more nutritious foods, or finding a job that isn't so exhausting, etc.

5. Many customers, when trying to decide which non-prescription drug is right for them, pick up a half-dozen products from our shelves (like Dimetapp, Coricidin, Contac, Sudafed, etc.). But these customers are absolutely unable to replace the products in the proper spot on the shelf. These customers seem to think that products for colds, coughs, sore throat, heartburn, constipation, diarrhea, gas, fever, etc. are randomly arranged on drugstore shelves. These customers do not realize how much time is consumed by store clerks in returning products to their precise location.

6. Many customers phone in the wrong prescription number and arrive at the pharmacy wondering why their prescription is not ready. I once had a customer who phoned in a prescription for his wife. When he arrived at the pharmacy and picked up the Rx, he told me that I had given him the wrong pills. It turns out that he

had mistakenly picked up the wrong bottle. He thus gave me the wrong Rx number on the phone. He did not recognize the pills I filled as one of the other medications his wife was taking. He made a big scene out of it, speaking loudly enough for several other customers to hear. He kept saying, "That's all right. Pharmacists make mistakes. Pharmacists are human." He seemed to take pleasure in accusing me of making an error, as in *Pharmacists think they're so important. I'll take him down a few notches.* I was never able to convince him that he had simply phoned in the Rx number for another of his wife's medications. I filled the Rx for the drug he meant to call in. Several other customers were looking at me the entire time, wondering whether they could trust me to fill their prescriptions. Yes, I've made mistakes in my career but this was not one of them.

7. Many customers get really mad at the pharmacist when we tell them that their insurance plan does not cover the drug their doctor has prescribed. The customers often seem to think that the pharmacist is intentionally trying to make life difficult. I once witnessed another pharmacist engaged in a heated exchange with a customer over the customer's obvious disbelief that the drug was not covered. Finally, the pharmacist used an explanation which I have since adopted myself: *This is between you and your insurance company!* This explanation is, in effect, saying, "Look buddy. I don't want to get in a big fight with you. You need to contact your insurance company." I have yet to see a customer who had an answer for that.

8. Many customers have been thoroughly conditioned by Madison Avenue to want a pill for every ill. They seem to think that, for each medical condition, surely there must be a safe and effective drug. I wish customers would, instead, seek an understanding of their body and ask themselves what steps they might take to prevent diseases before they occur.

9. A few customers describe their symptoms (e.g., jock itch) to the pharmacist and then ask the pharmacist for a recommendation for a non-prescription product. Shortly thereafter, the customer leaves the store without purchasing that product (e.g., Lotrimin), or

any other product, but the customer returns later and steals that product.

10. Many customers treat us like we're a clerk at McDonald's. I suspect that pharmacy drive-thru windows imply to customers that prescription drugs are similar to hamburgers. So pharmacists shouldn't be surprised when pharmacy customers behave the same as McDonald's customers.

11. Many customers seem to interpret their doctor's illegible handwriting as a sign of intellectual brilliance. Their reaction is "Wow! My doctor is so brilliant that even the pharmacist can't read his handwriting!" Customers should be offended that their doctor doesn't make the effort to write clearly so that there is no chance the pharmacist will misread the Rx.

12. Many customers get mad when we tell them there are no re-fills remaining on their prescriptions. The customers yell, "No!! My doctor said I could have unlimited refills!!" The customers do not understand that state law requires the pharmacist to check with the doctor after a certain period of time, depending on the type of medication.

13. Many customers seem to think they're the first to mention that "child-proof" caps are actually "adult proof." They jokingly say, "I have to get the kids to take the lids off for me!" These customers laugh approvingly at their powers of perception, not knowing that we've heard that observation a thousand times.

14. Many customers ask me to recommend a laxative. I often ask myself: *I became a pharmacist so I could spend my time recom-mending laxatives?* Customers don't seem to be eager to learn that laxatives are usually unnecessary, that fiber can decrease constipa-tion, and that overuse of laxatives can cause the bowels to depend on these drugs.

15. Many customers don't seem to realize that if they would just lose some weight, they might not need so many pills for hyperten-sion or type 2 diabetes. Customers want to be able to eat all they desire and then swallow a diet pill that allows them to look great in a swimsuit.

16. Many customers blame the pharmacist when the customer's insurance co-pay increases. Customers should realize that the co-

pay is not determined by the pharmacist. The co-pay is transmitted to the pharmacist immediately upon the pharmacist billing the prescriptions on-line.

17. Many customers wait until the pharmacist has completed filling that customer's prescriptions before telling the pharmacist that they have insurance coverage. This necessitates the laborious task of running each prescription back through our computer.

18. Many customers seem to think that generic drugs have something to do with genes since they call them "genetic" drugs. Many customers are unconvinced of the equivalence of generic drugs. They say, "No! I want the real thing!"

19. Many customers inexplicably think they need to speak with the pharmacist even when phoning in Rx numbers for prescriptions that need to be refilled. Pharmacists prefer that customers give these numbers to a tech or clerk.

20. Many customers phone in several prescription numbers and then arrive at the drive-thru window ten minutes later and can't understand why the prescriptions aren't ready. They should have asked us on the phone (or we should have told them) how long it would take. Drive-thru windows certainly create the expectation of instantaneous service at pharmacies. Many pharmacists feel that the drive-thru window is the worst thing that ever happened in our profession and that it is symptomatic of everything that is wrong with our health care system today, i.e., speed is the top priority. Quantity is valued more highly than quality.

21. Pharmacy customers rarely know when they have been well served. Customers rarely understand the significance of a pharmacist who catches a potentially serious drug interaction or a dose that's too high or a contraindication. Customers only care about how quickly their prescriptions are filled.

22. Many customers hand us several prescriptions, wait until after we've filled those prescriptions, and then inform us that they just want half the quantity the doctor specified on each prescription. Consequently we have to re-do each prescription.

23. Many customers are very interested in learning about their medications but are not interested in waiting in line while other customers ahead of them get that same type of information.

24. Many customers think that it is entirely reasonable to go their doctor for an antibiotic for the common cold. They do not understand that antibiotics are ineffective against viruses.

25. Many customers don't seem to be embarrassed easily. They routinely approach the pharmacy and ask what we recommend for gas—with several other customers hearing the conversation.

26. Many customers at the drive-thru window honk their horns, expecting prescriptions to be filled as quickly as McDonald's fills burger orders.

27. Many customers equate power with effectiveness. They frequently ask us "What's the strongest thing you have to knock out this cough?"

28. Many customers leave their doctor's office with a prescription but without a clear understanding of what the drug is used for.

29. Many customers discard our drug information leaflets without reading a single word.

Here is a rather common scenario. A customer phones the drugstore from home or comes into the drugstore and says that he needs to get his prescription(s) refilled right away because he's on his way to catch a plane and he forgot to have them refilled beforehand. Most pharmacists hate situations like this. We're running an hour or so behind and this customer expects us to put his prescriptions ahead of everyone else's. Other customers who have been waiting patiently in the store are equally turned off by these customers. I once saw a coffee mug in a pharmacy imprinted with a message pharmacists love: *Poor planning on your part does not necessarily constitute an emergency on my part.* In other words, just because you didn't remember to have your prescriptions refilled in a timely manner prior to your trip doesn't necessarily mean I'm going to drop everything to refill your prescriptions ahead of everyone else. Of course, our corporate bosses require that we keep messages like this out of sight of our customers. The corporate bosses don't like to see any negativity in the drugstore. Our bosses prefer the model of the pharmacist as affable automaton who absorbs an endless number of indignities without complaint.

Here's another common scenario: All four phone lines are for the sole pharmacist on duty. Customers are honking their horns at the drive thru-window. They're clanking their keys on the counter, clearing their throats, and asking how much longer it will be. ("Why does it take more than a couple of minutes to put a few pills in a bottle?") They're bombarding me with questions like the following (many of which should clearly be directed at the non-pharmacy personnel but the pharmacist and techs are more visible):

• What aisle is the motor oil on?
• Do you have any Coke or Pepsi products on sale this week?
• What are the possible side effects with the medication?
• What kind of dressing should I put on this cut?
• Where are your hearing aid batteries?
• Can you recommend a laxative for my three-year-old?
• What do you recommend for gas?
• What's good for lice?
• Where are your pregnancy tests? Which one is the most accurate?
• What do you recommend for poison ivy?
• What do you recommend for sunburn?
• What's the difference between all the products for yeast infection [Monistat, Femstat, Vagistat, GyneLotrimin, etc.]?
• Why hasn't my insurance company reimbursed me for the drugs I got two months ago?
• What do you think of DHEA (melatonin, zinc, chromium, etc.)?
• My doctor says I need to start taking calcium. Which brand do you recommend?
• Do you have any more diapers in the stockroom? You're out of the ones I usually buy.
• Why is my prescription so expensive?
• Why doesn't Medicaid cover my prescription?
• Can I use your phone to call a cab?
• Can you recommend a good multivitamin?
• I don't seem to have any energy. Can you recommend a vitamin for energy?
• What do you think of amino acid supplements for weight lifters?
• What's good for sleep?

• I'm in a hurry. Can you fill this prescription right away?
• Your Coke machine outside stole my money and didn't give me a drink. Who do I need to see?
• How come the generic is less than half the price of the real thing? Is it just as good?
• Can you leave those child-resistant safety caps off my prescriptions? I have to get the kids to take them off for me. [Customer laughs as if he is the first person to make this observation.]
• Is there anything cheaper over-the-counter that would be just as good as what my doctor prescribed?
• Can I just get half the prescription? I'll come back and get the rest on Friday when I get paid.
• Do you have a restroom I can use?
• My doctor was supposed to phone in my prescription. Is it ready?
• What's the best vitamin for a six-year-old who just won't eat?
• My doctor says I need to start taking iron. Which one do you recommend?

When customers describe their symptoms to me and ask me to recommend a non-prescription product, I have found that these customers don't usually like it when I give them an assortment of alternatives. Customers seem to think that each symptom has a precise solution, just like each math problem has a precise solution. Customers want a definitive answer like *two plus two equals four*. Customers interpret a variety of solutions as tantamount to my not really knowing what product is best for their symptoms. Customers like pharmacists who immediately and confidently recommend one specific product. Customers view this pharmacist as more intelligent than the pharmacist who provides a number of alternatives. Customers do not realize that many pharmacists are just "throwing a solution" at the customer so he or she will go away.

For example, a customer may ask, "What do you recommend for colds?" The pharmacist then answers quickly: "I recommend Sudafed. It's on aisle two." Many of these short-answer pharmacists view all customer questions as annoyances. Of course, some pharmacists hurriedly throw a drug name at customers because we are overwhelmed with a huge pile of prescriptions and we truly don't have time to give your question the time it deserves. For example, before recommending a product for colds, the pharmacist should ask whether you have any conditions that may make specific products unadvisable, such as high blood pressure or enlarged prostate.

Say a customer describes symptoms that sound like heartburn. There are a wide variety of ways this can be treated with non-prescription drugs. At the most basic level, the pharmacist could recommend the safest products, i.e., antacids like Tums, Rolaids, Maalox, or Mylanta. At the next level, the pharmacist might recommend stronger non-prescription products which may have more side effects, i.e., H2 antagonists like Tagamet HB, Pepcid AC, or Zantac 75. The next level above the H2 antagonists is the non-prescription proton pump inhibitors like Prilosec OTC, Prevacid 24HR, Zegerid OTC, and the house brand omeprazole. Proton pump inhibitors are the strongest of these three categories and carry the highest potential for side effects, including a distressing rebound hypersecretion of acid upon discontinuation of these drugs.

Alternatively, the pharmacist might describe ways in which heartburn can be prevented: by not overeating; by not lying down too soon after eating; by maintaining proper body weight; by raising the head of the bed six inches; by avoiding coffee, alcohol, fats, chocolate, and smoking; etc. A thorough pharmacist should also mention that the symptoms of heartburn can be mistaken for other conditions (e.g., angina).

In my experience, most pharmacy customers don't like such detailed answers. They want the pharmacist to confidently name one product only. I have had many instances in which I tried to give customers several alternatives only to have them reply forcefully and in a somewhat irritated tone: *SO WHAT DO I NEED!!??*

Normally, the best advice from pharmacists would be to give all the preventive measures a serious try. Only if all these preventive measures fail should the customer try a drug. But very few pharmacy customers want to give serious consideration to non-drug preventive measures. The fact that these customers are in the drugstore means they're leaning heavily toward a quick-fix solution. In my experience these customers will be disappointed in a pharmacist who does not have a similar outlook, i.e., a pill for every symptom.

Pharmacy customers make unusual requests

Here are a few brief anecdotes illustrating that pharmacy customers sometimes make unusual requests.

One day a customer approached the pharmacy with some produce he had just purchased at the supermarket next door. He said he suspected that the scales at the supermarket were inaccurate so he asked me to weigh the produce for him. He said he heard that pharmacy scales are very precise. I told him that our pharmacy scale could weigh—at most—a few ounces. There was no way I could weigh his produce which required a scale capable of measuring pounds.

On another day, a customer stood a few feet in front of the pharmacy counter and proceeded to take off the top of his electric shaver. He then blew really hard to clean the shaver. Tiny hair particles spread around the adjacent area. He then handed me the top of the shaver and asked me whether we carried the appropriate replacement blades/heads. How could he not realize how unsanitary it was to clean his electric shaver in the store by blowing?

One day a customer asked me if we had a laxative for one of his farm animals (a horse, I think). I didn't have the courage to ask him how he determined that this farm animal was constipated. I told him that I didn't know whether the laxatives we sold were safe for animals. I also told him that I didn't know what dose he would need to give to the animal.

One day a lady asked me whether the print on the tablets her doctor prescribed posed any harm. Did the ink used to print the drug name and identification number on the tablets pose any harm to her system when she swallowed the tablets? I assured her that the ink was harmless even though I had no direct knowledge to make that statement.

One day a man mentioned to me that he knew that Benadryl could cause drowsiness. He asked me what dose of Benadryl would be needed to put his mother's cat to sleep permanently. He told me that the cat was old and sick. I told him the truth: I had no idea what dose would be needed to kill the cat. I didn't tell him that I wondered whether what he planned to do was legal.

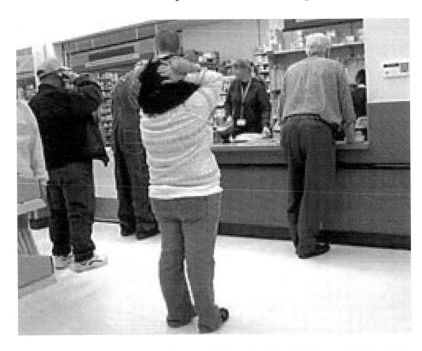

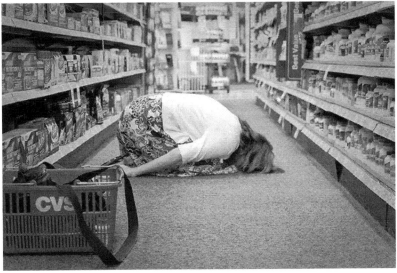

35

Did this customer intentionally contaminate a medication so he could sue us?

Here is an unusual story about an unusual pharmacy customer. I had just graduated from pharmacy school and I began work for a major chain in a small town in West Virginia. My boss told me that one of the pharmacy customers was in the process of suing the chain because a mold had grown in his pint bottle of potassium chloride liquid. Everyone seemed to know everyone else in this town. This customer had contacted a small law firm with only two attorneys. It turns out that both attorneys routinely came into our drugstore and routinely spoke with one of the pharmacy techs. My district supervisor brought me up to date on the lawsuit. He told me that the customer was going to bring me the bottle of potassium chloride liquid that contained the mold. I was to pack it carefully in a box and mail it to the manufacturer with a letter requesting that they inform us what foreign substance was in the bottle. A few weeks later, I received a letter from the manufacturer stating that, yes, there was mold in the bottle.

This was all very bizarre because no professor in pharmacy school had ever told us to watch out for the possibility that liquid medications from major manufacturers were prone to contamination with mold. Like I said, I had been out of pharmacy school for only a few months so I wasn't confident how I should handle the situation. Why had I never heard of mold growing in liquid medications? One day one of the two techs mentioned to me something like, "You know, Dennis, Mr. Smith is kinda strange. He's a retired chemist." So I began thinking: *What's really going on here?*

It turns out that the bottle that Mr. Smith had given me to send to the manufacturer was not the bottle in which we had originally dispensed the medication. I finally concluded that Mr. Smith had purposely succeeded in growing mold in that nearly empty bottle of liquid potassium chloride in an attempt to sue the drugstore chain. My district supervisor appeared to be accepting the customer's story at face value, not suspecting anything out of the ordinary. My district supervisor appeared to believe that the manufacturer had failed to adequately prevent mold growth in this product. So I told my district supervisor, "This whole thing is very strange. Mr. Smith apparently transferred the potassium chloride to a different bottle and, as a retired chemist, succeeded in growing mold in that bottle." I called one of the lawyers representing Mr. Smith and said something quite similar to what I had told my district supervisor. I said something like "Surely we're not responsible when a customer transfers a medication to a different container. He's a retired chemist and he appears to have undertaken a project of growing mold in this bottle in an effort to sue us." The lawyer listened carefully and, for some reason, the lawsuit against my employer did not proceed any further. I'm guessing that the lawyer had similar questions about the mental stability of Mr. Smith, but I don't know that for sure. Anyway, that lawyer and his partner continued to shop in that drugstore as did Mr. Smith. They all acted like nothing had happened.

I didn't hear anything more about Mr. Smith until a few months later when he returned the unused portion of a package of non-prescription sleeping pills and asked for a refund. I recall he said something like "It didn't work." Or "It didn't put me to sleep." He was conceivably telling the truth that the sleeping pill didn't put him to sleep. But most customers do not return products to the drugstore and ask for a refund, claiming that the product doesn't work (even though that is a potentially realistic scenario). What if every customer asked for refunds on non-prescription medications that didn't work for them (like products for colds, coughs, acne, warts, backache, etc.)? I can't recall whether we gave him a refund for the non-prescription sleeping pills. I assume we did if for no other reason than to keep him happy.

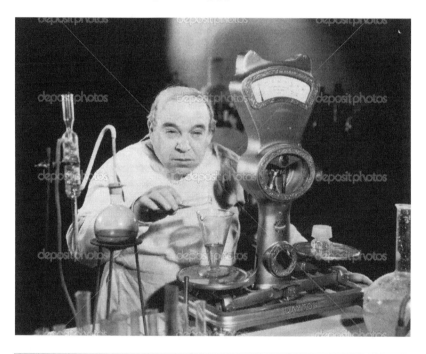

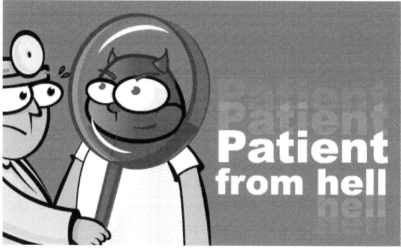

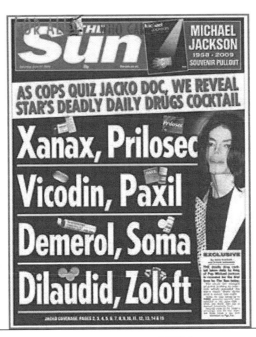

PART VIII

DRUG ABUSE, DRUG DEALING, THEFT, SHOPLIFTING, ROBBERIES

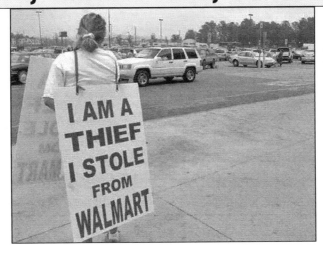

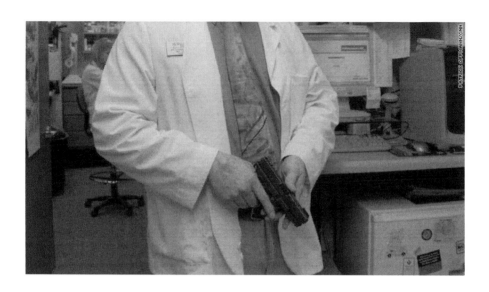

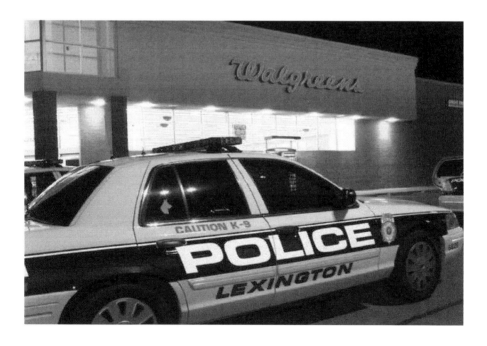

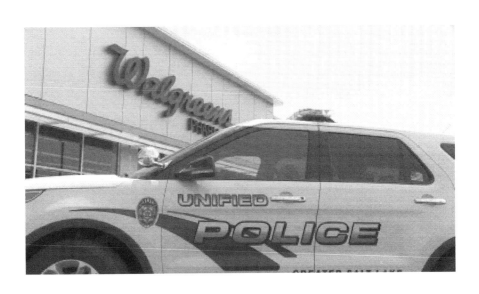

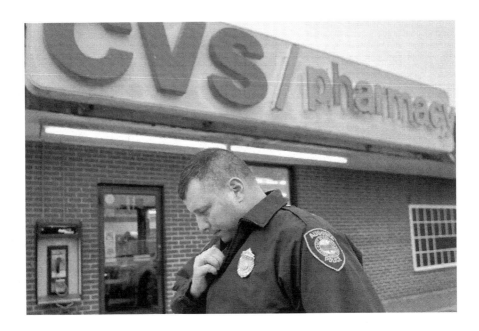

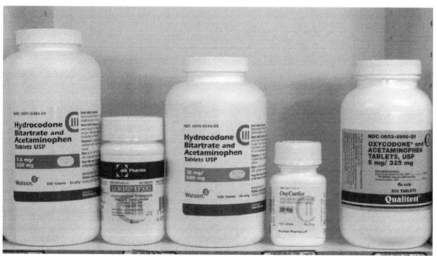

Drugstores are robbed frequently for these popular narcotics containing hydrocodone and oxycodone.

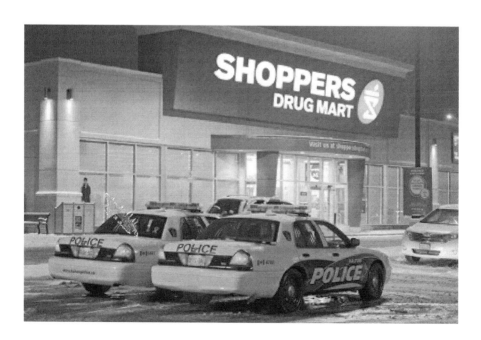

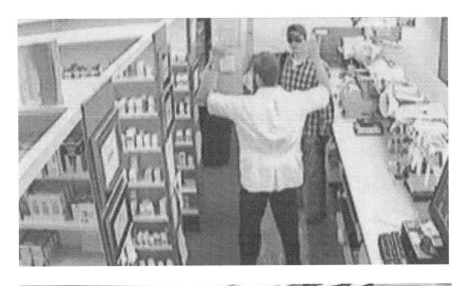

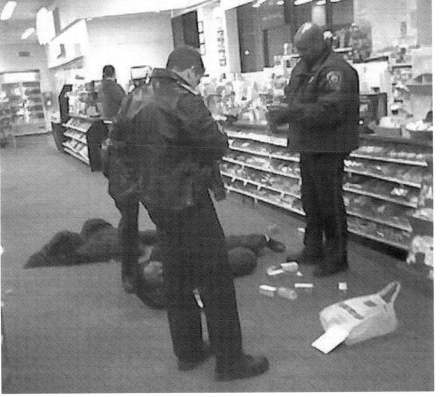

36
Dishonest pharmacists, technicians, and customers

During the first half of my career, pharmacists and technicians were required to take a polygraph (lie detector test). I took a polygraph twice in my career: before being hired by Rite Aid and before being hired by Revco. On both occasions the polygraph examiner asked many variations of "Have you ever stolen anything at work?" One examiner prefaced this by explaining that he was not concerned with, for example, employees discovering (at home) store ink pens in their shirt pockets or smocks.

The polygraph was, needless to say, a very demeaning experience. In the second half of my career, the polygraph was dropped for pharmacists but prospective technicians and clerks were required to take a written test to determine their honesty. I recall that we went through a period of a year or so when the majority of the clerks and techs who took the written test were deemed a risk and therefore not recommended for hire by the company that developed the test.

I vaguely recall that one question on the written test was something like this: "Since everyone steals little things like candy bars every now and then, do you admit that you've stolen inexpensive things like that from stores you've worked in?" This question was obviously loaded in suggesting that everyone steals. It turns out that, in fact, not everyone steals. If a prospective clerk or tech answered that question in the affirmative, he or she would not be recommended for hire by the developer of the test.

One day I did something that was against company policy. We needed a technician for the pharmacy and it so happens that one applicant for that position was previously a sales clerk at that store. I thought I knew her well enough to predict that she would make a good pharmacy tech. I coached her before taking the test by saying, "The written test considers stealing anything—regardless of its value—to be wrong and reason to recommend against hiring. It considers stealing one cent to be just as bad as stealing something worth a hundred dollars. Don't be trapped into admitting that everyone steals small things occasionally." It turns out that she passed the test but, unfortunately, she was a lazy technician. I never in my career mastered the ability to accurately predict—from a job interview—how an applicant would actually perform on the job. Some applicants who I felt would be great often turned out to be a disappointment. On the other hand, I've seen many applicants hired by other pharmacists and managers who turned out to be good employees, even though I would not have predicted that from my initial impression of those applicants.

During the first half of my career when pharmacists were required to take the polygraph, I knew many pharmacists who were adamantly opposed to it. Most said it treated pharmacists as common criminals. There's no doubt that it was a very demeaning experience that I dreaded but I will grudgingly agree that the chains need some way to weed out pharmacists and techs who abuse or steal drugs.

I don't know whether smoking marijuana leads to using "hard" drugs, but I do know that many of my pharmacy school classmates were frequent users of marijuana. I've often wondered whether some of them succumbed during their careers to the temptation of having so many drugs at their fingertips. Clearly drug abuse is a significant problem among pharmacists. State boards of pharmacy routinely discipline pharmacists after uncovering evidence that those pharmacists are drug abusers or drug dealers. The disciplinary actions are often publicized in board of pharmacy newsletters sent to pharmacists.

I filled in regularly at one store which had a pharmacist who I thought was a great guy, very friendly, easy-going. The store manager at that store gradually began to notice that the number of "overrings" on the pharmacy cash register was greater on days that pharmacist worked. I can't remember the details but I know that pharmacist was fired for bogus overrings. He apparently pocketed cash equivalent to the amount of each phony overring.

My district supervisor once hired a pharmacist who, according to the grapevine, was fired from her previous employer after she was found to be stealing Viagra and mailing it to her relatives in her home country. Polygraphs were not being administered when my district supervisor hired her.

Here's the problem, in my opinion: During the second half of my career, the big chains seemed to have a playbook that consisted entirely of burning out pharmacists and then claiming there was a shortage of pharmacists in America. As a consequence of such a high turnover in pharmacists, the big chains sometimes hire pharmacists who would not have been considered years ago. In the first half of my career, it was not unusual to find a pharmacist who had been with the same chain for ten years. Toward the second half of my career, a pharmacist who had been with the same chain for five years was considered a veteran.

Shoplifting is a tremendous problem in all types of stores across America, including drugstores. I was at a meeting of Revco pharmacists one day when a high-ranking Revco official stated that internal pilferage (i.e., by store employees) is greater than shoplifting by customers. I find that hard to believe but I assume he knew what he was talking about.

Another term for pilferage is "shrink." Chain drugstores bring in inventory crews maybe twice a year. After inventorying every item in the store and examining store sales, the store manager is presented with a "shrink" report. I recall that store managers were said to be doing an acceptable job when "shrink" was kept below three percent, i.e., when pilferage is kept below three percent of gross store sales. When pilferage was determined to be excessive, management would be instructed to take various preventive measures such as hiding security cameras behind lighting panels in the ceiling over cash registers (to see if any store employees were pocketing cash after bogus transactions).

I worked in only one drugstore that had a security guard. This was at the Revco in Heritage Square in Durham, North Carolina. Revco contracted with a security firm in Durham to supply our store with a security guard. That security guard worked 40 hours per week even though the store was open 80 hours per week. So, even at this store, there was no security guard present half the time the store was open. As best as I can recall, Revco decided to discontinue the practice of having a security guard in that store after this security guard was caught (by the store manager) stealing cartons of cigarettes. This store was in a high-crime area so the need for the security guard was obvious. There was a dollar store located directly adjacent to this Revco. The security guard at the dollar store would frequently come into our store on his breaks because he liked talking to our female clerks who ran the cash registers. I remember one day this security guard—during a break from the dollar store next door—actually caught someone in our store shoplifting a huge supply of deodorant products (a popular target for shoplifting, I later learned). I recall this guard from the dollar store next door telling me something like *Man, you need a security guard back in this store!* (after ours had been fired for stealing cigarettes). I agreed but unfortunately I was never in a position to approve the hiring of a security guard. Perhaps the reason for discontinuing the security guard contract in that store had something to do with the fact that Revco was apparently given a rent subsidy by some local or federal governmental entity in return for locating this store in a high-crime area. I had an occasion to speak with one of the management people at the security company that supplied us with the guard. This management person told me, "If it was up to me, I wouldn't put 'em in retail." His overtly racist statement implied that black security guards should be used only in situations like football games, basketball games, and concerts, as opposed to retail stores where there's lots of stuff to steal.

This store was very close to the interstate highway that runs through town. The back of the store is easily visible from that highway. One day I asked my district supervisor why all the stores—except ours—visible from the highway had a sign on the back door, making it easier for delivery trucks to determine which door belonged to which store. My boss told me that that was a conscious decision. He didn't want people driving down the interstate thinking, "Wow! Look how easy it would be to rob that pharmacy and then have an easy get-away on the interstate highway!"

I filled in at Revco in Hillsborough, North Carolina, for a pharmacist who was robbed at gunpoint by a person demanding drugs. That pharmacist was taken hostage for a few hours but somehow managed to escape. The incident caused the pharmacist to abandon retail pharmacy completely. After a week or two recovering from this traumatic event, he began a new career as a hospital pharmacist at Duke University Medical Center, safely away from anyone who might be intent on robbing a drugstore.

When I worked at one of the Rite Aid stores in West Virginia, the pharmacist who had worked in that particular store before me was licensed to carry a gun. Apparently he had been threatened by someone. My boss at that time told me that he (the boss) wasn't too happy that this pharmacist had a gun under his pharmacy smock every day at work. Due to confidentiality, I never found out the precise reason for that pharmacist leaving Rite Aid. I think it involved more than the gun.

When I worked at Revco in Oxford, North Carolina, one evening I happened to notice a man standing somewhat off to the side of the pharmacy looking closely at the prescription department shelves behind me. It is not unusual for customers to look at me or at our prescription department shelves while waiting for their prescriptions to be filled. But most of these customers seem to have a glazed look in their eyes, almost as if they were half-asleep and bored yet impatient while waiting for their prescriptions to be filled. This man was looking very closely at our prescription department shelves and I had an eerie feeling that something was wrong. Indeed, something was very wrong: The pharmacy was robbed late that night, long after all store employees had left. A big heavy rock was thrown through the exit door, shattering the glass. The store alarm indeed automatically notified the Oxford police, who arrived shortly. But the burglar (and, I assume, accomplices) had managed to get away after stealing a few bottles of controlled substances and our entire rotating Timex display which contained perhaps fifty watches. Apparently that suspicious-looking person from the night before was scanning our shelves in an attempt to locate the drugs he was interested in. I assume he knew that once the store alarm was set off, he needed to be out of that store in, say, less than a minute. My partner had been phoned in the middle of the night by the Oxford police. I was scheduled to work that morning. Upon arriving at the store shortly before opening time, I saw a big sheet of plywood covering the exit door. As the police investigated the burglary, my partner had placed that plywood over the exit door until morning when he phoned a glass company to repair the door. My partner told me he had been there ever since the police called him. My partner was checking our inventory to try to determine which drugs had been stolen. I did not tell my partner—or anyone else—about the incident that had occurred the night before, i.e., that I had observed a suspicious person looking intently at our prescription department shelves. I would have been blamed by my partner, by Revco district supervisors, and, I assume, by the Oxford police, for not taking more direct action by notifying the police of my suspicions. This incident occurred over fifteen years ago and I no longer work for Revco (now CVS), so I don't care if anyone knows now. The police told my partner that they had indeed arrived at the drugstore so soon after the alarm sounded at the police station that they (the police) were thinking the burglar or burglars were still in the store. They were not. After this incident, my district supervisor alerted all his stores to bolt the Timex display to the counter.

For a period of several months, I worked at a Revco in Durham at Wellons Village Shopping Center. We had several cashiers at that store who worked part-time while attending high school. One day, one of these young cashiers told me that she saw a young man steal a pair of sunglasses. The cashier implied to me that I needed to confront that young man before he left the store. Even though I was very busy in the pharmacy, I felt that I needed to approach that customer to show this cashier that the company took shoplifting seriously. I approached the customer but he protested to me that he had purchased the sunglasses elsewhere. Of course, I had no definitive proof that he was lying so I didn't pursue the matter. When he got home, he evidently told his parents what happened. I got a phone call from his father who proceeded to read me the riot act for accusing his son of shoplifting. From that incident, I learned to be more careful and selective in deciding when to believe a cashier who claims to see a customer stealing something.

Shoplifting at that store was especially bad. For a period of a few weeks or months, the store manager initiated a practice of locking all entrance and exit doors whenever she spotted a shoplifter in the act. She then phoned the police. By locking all the doors, the shoplifter could not leave the store. The store manager did this a few times but apparently she was told to discontinue locking the doors. Preventing the escape of shoplifters by locking doors endangers other customers trying get away from what could be a potentially dangerous situation, i.e., the shoplifter could pull a gun while being detained by the store manager.

One summer at this store I worked with a pharmacy student who had graduated pharmacy school but had not yet taken his licensing exam. One day this pharmacy "intern" lit out of the store in a flash, in pursuit of a shoplifter. It turns out that this intern was an athletic and somewhat macho kind of guy. He told me that he caught the shoplifter a short distance away from the store but decided against calling the police.

At this store we had a few part-time cashiers from North Carolina Central University, a predominantly black school. One day I received a call from one of these cashiers, named Vernon. Vernon was one of the nicest people I have ever known. He said that he wouldn't be able to come to work because he was being held at the Durham police station. He said that apparently his car was similar in appearance to one that Durham police believed was involved in a robbery. Vernon was exceedingly upset because he said he had been stopped by the police, with guns drawn, and told to lie on the ground. Vernon implied that, as a black man in a Southern town, he was at a terrible disadvantage. Vernon asked me whether I could help him some way. I was absolutely covered with a huge backlog of prescriptions, but I wanted desperately to leave the store to try to vouch for the character of Vernon, who I genuinely felt was the last person in the world who would be involved in a robbery.

As much as I wanted to go to the police station, I felt my district supervisor would not see things as I did. Therefore, I decided to ask this same pharmacy intern to go to the police station. It turns out that somehow the police determined that Vernon was innocent so he was released just as our pharmacy intern arrived at the police station. Vernon told me that the experience of having guns pointed at him while he was on the ground was something he felt he would never forget. Vernon asked me whether I had any suggestions for what he could do to show his displeasure with the way he was handled by the police. Even though I do not doubt that the police did indeed think Vernon was potentially involved, I understood how upset he was. This incident left me with perhaps a modest insight into what can happen to a black college student, away from home, in a Southern town. I told Vernon, "North Carolina Central has a law school. Maybe you could go there and ask them if there is anything you could do." As best as I can recall, Vernon did speak with someone at the law school and I think he was told that there wasn't much he could do since the police did apparently genuinely think Vernon was a suspect. But I think Vernon was somewhat relieved to be able to discuss the incident with someone at the law school.

One afternoon when I was working at the Revco in Oxford, North Carolina, one of the (middle-aged) cashiers told me that she personally witnessed a customer putting a bag of candy in her handbag. This cashier implied that I was a wimp if I didn't confront the customer. So, even though I was busy with a pile of prescriptions in the pharmacy, I reluctantly approached the customer and asked her to open her handbag. The customer refused. There was a young girl with this customer, presumably her daughter. I would guess the young girl was around six years old. The woman handed the handbag to the young girl and told her to run home. Of course, this was an unacceptable turn of events because if I were to call the police, I would have absolutely no evidence. So I tried to grab the handbag from the woman and the young girl but I decided, *What the hell, this isn't worth it!* The child looked like she was ready to start crying and I feared that she would run out of the store and be hit by a car while running home and I would be held liable. So I let the customer leave with the young girl but I told her never to come in the store again. I remember worrying whether there were specific laws detailing the circumstances under which management is permitted to hold a customer in the store. I was afraid I was potentially in legal jeopardy for not following some guideline. Of course, Revco wanted store employees to do what we could to cut down on customer shoplifting, but I don't recall Revco ever giving us instructions on the specific circumstances that allowed us to detain shoplifters until the police arrived. On the one hand, I was worried about a lawsuit if I overlooked some technicality. On the other hand, I was thinking, "This is the South. They don't coddle criminals in this town." I never saw that woman in the store again but I did run into her one day at the post office. Upon seeing her in the post office, I recall thinking what an absurd world this is. The previous encounter was hyperstressful in the drugstore whereas the current encounter consisted of brief eye contact while standing in line waiting to mail a package.

Here's a short anecdote about the clerk who notified me that she saw this customer steal the bag of candy. As I said, this clerk implied to me that I was a wimp if I did not confront the customer. On another occasion a few months later, the tables were turned on this clerk. One day a policeman pulled up to our store with a suspect he had just apprehended. When this suspect was apprehended, he (the suspect) had in his possession a product that had a Revco price sticker on it. (This was before bar code scanners made price stickers unnecessary.) The policeman told me that the suspect claimed he had just purchased the product at our store. The policeman suspected that the product had been shoplifted. The policeman asked me if it would be okay to ask the sole clerk on the cash register whether she recalled ringing up a sale for that man. I said that was fine so the policeman asked that clerk if she would agree to look at the man in the back of the patrol car to see whether she recalled seeing him and ringing up the product. This same clerk had, a few months earlier, implied that I was a wimp if I did not confront the customer she claimed to have seen stealing a bag of candy. This was now an opportunity for this clerk to make a stand against shoplifting. But the clerk told the policeman, "No. I don't want to get involved." So the policeman drove away, unable to verify whether the suspect had indeed stolen the product from our store. I'm sure this clerk had forgotten the event several months earlier when she implied I was a wimp if I did not confront another shoplifter. I do not blame this clerk for refusing to help the policeman make a case against the suspect. This clerk probably feared retribution from the suspect. I'm only pointing out this clerk's hypocrisy.

I worked for Rite Aid in Hurricane, West Virginia for part of 1976 and 1977. One day the non-pharmacist store manager got a call from the Hurricane police department. An informant apparently had tipped them off that a burglar was planning to enter our store overnight via the roof air shaft, apparently to steal drugs from the pharmacy. The police told the non-pharmacist store manager that a few undercover policemen wearing plain clothes would enter the store intermittently throughout the evening in a very non-conspicuous manner, in case our store was being watched by the burglar. Sure enough, throughout the evening, a total of three or four people wearing unremarkable clothes entered the store and proceeded to the stockroom. Apparently the police had determined that the burglar's entry via the roof air shaft meant that the burglar would most likely set foot in the store first in the stockroom. Since the only restrooms in the store were in the stockroom, store employees (including myself) who went to the restrooms that evening witnessed the police preparations as they built barricades in the stockroom in anticipation of the overnight break-in. Interestingly, the barricades consisted entirely of big boxes of merchandise from our stockroom shelves. And even more interestingly, the biggest boxes contained baby diapers. I wondered how the police expected boxes containing baby diapers to stop bullets fired by the burglar. Later I concluded the boxes were mainly for hiding, not to stop bullets. Store employees viewed the entire situation as quite exciting and entertaining. There was almost a party atmosphere among store employees since excitement such as this is rare for a drugstore. Company regulations do not allow non-employees (including police) in the store without a store employee present (usually a manager, assistant manager, or pharmacist). Since he had to be present with the police in the store, the non-pharmacist store manager went home to get a portable television. He planned to watch television overnight in his office to avoid boredom. (I assume the Hurricane police were told by this manager that he would have to stay in the store, and apparently the police agreed.) If the burglar had been walking around in the store in an effort to determine whether everything looked okay for break-in overnight, surely the burglar would have sensed the party atmosphere among store employees and surely he would have sensed that something unusual was going on. Having three or four policemen with rifles in our stockroom was very exciting for store employees. Unfortunately, the store manager did not have the presence of mind to tell all the store employees to act as if nothing unusual was happening. Indeed, the store manager himself seemed to be caught up in the excitement. I am somewhat surprised that the police did not realize that the behavior of store employees risked making the burglar suspicious, if he happened to be walking around in the store as if he were a regular customer. At some time past the 9 PM store closing, only the store manager and the plain-clothed policemen remained in the store. The next day, all the store employees—including myself—were eager to hear what happened overnight. When I arrived at work the next morning, I was informed that, after several hours spent in the stockroom, the police decided to leave the store, apparently concluding for some reason that no break-in was likely that night.

Many customers tell the pharmacist that they deserve an early refill on their Vicodin or other similar pain pill containing the narcotic hydrocodone. These customers sometimes claim they were standing by their medicine cabinet and "accidentally dropped the pills in the toilet." Customers who are hooked on pain pills think up an endless number of clever stories in an attempt to convince the pharmacist to refill their narcotic pain pills earlier than would be expected from the doctor's directions. Say a doctor prescribes a twenty-day supply of narcotic pain pills and indicates that the prescription can be refilled once if needed. When the customer comes back to the pharmacy after, say, ten days, and requests a refill, our computer flags this as early and therefore suspicious. Pharmacists are not supposed to agree to early refills if we suspect that the customer is abusing the drug by taking it far more often than the doctor's directions indicate.

I suspect that nearly every pharmacy in America is plagued by customers making up ingenious stories to justify early refills on narcotic pain pills and anti-anxiety pills like Xanax and Ativan. Pharmacists talk among ourselves about this problem all the time. You would probably be surprised by the number of pharmacy customers in this country who are either hooked on prescription drugs or are headed in that direction. Many pharmacists privately refer to these customers as "druggies," a moniker that reflects the endless stories that our customers invent in an attempt to snow the pharmacist into allowing early refills.

Another headache for pharmacists is forged prescriptions. Maybe once or twice a year, I receive what is clearly a forgery. I suspect this occurs so often because doctors sometimes leave their prescription pads in an exam room and then the patient (a drug abuser or dealer) steals the prescription pad and begins forging prescriptions on that doctor's prescription pad. Pharmacists can usually recognize the handwriting of local doctors. Consequently, when we receive a prescription with unfamiliar handwriting or with something else that looks suspicious like...

• an unusually large quantity of narcotic pain pills
• an unusually large number of refills
• refills on Schedule II drugs which—by law—can't be refilled

...we usually phone the office of the doctor who wrote the prescription. The doctor either confirms our suspicion that we have a forged prescription in our hand, or, occasionally, the doctor says we are mistaken and it is indeed a legitimate prescription.

Some pharmacists alert the police when we receive a forged prescription. Other pharmacists don't want to get involved. Some pharmacists feel that it is not our job to be policemen, so these pharmacists just hand the prescription back to the customer and say "We don't stock this drug." I've seen a few macho male pharmacists hand the prescription back and make some comment like "You ought to be glad I'm not calling the police." The customer/abuser/dealer then high-tails it out of the drugstore.

I once received a call from someone who said he was a detective on the local police force. He sounded quite polished and said that the police department had a few incidents recently in which pharmacies had been robbed overnight and the narcotic Percocet was stolen. This so-called detective then asked me whether we stocked Percocet in containers of 100 tablets or in containers of 1000 tablets. This sounded like a highly unusual question so I told this so-called detective, "No, we don't dispense enough Percocet to stock it in the 1000-tablet container." I suspect the caller was actually a fairly sophisticated drug abuser or dealer who was planning to rob us some night if I had been naïve enough to tell him that we indeed stocked Percocet in the 1000-tablet container. I considered calling the police department after this incident but I was very busy and it all seemed so bizarre that I didn't notify anyone. My hope was that, by informing the caller we stocked Percocet only in the small container, he would be prompted to look for another drugstore to rob. Unquestionably, I should have followed up with the police. But I was covered up with prescriptions and I simply didn't have the time to get involved. Many pharmacists feel that drug abusers and dealers are so numerous that we, as pharmacists, are never going to solve this problem that is so deeply rooted in our society. Why should we as pharmacists endanger our lives by helping to nail such dangerous criminals?

I once worked in a town of around ten thousand people. One day someone called me and identified himself as Dr. Kaplowitz. He proceeded to act as though he was phoning in a prescription for one of his patients. I hadn't worked in that town very long but I seemed to recall having spoken with Dr. Kaplowitz on the phone once or twice before. I seemed to recall Dr. Kaplowitz being quite self-confident, quite forceful, bordering on arrogant. This person who claimed to be Dr. Kaplowitz was none of the above. He said something like "I'm thinking about prescribing Vicodin for Jane Smith or maybe Lorcet. What do you think?" Such uncertainty is—or should be—a definite tip-off to pharmacists. I've never in my career had a physician call me who was so unsure of himself. An hour or two later, "Jane Smith" called and asked me whether the prescription phoned in by Dr. Kaplowitz was ready. I told her simply, "No. Dr. Kaplowitz did not call." I should have called the real Dr. Kaplowitz and told him that someone was pretending to be him, but it was a very busy day and I felt that surely no pharmacist in America would be fooled by such an amateurish imposter.

Many drug abusers approach the pharmacist and imitate a cough, hoping we'll sell them a cough syrup containing the narcotic codeine. Codeine can be habit forming so government regulations place this drug in a special class called "exempt narcotics." Pharmacists are allowed to sell these codeine-containing cough syrups to customers without a doctor's prescription. What usually happens is this: A customer describes his or her cough symptoms to the pharmacist or actually imitates a cough. If the pharmacist thinks the customer is telling the truth (admittedly a subjective assessment on our part), i.e., the customer does indeed appear to have a real cough, the pharmacist can sell one of these codeine-containing cough syrups. My guess is that every pharmacist in America has seen many people who are hooked on these products. Or these customers simply like the feeling that these products provide.

Many customers approach the pharmacist and state that they need to purchase needles for their diabetic grandmother's insulin injections. Here again, if the pharmacist believes the customer is telling the truth, the pharmacist can sell the needles. Drug addicts very frequently use the "for my grandmother" story to obtain needles to inject themselves with illicit drugs—not insulin. When pharmacists are suspicious of the customers' demeanor or appearance, we decline to sell the needles. We often lie by saying, "We're out of needles."

Pharmacists hear endless stories from customers seeking needles, codeine-containing cough syrups, and early refills on their narcotic pain pills. This procession of phony stories from customers convinces pharmacists that drug abuse is a tremendously huge problem in America. Many pharmacists become jaded toward almost anyone who has prescriptions filled for drugs like Vicodin and Percocet. Many pharmacists seem to assume that nearly everyone who is on these drugs must be a drug abuser or drug dealer who has been successful in snowing their doctor into writing such prescriptions. When pharmacists see customers with prescriptions for narcotic pain pills, some pharmacists assume these people have been "doctor shopping," i.e., going around to various physicians in the area looking for one who will write narcotic prescriptions. But pharmacists should keep in mind that there are many people who have a legitimate need for these drugs. My mother died from colon cancer that spread to her liver. During the final two months of her life, she unquestionably needed the Percocet that was prescribed by her oncologist. She was the last person in the world who would want to take Percocet unnecessarily. I was fortunate that I was able to stay with her for the final few weeks of her life. I recall taking one of her prescriptions for Percocet to a nearby pharmacy. It was at night and the pharmacist on duty was alone in the pharmacy. When I handed the Percocet prescription directly to the pharmacist, I detected that skeptical look in his eye assuming my mother must be a drug abuser. I wanted to say to him, "You asshole. She's dying from cancer."

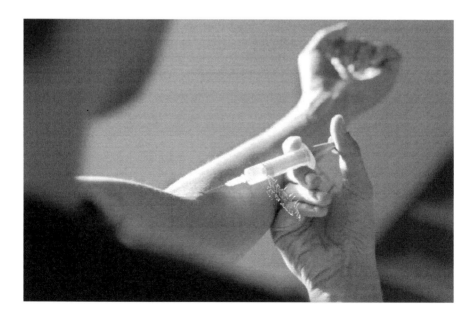

PART IX

CHAIN DRUGSTORES

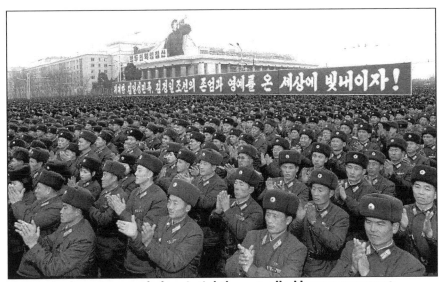

The chain drugstore workplace is tightly controlled by management. Individuality is not encouraged.

37
The chain drugstore culture

Intense focus on sales volume

In my 25-year career as a pharmacist, I've worked for three major drug chains, including the Rite Aid chain from 1975 to 1978. The focus on sales volume was always intense with each of the drug chains I've worked for. But the focus on sales volume at Rite Aid was extremely intense. I remember that the number one question my Rite Aid supervisors asked me (on the phone and in person) was some variation of this: "How is prescription volume looking this week?"

Back in the 1970s most of the sales figures that pharmacists and store managers sent to corporate headquarters were handwritten. Today, sales figures are transmitted to the corporate office electronically. I remember that on our weekly handwritten sales recap that we sent to our Rite Aid district office, the most prominent figures we submitted were the number of prescriptions we filled during the current week and also the number of prescriptions we filled during the same week the previous year. The previous year's numbers were obtained from a notebook we maintained containing weekly sales figures. The form, completed at the end of each week (i.e., Saturday), looked something like this:

• Number of prescriptions filled this week
• Number of prescriptions filled same week last year
• Dollar value of prescriptions filled this week
• Dollar value of prescriptions filled same week last year

Comparing the current week to the same week during the previous year was an important yardstick used by our Rite Aid bosses to determine whether our store was on an uphill trajectory or a downhill trajectory. Pharmacists working in stores on a downhill trajectory needed to have a logical explanation for the decline (e.g., a competitor recently opened a drugstore down the street), or else endure being blamed for killing the store. Pharmacists can directly affect the success of pharmacies by obvious things like being too slow in filling prescriptions, being out-of-stock of too many drugs, or being rude to customers.

I had several different district supervisors during my three years at Rite Aid. All of them seemed to have been programmed to ask that same question: "How are prescription numbers looking this week?" The obsession with sales figures led to efforts to inflate these numbers by whatever means necessary, legal or borderline legal.

For example, pharmacists were encouraged to give an additional refill or two on prescriptions. Say a doctor specified five refills on the prescription he wrote. For "maintenance" drugs (those that treat chronic conditions like hypertension, arthritis, depression, type 2 diabetes, etc.), Rite Aid's corporate attitude seemed to be that one or two additional refills wouldn't hurt anyone. Let me emphasize that we were not encouraged to exceed the specified number of refills for controlled substances or antibiotics. Exceeding the specified number of refills with controlled substances would have been (and still is) a serious violation of the law.

With maintenance meds, the corporate attitude seemed to be "John Smith isn't going to be cured of his hypertension any time soon so an additional refill or two is no big deal." Of course, the pharmacist was encouraged to phone the doctor for authorization for additional refills when the customer ran out of refills. But pharmacists working in seriously understaffed stores frequently take the course of least resistance: giving an additional refill or two without calling the doctor for authorization. It's much easier for the pharmacist to go ahead and refill "maintenance meds" an additional time or two than always call the doctor.

There are many pharmacists who would never consider exceeding the number of refills specified by the doctor. Other pharmacists have a much more relaxed attitude toward exceeding the specified number of refills (on medications that customers will likely use for a long time). Rite Aid encouraged a more relaxed attitude toward refills compared to the other two drug chains I've worked for. This was Rite Aid back in the 1970s. I am not qualified to say whether a similar attitude exists today at Rite Aid pharmacies.

The obsessive focus on prescription volume led to an interesting situation. For example, whenever a customer asked the pharmacist to recommend a multivitamin, our supervisors recommended that we walk to the sales floor, recommend a product, then carry that product (One-A-Day, Theragran, Myadec, etc.) back to the pharmacy and make a prescription out of it. We were to ask the customer for the name of his doctor and then act like we had just received a prescription from that doctor for the multivitamin we were recommending. We would type a label instructing the customer to, for example, "Take one tablet daily." We would then slap that label on the product. Magically, we could then record this as an additional prescription.

Say we filled 150 prescriptions daily on average. Say we made five separate recommendations each day for multivitamins. These additional five recommendations would allow us to report an additional five prescriptions filled each day, or thirty-five per week. So, say we filled a thousand prescriptions in a certain week. This tactic would allow us to report to our district headquarters that we actually filled 1,035 that week. The inflated figure was obviously phony but it played well in the numbers game that obsessed our supervisors. This practice let us know that prescription volume should be the number one priority for chain pharmacists. Pharmacists understood quite clearly that the numbers we reported each week were how our bosses judged us. Most pharmacists got the message and wanted to report numbers that pleased our bosses.

Tightly controlled workplace

The chain pharmacy workplace certainly has many more rules regulating personal behavior than does pharmacy school. Workplace regulations I have personally seen enforced during my career:

• No personal reading material allowed in the pharmacy (like *People* magazine, a favorite among female pharmacists).
• No radios allowed in the pharmacy.

• No chairs allowed in the pharmacy.
• Pharmacists and techs must not sit on stools while entering prescriptions into pharmacy computer. Sitting on stools creates the impression of laziness.
• Pharmacists must answer the phone within three rings and routinely return to any callers on hold to tell them the status of their call.
• Bottles on shelves must be straight as "little toy soldiers."
• No notes (like the phone number to the local sub shop) taped to walls, including walls outside the view of customers. Notes on the pharmacy walls create a cluttered appearance. If you want notes, get a notebook.
• Male pharmacists must wear a tie, a name tag, and white jacket.

Countless times I've watched pharmacists forcefully and confidently advising customers about the importance of taking prescribed medications religiously for elevated blood pressure and elevated cholesterol, while I've rarely seen pharmacists forcefully and confidently advising customers about the importance of maintaining ideal weight, eating nutritious foods, and otherwise having a healthy lifestyle, all of which might lessen the need for such drugs. Of course, pharmacists rarely have time for in depth conversations ("consultations") with our customers. Even though it's never verbalized, it is clear to most pharmacists that our employer doesn't want us advising customers about non-drug approaches to illnesses. Non-drug approaches circumvent the drugstore.

In my opinion, there is no greater contradiction in pharmacy than the perspective of the big chains (that pharmacy is mainly a distributive enterprise) and the perspective of pharmacy schools (that pharmacy is a cognitive enterprise). The culture in chain pharmacy is nearly opposite that in pharmacy school. From my perspective, pharmacy professors do not adequately prepare students for the transition from pharmacy school to the real world. Professors do not alert students about the culture shock we experience when we find ourselves ringing up diapers, deodorant, and suntan lotion at the pharmacy cash register along with prescriptions.

Fortunately, some pharmacists are able to take the more demeaning aspects of our job in stride. One recent pharmacy graduate commented to me, "I'll happily ring up groceries all day for what I'm being paid."

I have heard many pharmacy students say that their professors ridicule retail pharmacy (as opposed to hospital pharmacy) for being intellectually unsatisfying, not what pharmacy is really about, physically exhausting grunt-work in a factory. I've never worked in a hospital pharmacy so I am unqualified to say whether hospital pharmacy is more satisfying.

I wish someone would do a study comparing academic performance in pharmacy school versus satisfaction with chain pharmacy. My theory is that the higher the pharmacy student's grade point average, the less he or she is satisfied with chain pharmacy. Perhaps the intellectually curious students find the chain pharmacy environment to be deeply unfulfilling, vacuous, assembly-line piece-work/production-work. Perhaps the best students in pharmacy school are profoundly uneasy in the retail environment in which speed in filling prescriptions is valued much more highly than drug knowledge. Perhaps the pharmacists who were slackers in pharmacy school are more satisfied with monotonous, repetitive, robotic chain pharmacy.

Our chain pharmacy bosses certainly do not value highly those pharmacists who want to spend a lot of time examining potential drug interactions, phoning doctors about potential problems, advising customers, etc. The corporate bosses feel that pharmacists who want to spend their time discussing drugs should leave the retail environment, become a member of the pharmacy school faculty, and teach full time.

Professors in pharmacy school tell us that pharmacists will be paid for our drug knowledge. The drugstore chains have an entirely different outlook: We are paid for our labor. Supervisors with the drug chains relate to pharmacists below them completely in terms of sales—not health. Having a supervisor engage us in a conversation about some drug treatment would be unimaginable. Supervisors talk to us about three things: sales, sales, and sales. The most important question to supervisors is: Are the pharmacy sales figures up compared to the same period last year?

A district supervisor for a competing drug chain took me out to lunch one day in an effort to fill a slot in one of his stores. During our surprisingly frank discussion (perhaps this was his way of letting me know what kind of pharmacists he likes), he told me that most pharmacists just out of school have some unrealistic expectations of what it's like working in a drugstore forty hours a week. He told me that most of them leave the ivory towers of the universities with a "know-it-all" cockiness and that they take too long to learn (some never learn) that their job is just like "flipping hamburgers at McDonald's" all day long. He said that few graduates understand that, in the real world, they're being paid for their labor. He said they don't know that pharmacy (as practiced by the big chains) is one of the few professions where licensees are paid mainly for their labor. Whereas doctors, lawyers, professors, etc., are paid for using their heads, chain pharmacists are mainly paid for using their hands and feet. He said that the average chain pharmacist in this country fills somewhere between 100 and 200 prescriptions in an eight- or twelve-hour day and that this puts chain pharmacists in the category of piece-workers. He acknowledged that this is demeaning and that he was not pleased that our profession had degenerated to this. But he said he was tired of hiring pharmacists who didn't seem to be able to accept reality and perform accordingly.

This economic perspective in the drugstore quickly replaces the drug therapy perspective we had in pharmacy school. In fact, the economic perspective pretty much colors our attitudes and outlook in the drugstore. In cities where our chain has more than one outlet, pharmacists frequently spend a lot of time on the phone with pharmacists at the other outlets. We call these local pharmacists often to see if they have various drugs on hand that we're out of. Occasionally, when we can steal a minute or two, we talk about whatever is on our minds. In my experience, the most frequent topic between pharmacists is "How's business?"

The competitive drive being what it is, the pharmacist at the higher-volume store very often lords this fact over the pharmacist at the lower volume store. The importance of sales has been so thoroughly hammered into our heads that we use it as a yardstick to gauge our success as pharmacists. Superior prescription volume is a reason to feel superior to a another pharmacist. Superior knowledge about medicine or health or prevention is rarely the basis for such egotism. Success is, unfortunately, not measured in terms of the quality of the answers that the pharmacist gives to customers' questions. I've never seen a pharmacist criticized by a supervisor for giving poor or mediocre advice to a customer. On the other hand, supervisors are very often critical of pharmacists who are slow in the dispensing of prescriptions.

The unit malfunctioned

One day my partner and I were in the pharmacy and a customer walked up to us and said, "These don't look like my usual pills." We examined the contents of her bottle and, sure enough, the "floater" pharmacist who had worked the day before had given her the wrong pills. This floater had worked the last day of my partner's vacation. This floater had mistakenly dispensed Premarin 2.5 mg instead of Provera 2.5 mg. This was not a major error since these are both female hormones, yet it was indeed an error. After he gave the customer her correct pills, my partner said to me, "The unit malfunctioned yesterday." My partner has grown attached to the word "unit" as a way of expressing how our employer has turned pharmacists into robots. I usually use the word "automaton," but my partner thinks the word "unit" more closely captures the absurdity of our work environment. My partner uses the word "unit" to compare pharmacists to mechanical devices in the pharmacy like fax machines, cash registers, and laser printers. Commenting further on this floater's error, my partner said, "That's what Revco [our employer, a big drug chain that was sold to CVS] wants. They want us to *run 'em thru* [fill prescriptions at lightning speed]." My partner did not apologize to the customer for the floater's mistake. He just thanked the customer for coming back. My partner is tired of apologizing for errors that he feels are inevitable in the chain's "speed is all that matters" culture. He's tired of incurring the wrath of customers for errors made by other pharmacists in an impossible system.

Speaking with customers is discouraged even though management claims otherwise

My employer says that we should talk to customers, but most pharmacists are highly skeptical that the corporation really means it. I have heard numerous supervisors ridicule various pharmacists for spending too much time talking to customers. Talking with customers sure slows things down. For example, a customer might say she's experiencing a certain symptom and then want to know whether it could be a side effect of the drug she's taking. This would require me to pull out the professional insert or consult the *Physicians' Desk Reference* or *Facts & Comparisons* to search carefully to see whether that symptom is listed as a possible side effect of the drug.

Older pharmacists have told me that when they graduated from pharmacy school, they were forbidden to discuss medications with customers. They were supposed to refer the customers with their questions back to the doctor who prescribed the medication. These pharmacists weren't even allowed to put the name of the drug on your prescription label. Even though that was not good for teaching customers about their medications, it certainly made life simpler for those pharmacists. Not having to answer customers' questions sure would make my job easier and I would have less legal liability.

Mystery shoppers

My employer periodically sends around "mystery shoppers" for secret undercover evaluations of store employees and store management. The mystery shopper does not identify himself or herself. He or she checks things like: whether another cashier is called when there are over three people in line at the cash registers, whether all employees are professional and courteous to customers, and whether employees greet customers and make eye contact. The mystery shopper also checks the amount of time it takes the pharmacy staff to fill prescriptions—as if we were not already working as fast as we can, in fact, already at unsafe speeds. In most of the stores, we usually have to fight our urge to go to the bathroom or eat. We fight like hell just to keep up with the prescription flow. Yet management acts as though we're leisurely viewing *Playboy* magazine all day long.

Pushing non-prescription drugs

An important part of the pharmacist's job is to help move the non-prescription drugs in the store. This isn't too difficult. Customers have been well-programmed from radio, television, and magazine advertisements to interpret every discomfort as the need for a product from the pharmacy. As Ivan Illich (author of *Medical Nemesis: The Expropriation of Health,* New York: Pantheon, 1976) would say, the customers have been trained to *need on command.*

Selling non-prescription drugs is one of the parts of my job that I hate the most because I need to leave the prescription department to show the customer the product I recommend. In the prescription department, at least there is the mystique from not seeing or knowing precisely what the pharmacist is doing. But on the sales floor I feel surely the customers see me purely as a merchant trying to move products. I usually recommend the most popular product for each particular ailment. For example: Dimetapp for colds, Robitussin for coughs, Sucrets for sore throat, Preparation H for hemorrhoids, Mylanta for excess acid, Centrum for a vitamin, Advil for mild pain, Neosporin for minor cuts or abrasions, Donnagel for diarrhea, Metamucil for constipation, Cort-Aid for poison ivy.

I recommend only well-know products because, if the customer doesn't find any benefit from that product, I have a big company like Proctor & Gamble or Bristol-Myers Squibb behind me. This way the customer can't say, "The pharmacist recommended some dumb product that didn't do me any good." By recommending a well-known brand name, I have the entire hype department of a multi-national drug company supporting me. This way the customer would be challenging the mountain of hype from that company. The customer can't claim I recommended some unheard of product.

My instructors from pharmacy school would surely feel I am disregarding their fancy justifications for the various products. And they would be right. I feel it is amazing how thoroughly the drug companies have done their job of selling Americans on the pill-for-every-ill concept. It is apparent to me that many people believe whatever marketing pitch they hear on television. I feel sorry for many customers because of their simplistic understanding of health, yet, at the same time, I am amazed they are so confident that their single-minded pursuit of quick-fix solutions is logical.

Occasionally when someone describes some innocuous symptoms and then asks me what we have for it, I say, "I don't know of anything that would be good for that." Invariably the response is, "Well, thanks anyway" and the customer has this expression on his face: *This Is A Dumb Pharmacist.* So I have come to the conclusion that I'd better make a recommendation when asked.

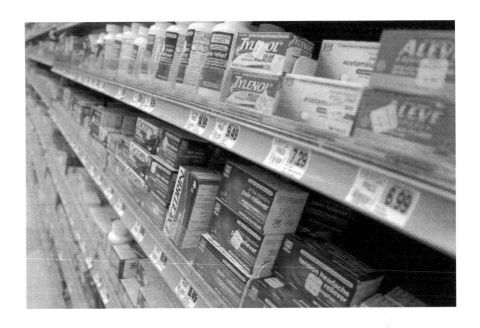

Quick-fix medicine is not fulfilling

Pharmacy professors tell students that pharmacy is very fulfilling because pharmacists help people with health problems. In my opinion, helping people find a quick-fix solution is not fulfilling. Dispensing products as fast as my hands and feet will allow is not fulfilling. Giving advice can be more fulfilling but, too often, we don't have enough time to give advice. Most customers aren't interested in gaining the insight that might allow them to prevent their problem whether it be depression, insomnia, vaginal yeast infection, jock itch, type 2 diabetes, elevated cholesterol, elevated blood pressure, constipation, diarrhea, heartburn, headache, etc.

How can pharmacists find it fulfilling when our days are spent dispensing Botox for facial wrinkles, Paxil for shyness, Vaniqa for female facial hair, Ritalin for hyperactivity, Anafranil for excess handwashing, DDAVP for bedwetting, Sarafem for premenstrual dysphoric disorder, Xanax for panic attack, Imitrex for migraine, Sonata for insomnia, Rogaine for baldness, TriCyclen for female acne, Renova for wrinkles, Nexium for acid, Imodium for diarrhea, and Meridia for obesity? Most of these conditions are preventable or treatable without drugs or they're conditions for which Big Pharma has succeeded in making the public feel inadequate (e.g., baldness, female facial hair, wrinkles, impotence, shyness).

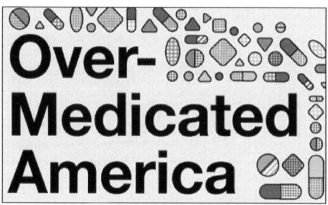

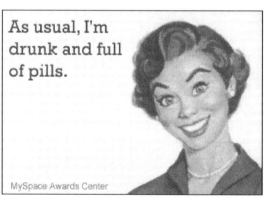

As usual, I'm drunk and full of pills.

MySpace Awards Center

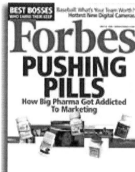

Forbes
PUSHING
PILLS
How Big Pharma Got Addicted To Marketing

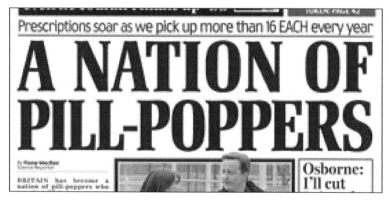

Prescriptions soar as we pick up more than 16 EACH every year

A NATION OF PILL-POPPERS

Osborne: I'll cut

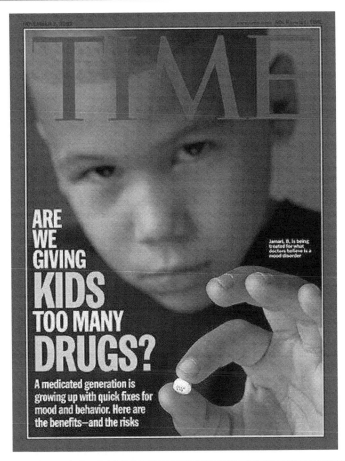

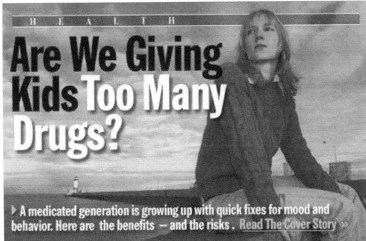

We're just a number

A medical sociologist once told me "The socialization process in medical school is stronger than a prison." In my opinion, pharmacists go through a similarly powerful socialization process with the big pharmacy chains. Socialization into the corporate culture involves a loss of individuality. Several pharmacists have told me that they feel more like a number than a person as we fill prescriptions at some mega-chain that has absolutely no concern for us as a human being.

Most people are surprised to learn just how *mega* the mega-chains are. Here's a ranking of the chains by number of pharmacies in 2012 (*Drug Store News*, April 2013, http://4.bp.blogspot.com/-PbFjAXL6ckw/UXXiQuLDp_I/AAAAAAAAEII/iFzleilUM6o/s1600/PoweRx_Top20_DrugStoreNews_April2013.png):

Chain drugstores by store count–2012

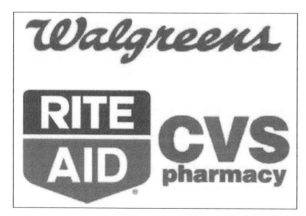

1. Walgreens—7,941 pharmacies
2. CVS—7,402 pharmacies
3. Rite Aid—4,623 pharmacies
4. Wal-Mart—3,943 pharmacies

Having so many stores means that corporate is obsessed with standardization, predictability, uniformity, and control. It means that each outlet of Chain X should be indistinguishable from the others, that pharmacists should be interchangeable in the various locations, and that the shopping experience at each store should be identical. Efficiency dictates that interactions between customers and employees be limited. The fast food model requires socialization into the overarching corporate ethos and a homogenization of pharmacists that leaves little room for those who yearn to find their own path. Students in pharmacy school who hope for creativity in their career will almost certainly be sorely disappointed with the rigid and regimented chain culture. The chain drugstore requires achieving control through automation or de-skilling of the workplace because people are inherently unpredictable and inefficient. The big chains want to routinize and mechanize the workplace as much as possible so that unskilled workers can replace skilled workers.

The big chains view pharmacy as a business, not a profession. The chains aggressively fight unions. Pharmacists working for the big chains occasionally go on strike, illustrating that labor/management issues are just as important in chain drugstores as they are at General Motors, Ford, and Chrysler. Pharmacy unions fight for better pay for pharmacists, but the unions also fight for things that many workers in our society take for granted, like meal breaks and bathroom breaks. In drugstores that have only one pharmacist on duty at a time, having that pharmacist leave for a few minutes to eat lunch or go to the bathroom causes an impatient public to complain about poor service. The chains see pharmacists as wage laborers who provide a product, rather than professionals who provide a service (screening for drug interactions, checking dosages, advising customers about proper use of medications, etc.).

A never-ending loop of happy drug messages on the store audio system

Chain pharmacists have surprisingly little control over the environment in which we work. For example, many of the big chains produce their own advertising messages at the corporate level which are then piped into each store. This bathes customers and store employees in a never-ending loop of pill-for-every-ill messages...all day, every day. To me, the effect is much more irritating than background music like Muzak. That's because these in-store messages usually have some annoyingly cheerful announcer pretending he's Ron Radio. I often wonder whether our corporate bosses ever considered the effect that constant repetition of these messages has on store employees. The corporate bosses seem to feel that store employees are no more adversely affected by this verbal pollution of our workplace than the products sitting on our shelves. A bottle of Robitussin cough syrup and a tube of Preparation H are unaffected by this noise pollution but I don't think the same can be said for human beings. I often feel like a lab rat being tested to see how many advertising messages I can withstand without developing some drugstore equivalent of *going postal.*

It seems to me that this constant assault by advertising messages has a numbing and dehumanizing effect on store employees. It is as if the corporate bosses have no respect for store employees as human beings. I often wonder whether our customers are similarly annoyed by these messages. Surely this continuous repetition of messages about drugs convinces customers (and, yes, pharmacists) that pills are the answer to every health problem. To the best of my recollection, none of these messages have dealt with the importance of proper diet, proper weight, exercise, etc., because such approaches circumvent the drugstore.

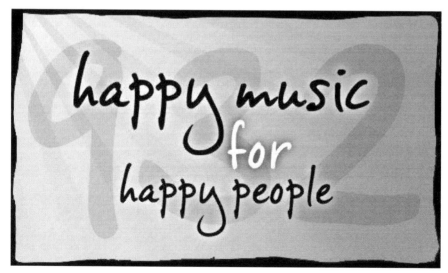

Should drugstores sell candy, cigarettes, and alcoholic beverages?

Three of the leading substances causing disease in America (sugar, tobacco, and alcohol) are readily available in drugstores. When your drugstore chain advertises that it cares about your health, ask yourself how that is possible if that chain sells cigarettes, alcoholic beverages (beer and wine), and candy. Sugar, alcohol, and tobacco are either addicting or cause craving. Obesity, dental cavities, alcoholism, and lung cancer can be the end result of the excessive use of products easily obtainable in most drugstores.

Drugstores sell alcoholic beverages while the pharmacist fills prescriptions for Antabuse, a drug that helps alcoholics quit. Drugstores sell cigarettes while the pharmacist fills prescriptions for people with lung cancer. Is it not hypocritical for drugstores to sell cigarettes and also sell nicotine gum and patches to help you quit smoking?

Americans associate holidays with candy. The drugstore aisles overflow with candy each Halloween, Easter, Mother's Day, Valentine's Day, and Christmas. As everyone knows, candy causes dental caries and contributes to obesity, which in turn contributes to type-2 diabetes and hypertension. Is it hypocritical that we sell candy in the front of the store and fill prescriptions (Xenical and Meridia) for obesity in the pharmacy? We also fill countless prescriptions for acetaminophen w/codeine and penicillin VK as a result of the dental caries caused by candy.

Is it strange that many public schools are prohibiting soft drink and candy vending machines while pharmacies sell lots of soft drinks and candy? Is it time to jettison the idea that people should bring a box of candy when they visit friends or relatives who have recently been discharged from the hospital? Is it time to re-examine our cultural practice of celebrating special occasions by buying a box of candy at the drugstore for one's spouse, girlfriend, or mother?

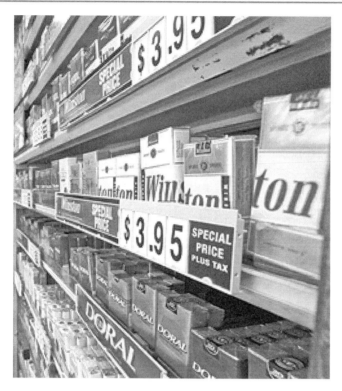

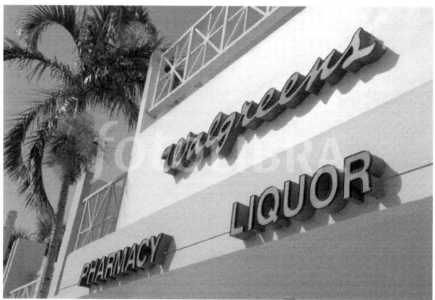

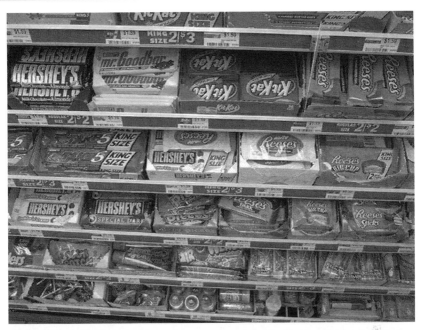

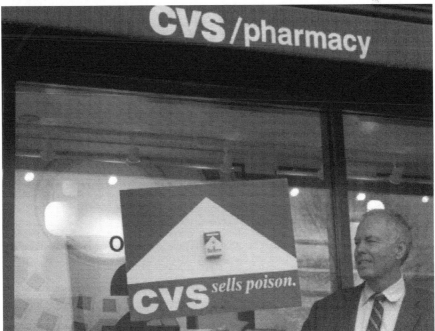

Should drugstores sell tobacco products?
http://www.toxic-tobaccolaw.org/13news.shtml

38

Would somebody please clean the men's restroom?

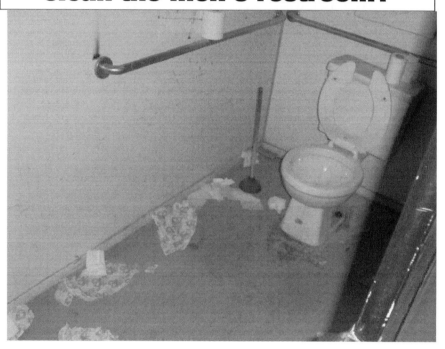

Would you eat in a restaurant with filthy restrooms? People assume that if the restaurant restrooms are filthy, chances are that the kitchen is unsanitary and the staff is ambivalent about cleanliness. Many customers react the same way to restrooms in drugstores. I've often wondered how customers react when they see the filthy restrooms at some of the drugstores I've worked in.

The cleanliness of the restrooms tells a lot about the way in which the drugstore is run. In many stores, the restrooms are always clean. In other stores, the restrooms are usually filthy, unless it happens to be just a day or two after the weekly or twice-a-month contract floor cleaners did their work. These floor cleaners clean the restrooms as part of the floor cleaning contract.

At many stores in which there is an ongoing conflict between the pharmacists and the store manager, the cleaning of restrooms becomes an issue of power and status. The store manager feels that he has more power than the pharmacists since the store manager controls more square footage than pharmacists. At stores in which there is not, say, a male part-time high school student who can be assigned the job of cleaning the restrooms, this task can fall on the shoulders of the only other non-pharmacist male in the store, i.e., the store manager. The store manager doesn't want to clean the restrooms himself because he fears he would suffer a diminution in status in the eyes of the pharmacists. So if there is no other male in the store other than the store manager, the restrooms are often left filthy until the scheduled arrival of the contracted floor cleaners.

I've worked in stores in which the store manager kept the restrooms locked, forcing customers and employees to ask for the key for entry. This allowed him to screen the people who could use the restrooms. The store manager didn't want to make it too easy for customers to enter the restrooms.

Some store employees tell customers "We don't have public restrooms." I recall seeing a memo from corporate stating something like, "Keep in mind that many of your customers have medical conditions which may require them to have access to restrooms. Therefore, restrooms should be made available to customers." Of course, this memo didn't address the fact that many customers leave a filthy mess in the restroom that store employees must clean up. It's easy for corporate to tell us to keep the restrooms available to the public. That's because the corporate hotshots don't have to clean the restrooms themselves. I'd love to see the corporate suits cleaning restrooms.

I worked in one store in which the store manager did not keep toilet paper in the restrooms. (Employees and customers had to request it beforehand.) I asked him about this once and he said that he was tired of finding whole rolls of toilet paper dumped in the toilet. I never understood why customers would be so angry or crude as to dump a full roll of toilet paper. Were they protesting the way they were treated by store employees? Were they angry at our prices? Were they upset having to wait for their prescriptions to be filled?

At most stores in which I've worked, the women's restroom is cleaner than the men's restroom. Perhaps male anatomy (standing versus sitting) makes it inevitable that the men's restroom will be less clean than the women's restroom. It is possible that women have been socialized into keeping clean restrooms whereas men view the cleaning of restrooms as beneath them, a feminine activity. Some men seem to view filthy restrooms as a macho thing. These men seem to feel that concern about restroom cleanliness is for women only.

I worked in one store in which the sales floor area was always well-maintained and the products on the shelves were always straightened ("front faced"). But the men's restroom was always filthy. That was in a store with a lazy male manager but a very hardworking female who essentially functioned as the floor manager. She kept the store shelves well stocked and clean and she made sure that the women's restroom was always in good shape. Understandably she didn't touch the men's restroom. Surely it is not fair to ask female employees to clean the men's restroom.

Like many pharmacists, I've often needed to stay after store closing to get caught up before going home. This means I have often been in the store by myself. I confess that, under these circumstances, I've often utilized the women's restroom because the men's restroom is simply too gross and I'm too lazy or too tired or too fed up with the store manager to clean the men's restroom myself.

The only period during which I've routinely cleaned the men's restroom myself was back in the days when the pharmacist was the store manager. I happened to be the manager of a new store in Burlington, North Carolina. With the exception of the other pharmacist, I was the only male in the store. Knowing the other pharmacist as I did, I'm sure there's no way that he would have cleaned the restroom himself. Most male pharmacists would rather kill themselves than clean a drugstore restroom.

39

Chain drugstores are intellectually deadening

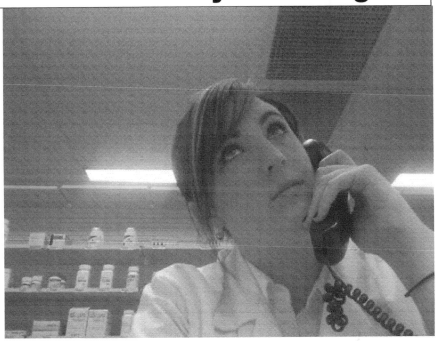

Customers probably think that chain drugstores are centers of lively and passionate discussion about the safety and effectiveness of prescription and non-prescription drugs. Is there indeed a frank discussion among chain pharmacists about the pros and cons of various drugs?

In my experience, the chain drugstore environment is almost exclusively focused on production, i.e., numbers of prescriptions and numbers of dollars. It is quite unusual for pharmacists to engage in significant discussions among themselves about drugs.

Many pharmacists entering the real world after pharmacy school are shocked to see that the focus of their job in the chain drugstore is almost the exact opposite of the focus in pharmacy school. In pharmacy school, the study of drugs was our primary focus. At the chain drugstore, filling prescriptions as fast as we can is our primary focus.

In my 25 years as a chain pharmacist, I rarely saw pharmacists at work engaging in the types of drug therapy discussions with other pharmacists that would make our pharmacy school professors proud. Conversations among pharmacists usually focused on everything *except* pharmacology: plans for the weekend, plans for an upcoming vacation, family matters, difficult bosses and co-workers, understaffing, attitudes of local doctors, the pros and cons of working for CVS versus Walgreens versus Wal-Mart versus Rite Aid, the fact that the non-pharmacist store manager too often doesn't have a clue about the stresses pharmacists feel as a result of understaffing, and last—but certainly not least—attractive female customers.

It is clear to pharmacists soon after graduation from pharmacy school that drug chain supervisors do not think highly of pharmacists who are overly fixated on the "drug therapy" side of pharmacy. In fact, engaging our district pharmacy supervisor in a discussion about some drug therapy is very difficult for me to imagine. District pharmacy supervisors (who are, by the way, usually pharmacists themselves) are clearly primarily interested making sure that Rx volume in each of his stores is on the upswing.

It is also my experience that chain pharmacists rarely discuss among themselves significant events like the FDA adding critical black box warnings to the official prescribing information, or the FDA taking the drastic step of removing drugs from the market.

Ever since I entered pharmacy school in 1972, I've been hearing that the model of the pharmacist as drug expert will become the dominant model. However, the big chains are unyielding in their disdain for this "clinical" orientation of newly-graduated pharmacists. The big chains want pharmacists who can fill prescriptions at lightning speed. The big chains certainly don't want pharmacists who spend too much time discussing drugs with customers, calling doctors about potential drug interactions, or otherwise functioning as the public expects. The big chains view prescriptions like any other commodity in the marketplace. Shortly after graduation from pharmacy school, young pharmacists working for many of the big chains become shocked, saddened, and disillusioned when they fully comprehend the fact that they are no more than highly paid piece-workers on a production line based on McDonald's, complete with a two-lane drive thru.

When I was in high school and college, I thought I'd like to work for a big corporation. I was completely invested in the idea that corporations are efficient, exciting, and meritocratic. I felt sure that working for a corporation would be an interesting experience. When I graduated and began working for the big drug chains, I found a reality that was far different from what I had expected. I discovered that efficiency in the chain drugstore industry means mind-numbing and exhausting repetition: filling an endless river of prescriptions as fast as my hands and feet would allow. Efficiency in the chain drugstore means a never-ending quest by the corporation to figure out more ingenious ways to squeeze more production out of pharmacists and technicians.

Instead of being intellectually challenging, I found the big drugstore chains to be intellectually deadening. In my opinion, the big chains would be more accurately described as anti-intellectual:

• The big chains are completely uninterested in issues like whether Big Pharma exerts too much pressure on the FDA.
• The big drug chains aren't interested in safety issues surrounding drugs.
• The big chains aren't interested in examining, monitoring, or reporting the short term or long term adverse effects of drugs.
• The big chains aren't interested in discussing whether Americans are overmedicated. In fact, the big chains clearly *want* Americans to be overmedicated.
• The big chains aren't interested in the profound social implications of the mass prescribing of antidepressants to adults and, increasingly, to children.

• The big chains aren't interested in the tremendous overprescribing of antibiotics for the treatment of the common cold. The big chains aren't interested in the severe problems that the overprescribing of antibiotics causes in the development of drug resistance.

• The big chains aren't interested in the field of prevention—because prevention usually means finding alternatives to drugs.

• The big chains aren't interested in examining the striking age-adjusted variations in the incidence of diseases around the world and learning what this tells us about the powerful potential of prevention.

• The big chains aren't interested in pollution, in the ubiquity of toxic substances (including carcinogens) in our environment, in pesticide residues on fruits and vegetables, in cancer clusters around factories that discharge hazardous materials into the air and water.

• Clearly the big drugstore chains are more interested in the treatment of cancer than in its prevention.

• The big chains are opposed to any type of prevention that circumvents the drugstore.

• The big chains aren't interested in discussions about whether drugs are overprescribed.

• The big chains aren't interested in discussions about whether drug advertisements on television prompt consumers to ask doctors for drugs that may be unnecessary.

• The big chains aren't interested in the controversy surrounding the widespread prescribing of drugs like Ritalin for children who do poorly in school because they don't pay attention ("attention deficit") or won't sit still ("hyperactivity").

• The big chains aren't interested in the consequences of the overprescribing of post-menopausal estrogens, including increases in stroke, heart disease, and breast cancer.

• The big chains aren't interested in whether Big Pharma exaggerates the benefits of drugs and minimizes the risks.

• The big chains aren't interested in examining the extent to which the placebo effect accounts for so much of the benefit that patients receive from pharmaceuticals.

• The big chains aren't interested in examining whether our health care system should be based on prevention rather than pills.
• The big chains aren't interested in a social critique of pharmaceuticals.
• The big chains aren't interested in the many booklength exposés of the pharmaceutical industry.

So why would any intellectually curious pharmacist want to work for the big drugstore chains? How could the complete mercantile focus in the drugstore appeal to any pharmacist who is interested in examining drugs in a broader social, cultural and even political context? How can a pharmacist who is a strong advocate of prevention be happy amidst the commodity fetishism that describes our daily existence in the drugstore? The big chains want pharmacists who fill prescriptions fast and who do not have doubts about the pill-for-every-ill focus of modern medicine.

Thousands of times in my career I have made recommendations for non-prescription products in response to customers' requests, even though I'd never use those products myself. Thousand of times I've made recommendations for products for colds, cough, insomnia, constipation, diarrhea, etc., even though I'd never take those products myself. Countless times I recommended Centrum when customers asked me to recommend a vitamin even though I don't take vitamins myself. In my opinion, one's focus should be on eating a nutritious diet rather than on attempting to fine-tune one's vitamin intake based on the latest magazine article or TV story that extols the virtues of vitamins. For whatever symptoms a customer describes to me, there's absolutely no chance that I would make a recommendation for a non-drug approach if my district supervisor is standing anywhere near me.

Soon after graduation from pharmacy school, I concluded that customers want definitive answers when they ask the pharmacist: "What's good for..." (cold, cough, sore throat, backache, muscle aches, hemorrhoids, constipation, heartburn, dry eyes, minor cuts/abrasions, acne, diarrhea, insomnia, lack of energy, etc.). Customers do not like it when pharmacists answer these questions by suggesting lifestyle changes, dietary modifications, weight loss, adequate sleep, exercise, etc. Customers like pharmacists who force-fully and confidently answer, "You need X" (Sudafed, Robitussin, Myoflex, Preparation H, Pepcid AC, Sleep-Eze, Sucrets, Kaopectate, Metamucil, etc.).

EAT.
SLEEP.
PHARMACY.
REPEAT.

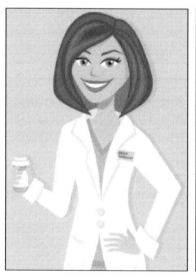

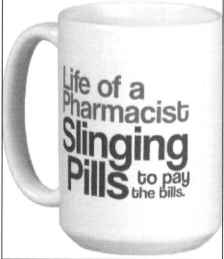

40

Why I resist wearing a white coat

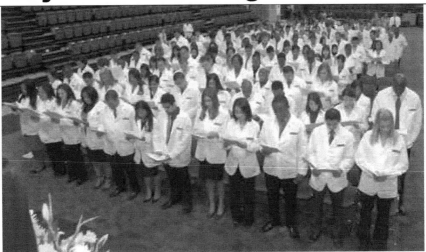

In pharmacy school, students were required (or highly encouraged) to wear our white coat during lab exercises. As best as I can recall, this was because, in some lab exercises, we handled chemicals that were potentially hazardous and thus the white coat could protect our skin and clothes. But the primary reason that we wore a white coat in our labs seemed to be because our professors viewed lab exercises as simulating real world pharmacy and the professors wanted us to get used to a "professional" appearance. Perhaps one third of the students in my class wore their lab coat all the time (i.e., in lecture halls *and* in the labs). These students seemed to be proud wearing their white coat. I resisted wearing my white coat because I never accepted the pill-for-every-ill outlook in pharmacy school and at CVS, Rite Aid, and Revco.

In the drugstore, wearing the white coat sent a subtle message to our bosses that we were loyal team players. Not wearing a white coat implied that a pharmacist was somehow rebellious and marched to the beat of his own drummer. I never felt comfortable wearing a white coat because it made me feel that I had sold out to the entire belief system of quick-fix medicine: suppressing symptoms with drugs, minimizing potential hazards of drugs, ignoring the powerful potential of prevention, placing the treatment of disease with drugs ahead of the prevention of that disease, accepting the hierarchical power structure which gave (oftentimes immature) supervisors power over pharmacists.

As someone who maintains a skeptical view toward the commodification of health, I am uncomfortable wearing the uniform that implies I am a team player in that enterprise, that I have accepted the goals and outlook of that enterprise, that I am part of a conspiracy to convince our customers that pills are better than prevention, that my primary allegiance is to the belief system I was taught in pharmacy school, that I accept The World According to Big Pharma. To me, wearing a white coat or uniform implies embracing the collective outlook of a group, being proud to be a member of that group, accepting the ideals and beliefs of that group. The word "uniform" comes from "one" plus "form." The chains would love for all pharmacists to look alike with a crisp white uniform and think alike—affable airheads who don't mind filling prescriptions at unsafe speeds at the pharmacy version of McDonald's.

My white coat increased the distance between me and customers. A white coat is somehow like a barrier. It says to customers, "I am the pharmacist. I am the drug expert. You are ignorant of drugs."

Here's an anecdote about white coats: The big chains had many rules for everything we did in the pharmacy (such as: no food in the pharmacy refrigerator, no radios or personal reading material in the pharmacy, no sitting on stools while using the pharmacy computer, products on our shelves should be "straight as little toy soldiers," phone-answering dialog should be "Thank you for calling Revco. This is [pharmacist's first name]. Can I help you?") But the corporate demand that really got under my skin was the requirement to wear a white coat.

District supervisors visit the pharmacy for perhaps an hour every two weeks. Too many district supervisors don't have a clue how pharmacists act toward customers when they (the district supervisors) are not in our store (i.e., the vast majority of the time). I have known many pharmacists who are very rude to customers and store employees. I have often thought that the first thing these district supervisors need to do is confront that pharmacist about his or her attitude toward customers or other employees. Every pharmacist knows that many pharmacists become a different person when our district supervisor is in the store, but that pharmacist immediately reverts to being a jerk toward customers and other employees as soon as that district supervisor walks out the door. District supervisors only know what they see, and those pharmacists become little angels when our district supervisor is present.

Rather than address such major problems like the rudeness of certain pharmacists, our district supervisor sees only what's in front of him: a pharmacist is not wearing a white coat. The district supervisor walks into the pharmacy and the first thing he notices is whether the pharmacist is wearing a white coat. A district supervisor once told me, "You need to wear your white coat." I answered him by saying, "The air conditioner in this store does not work very well." This was a correct statement but his reply was simple, "Well, you still need to wear it." Clearly, adherence to corporate policy is more important than the personal comfort of pharmacists.

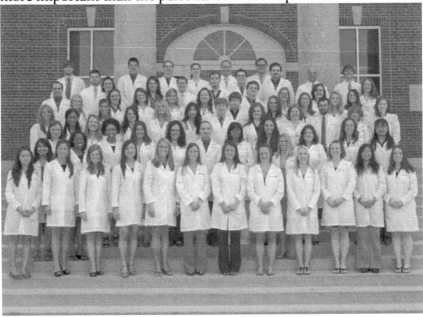

41

The chains' *Alice in Wonderland* view of pharmacy mistakes

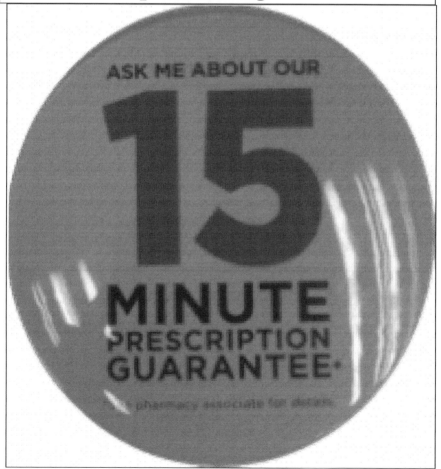

Alice in Wonderland is a well-known work of literary nonsense in what is called the "fantasy genre." In the world of pharmacy, a prominent example of the fantasy genre is the rationalizations given by chain spokesmen to reporters inquiring about pharmacy mistakes. Case in point: *USA Today* did a 3-day series (Feb. 11-13, 2008) on pharmacy mistakes. *The USA Today* series essentially placed the blame for pharmacy mistakes on the common practice of understaffing at the big chains. The big chains came out looking like they place high-speed production above accuracy.

Following a serious pharmacy mistake, spokesmen for the big chains are often interviewed by newspaper and TV reporters in the city in which the error occurred. Over the years, I've noticed that these chain spokesmen routinely make the following points, none of which—in my opinion—reflect the real world. These statements to the media are highly regrettable because, in minimizing the reality of serious mistakes, they perpetuate the current system of fast food pharmacy that guarantees errors. These explanations for pharmacy mistakes have an *Alice in Wonderland* quality about them because, quite often, the opposite is true. It is as if the chain spokesmen are living in some parallel universe.

Let's examine each of the chains' fantastical rationalizations individually. In soothing and reassuring tones, chain spokesmen say:

1. "Millions of dollars invested in technology will drastically reduce pharmacy errors."

In reality, the chains want a technological solution to a human problem. A major cause of pharmacy errors is understaffing but the big chains want the public to believe that errors are a technical problem with a technical solution, rather than a human problem that requires adequate staffing. Aside from the fact that some pharmacists are simply careless and would make mistakes regardless of the Rx volume, the primary problem in the pharmacy is the lack of an adequate number of properly trained techs and/or the need for more than one pharmacist on duty at a time. I know pharmacists who privately welcome the huge jury verdicts against chains in dispensing error cases. These pharmacists hope that the huge settlements will embarrass the chains into providing adequate staffing.

The big chains tell us that technology will make our lives easier. But the truth is that the big chains cut staffing commensurate with any efficiency gained by technology. The big chains dangle the carrot in front of us that technology will allow a more relaxed pace in the pharmacy. In reality, any gains in productivity brought about by technology will be met with an equivalent decrease in staffing. Indeed, the primary reason for adding technology in the pharmacy is to cut staffing.

---

2. "Every pharmacist will tell you that one error is too many."

This is one of the chain spokesmen's favorite red herrings. It is a clever way of implying that the chains are approaching the elimination of pharmacy errors, that the number of errors is minuscule. If the chains feel that one error is too many, how would they characterize the millions of errors that are estimated to occur each year across this country? In fact, chain pharmacy is nowhere near eliminating errors. Rather than decreasing, it's just as likely that the frequency of errors is actually increasing each year as the big chains focus on production rather than safety.

---

3. "There are no quotas. Scripts per hour are only guidelines which can be modified as needed in the store."

That's the most absurd statement I've ever heard in my life. Chain pharmacists have absolutely no power to increase R.Ph. staffing levels and thus lessen the burden of overwhelming and dangerous workloads.

---

4. "More errors occur when things are slow in the pharmacy because pharmacists are not focused."

This is the chains' favorite mantra. It is like saying speeding on an icy highway is good because the inherent danger forces us to be more careful.

5. "No pharmacist is pressured to fill prescriptions faster than he or she feels comfortable."

Yeah, Right! What about those computer systems that track the number of prescriptions not completed within 15 minutes of having been entered into the pharmacy computer? This data is compiled by corporate and often results in admonishments from our bosses to complete prescriptions more quickly.

6. "Safety is our number one priority."

Nope. Speed is the chains' number one priority. Indeed the entire chain drugstore concept is based on speed and volume, just like at McDonald's.

7. "There is no correlation between high prescription volume and errors."

The chains say that pharmacy mistakes occur in low volume stores and in high volume stores. The chains conclude, therefore, that there is no relation between volume and pharmacy mistakes. That is as illogical as saying that highway accidents occur at every speed, therefore there is no correlation between speed and auto accidents. It is like saying there should be no speed limits on highways because auto accidents occur at slow speeds as well as fast speeds. The reality is that speed kills on the highway and that speed in the pharmacy endangers the public safety.

Privately, chain management knows there's a correlation between volume and errors. But when reporters ask about such a relationship, chain management denies there is one. Using their tortured logic, we should be able to handle double, triple, or quadruple our current Rx volume without the hiring of additional techs or pharmacists.

If there were no correlation between volume and errors, why don't the chains expect each pharmacist to fill, say, three thousand prescriptions per shift rather than, say, three hundred? Clearly the chains do recognize that there are physical limits to human production. The chains claim that those limits are much higher than pharmacists believe.

Apparently speed causes errors in every human activity except the filling of prescriptions. I would like to ask chain executives to name any human cognitive activity in which speed does not increase errors. I can't think of a single one. Do you want your dentist rushing when he's making an impression of one of your teeth for the dental lab to prepare a crown? Do you want your heart surgeon rushing when he's giving you a triple bypass? Do you want your electrician rushing when he's re-wiring your circuit breaker panel? Do you want your automobile mechanic rushing when he's working on your brakes? Do you want your accountant rushing when he's doing your taxes? Do you want your pharmacist rushing when he's checking a counter full of prescriptions filled by rookie technicians?

Some of the contestants on the TV game show *Jeopardy* come up with some really stupid answers (or, more precisely, questions). Part of the reason is that those contestants are under heavy pressure because they're on television and there are two other contestants who are trying to buzz in first. Likewise, pharmacists are under tremendous pressure from customers and corporate management to fill prescriptions quickly. But somehow, according to chain management, being overwhelmed with prescriptions does not increase the occurrence of errors. Pharmacy is unique among human activities in that speed does not increase the occurrence of errors.

You've all heard that HASTE MAKES WASTE. Supposedly, this old dictum applies to every human activity except the filling of prescriptions. In the view of chain executives, HASTE MAKES MONEY.

42
When efficiency is all that matters

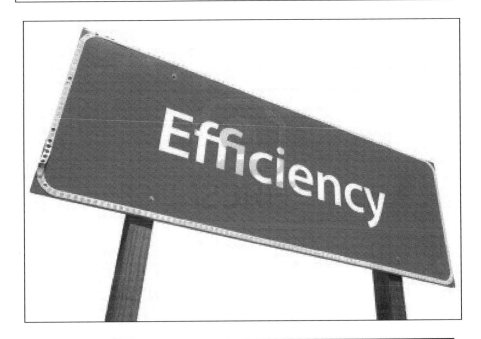

Efficiency and Productivity
Today's marketplace is ruled by survival of the fittest. It's time to get faster, leaner, smarter and more agile.

When I was in college, I used to think "efficiency" was an un-equivocal good. I was attracted by the chain drugstore model because I bought into the concept that chain drugstores are efficient. Even though I am often critical of chain drugstores today, I admit that they try hard to cut their unit cost for filling each prescription.

The chains enthusiastically embrace the latest technology to improve efficiency. When I first graduated, pharmacists had to write the Rx order each week by hand into a bulky order book. Later, the introduction of the Telxon allowed us to punch the product order number into this hand-held device. More recently, automatic replenishment freed pharmacists from the time-consuming and deadening task of eyeballing each product on our shelves on a weekly basis.

In the past, all the clerks in the drugstore punched time cards upon starting their shift, when leaving for lunch/dinner breaks or 15-minute breaks, when returning from those breaks, and when their shift was over. I vividly remember the extremely boring and laborious task of calculating each employee's time card into tenths of an hour each day. Now, each clerk simply punches his or her employee number into the high-tech cash register which doubles as a computer in automatically adding up each clerk's hours.

These advances in technology undoubtedly help the pharmacist. But technology can have a downside. Many pharmacy computers now have the ability to transmit data to our bosses about our speed and efficiency in filling prescriptions.

Many pharmacists feel that the chains care more about their technology than their employees. Pharmacists have been told routinely that improvements in technology will allow us more time to spend with customers. This has always been a bald-faced lie. The fundamental reason for the chains introducing the latest technology is to cut staffing. Staffing levels are cut commensurate with each technological advance.

Efficiency is what the chain drugstore is all about. The chain concept is meant to facilitate economies of scale. Mass purchasing of products allows lower unit costs. Chainwide computerization means that stores can be run more efficiently. In contrast, the basis for the independent drugstore is customer service. The chains want the public to think that we offer customer service that's as good as independents, but that is very often not the case. I've had bosses who ridicule pharmacists (behind those pharmacists' backs) for spending too much time talking with customers. The chains say they want us to speak with customers, but most pharmacists realize quickly that the chains don't really mean it. For example, the chains have always viewed patient counseling as a major drag on productivity that adds nothing to the bottom line.

The narrow focus on efficiency in chain drugstores comes at a huge cost to customers, to employees, and to society. Equating health with the efficient delivery of products comes at a tremendous cost that the big chains don't want to discuss. Search Google for "pharmacy mistakes" for one illustration of the many costs of placing speed and efficiency above everything else. Many pharmacists feel that the chains have made the cold calculation that it is more profitable to sling out prescriptions at lightning speed and pay any customers harmed by mistakes, rather than provide adequate staffing chainwide so that mistakes are a rarity rather than a predictable occurrence. I'd love to see a study that compares the per store error rate at chain drugstores versus independents.

When efficiency is all that matters in a business, the employees are viewed as machines rather than as human beings. Management at the big chains is endlessly disappointed that they are not able to remake the genomes of store employees so that those employees are robots. Pharmacists should realize that if the chains figure out a way to completely automate the pharmacy, we would be toast overnight.

When efficiency is all that matters, employees see that chain management views us only as a necessary evil to be barely tolerated until the chain can figure out a way to automate our jobs. Store employees resent not being treated as human beings, so they take out their resentment on our customers. If chain management doesn't care about us as human beings, why should we care about customers as human beings? Thus rudeness toward customers is not surprising in the chain drugstore model.

The narrow focus on efficiency in the drugstore has costs far beyond that of disillusioned store employees. Pharmacists know that we don't have time to do much more than throw a few words at our customers. Our customers end up not understanding their medications. Our society pays a heavy price for this assembly-line model that says that human health is directly proportional to the per capita consumption of pharmaceuticals. Our entire health care system is based on quantity rather than quality. In this model of health care, the concept of prevention becomes a quaint dream of the distant past. Americans remain ignorant of the non-pharmacological determinants of human health. This model based on efficiency promotes a quick-fix pill for every ill rather than a fundamental understanding of those lifestyle choices than can have a profound effect on one's health.

Very often, the pharmacy staff doesn't care enough to cultivate good relationships with local doctors and the receptionists who phone in prescriptions. I've seen floater pharmacists who are very rude to customers and doctors/receptionists because these floaters feel they'll just be working in that store for a day or two. So why care if customers, receptionists, and doctors are angered by the pharmacist's attitude? Many pharmacists feel that making customers angry is fine because we have too many customers to handle now with the ridiculous staffing levels.

The chains spend huge sums on marketing to attract customers into our stores. Too often, customers arrive to discover bright shiny new stores complete with two-lane drive-thru windows and...Guess what?...deeply discontented employees. These employees, in effect, spend their time discarding those customers brought in by the chain's marketing. A pharmacist once commented to me that the best place to locate an independent is beside a chain because the chain will draw people to that location with advertising and then the independent can thrive off all the unhappy customers discarded by the unhappy workers at the big chains.

I've seen so many instances in which the chains had to pay pharmacists time-and-a-half overtime because the chains can't keep pharmacists. The chains are forced into bidding wars to attract pharmacists who, very often, don't want any part of the reckless game known as chain pharmacy. From my perspective, the chains end up paying much more in labor costs than if they had just treated their pharmacists well to start with.

I don't know if I'm unique but many times I would have happily forgone a pay raise in favor of an increase in tech staffing. I don't think that increased salaries for pharmacists can make up for miserable tech staffing levels. Many pharmacists have felt that there has never been a true national shortage of pharmacists, just a shortage of pharmacists willing to work in the chains' dangerously understaffed pharmacies. Do the chains not care that a large number of their pharmacists are questioning why they chose pharmacy as a career?

I have often wondered how this model of routinely burning out pharmacists and training new ones can be profitable. The chains would rather keep hiring young eager graduates who are willing to work at unsafe speeds, burning them out, and endlessly repeating this cycle. Apparently this is more profitable than keeping existing pharmacists happy. It doesn't take long for pharmacists to realize that the pace is not compatible with his or her mental or physical health. From the chains' perspective, I assume this high turnover in pharmacists dramatically cuts down on pension responsibilities (assuming the company provides a pension).

When the chain I worked for was bought out by another large chain, most of the best pharmacists ended up going elsewhere. In my opinion, the new pharmacists who were hired to replace these veteran pharmacists were, very often, of a lower caliber (less professional, less customer-friendly) than the ones they replaced. As working conditions became more unbearable and the best pharmacists left, I found my bosses hiring pharmacists who never would have been hired in the past.

43

Customers often overhear pharmacists and technicians discussing private information

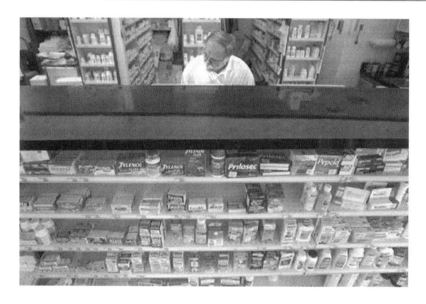

There is considerable disagreement among the various drug-store chains regarding how accessible the pharmacist should be to the public. Some chains construct the pharmacy so that the pharmacist is easily accessible for questions, recommendations for non-prescription products, etc. Customers routinely ask the pharmacist questions like:

What do you recommend for a cold?
What's the strongest thing you have to knock out this cough?

I don't have any energy. Can you recommend a vitamin?
What aisle is the motor oil on?
Do you have a restroom I can use?
Do you have any diapers in the stockroom? You're out of the ones I usually get.

Other chains feel that having the pharmacist so easily accessible slows down prescription filling. I doubt that the chains would admit it publicly but I think they probably would privately agree that constant interruptions from customers increase the occurrence of pharmacy mistakes. I once read a commentary by a pharmacist who said that if the chains expect pharmacists to work in high volume stores, management needs to get the pharmacist away from the public, i.e., the pharmacy should be constructed so that the pharmacist can't be interrupted by customers every fifteen seconds.

With federal HIPAA regulations, there's a great deal of concern over privacy in health care today, but spending a few minutes hovering near the pharmacy can reveal a lot of private information. Many pharmacies have a glass partition of some type separating the pharmacist from the public. In most of these pharmacies, there is often a consultation area, sometimes off to a side. But if there are three or four people standing in line waiting to speak to the pharmacist in the consultation area, those people can sometimes get an earful of private information listening in on the conversation between the pharmacist and the person at the head of the line.

Here's a common scenario: In many drugstores, the vitamins are shelved directly in front of the pharmacy, not by coincidence but by design. This allows pharmacists to answer customers' questions about vitamins and to make specific recommendations. In those stores where there's no partition between the pharmacy staff and the public, you could—if you were so inclined—spend a few minutes hovering around the vitamin section (or whatever products happen to be in front of the pharmacy). You might hear a lot of information that is private. You could hear pharmacists calling doctors offices to clarify poorly legible prescriptions. You might hear a pharmacist on the phone to a doctor's office saying, "I have a prescription here for Bob Smith. It looks like Viagra [for erectile dysfunction] but I just wanted to make sure." Or you could hear a pharmacist asking, "I have a prescription here for Mary Jones. It looks like either Prozac [antidepressant] or Prilosec [acid reducer]." Or you could hear the pharmacist saying, "Can we refill John Smith's Detrol LA [for bladder control]?" Listening in on pharmacists' phone conversations with doctors' offices might reveal that one of your neighbors has a yeast infection or herpes or that he/she takes pills for anxiety, depression, insomnia, etc. Equally disturbing is the possibility that you might overhear conversations between two young technicians talking about their boyfriends while filling your prescriptions. You ask yourself, *Shouldn't they be concentrating on my prescriptions rather than talking about their boyfriends?*

I filled in occasionally at one chain drugstore in Henderson, North Carolina, in which the pharmacy was specifically designed so that the pharmacist would be very easily accessible to speak with customers. It was an unusual triangular-shaped design in which the pharmacy actually juts out toward the sales floor. Customers could stand four feet away from me the entire time I was working on their prescriptions and they could easily observe me counting their pills if they so desired. There was no partition of any type between me and the customers. On one particular day, the pharmacy was terribly understaffed. It was only me and one technician who I would describe as a real scatter-brain. We were running far behind and things were extremely stressful. At one point, this tech said to me in a normal speaking voice, "I don't know if I'm coming or going." Comments like this between pharmacy staff are not that unusual. But what was unusual about this was that, as best as I can recall, there were perhaps seven or eight customers within fifteen feet of us, and perhaps three or four of them were within five feet. Judging by the expression on the face of one nearby customer, I am absolutely certain that she heard this tech's comment. This customer appeared quite concerned to hear what this tech said to me. The customer had every right to be concerned because the stress level in the pharmacy was incredible, a perfect opportunity for a mistake. Of course, I tried to act like I hadn't heard anything unusual, but in reality I wanted to strangle that tech for speaking loud enough for (at least) one customer to hear.

44

Do chain pharmacists fill prescriptions for "patients" or "customers"?

There are several politically correct terms in pharmacy.

Allow me to make the case for you that, in the real world, it is pretentious for chain pharmacists to refer to our clientele as "patients." Allow me to also make the case that the term "patients" is becoming less accurate for physicians' clientele as well.

You can tell a lot about a pharmacist by noting whether he or she uses the word "customers" or "patients." In my experience, the overwhelming majority of chain pharmacists refer to our clientele as "customers." Indeed, whenever a chain pharmacist refers to them as "patients," other pharmacists and techs are likely to roll their eyes or feel like doing so.

Can you imagine your district supervisor referring to your customers as your "patients"? Can you imagine one of your techs saying something like "We have six patients waiting"? Almost every tech I know refers to our clientele as "customers." Among pharmacists who actually work in chain drugstores, the term "patient" is used only when referring to a doctor's patient (e.g., "Dr. Smith's patient").

Many chain pharmacists feel it is pretentious for us to refer to our clientele as "patients." These pharmacists feel that since we don't even have time for meal or bathroom breaks, it is more accurate and honest to refer to our clientele as "customers." The term "patients" may represent the goals and aspirations of many pharmacists for our profession. Thus "patients" is the more politically correct term today. But many chain pharmacists feel strongly that we will never be able to change this profession unless we stop kidding ourselves about reality. Many chain pharmacists feel that our colleagues who use the word "patients" are living in a dream world and are thus incapable of recognizing the need to stand up to corporate bean counters and fight for better working conditions and staffing levels.

In my opinion, when chain pharmacists have bosses who only care about how fast we fill prescriptions, when we have customers honking their horns at the drive-thru window, when we have computer metrics that determine how fast we finish prescriptions, when we have corporate bosses who have complete disdain for pharmacists who spend too much time advising customers, when we're on hold endlessly with doctors' offices and insurance companies, when we have to sling out prescriptions at lightning speed because we don't have enough warm bodies in the pharmacy, when we eat lunch and dinner standing up, when we almost have to plead (to no avail) for adequate tech staffing, etc., etc., how can we honestly refer to our clientele as "patients"? In my opinion, chain pharmacy is strictly a business wherein cost-cutting is the core guiding principle.

With physicians now under intense pressure to see more patients in less time, the term "patients" is becoming less accurate for physicians' relationships with their clientele as well. Our health care system is pushing physicians away from a "doctor-patient" relationship to one that might more realistically be called a "doctor-client relationship," wherein some huge corporate entity controls so much of what a physician does that his autonomy is threatened along with his professional judgment and standing.

For example, if insurance companies push physicians to recommend an antidepressant medication for policyholders rather than talk therapy with a psychologist (because pills are less expensive than long-term talk therapy), do such physicians deserve to be called "doctors," or are they more like agents for the insurance company? Many pharmacists feel that we are unpaid agents for the many insurance companies to which we bill prescriptions.

A health professional who puts "Dr." in front of his name is expected to place the best interests of his/her clientele ahead of his/her own financial interests. But, like Wall Street, too many physicians are motivated by greed and therefore do not deserve to refer to their clientele as "patients."

With more and more health professionals losing personal autonomy and becoming mere cogs on some huge corporate wheel, employee physicians are often scrutinized by MBAs using production metrics (e.g., number of patients seen per hour) that are in many ways analogous to production metrics used by chains to evaluate pharmacists (e.g., number of prescriptions filled per hour).

When the relationship between pharmacists and our clientele is primarily economic, the word "customer" seems to be more appropriate. Since pharmacists don't have nearly enough staffing in the pharmacy to allow us to spend much time with our clientele, are we being honest with ourselves in referring to them as "patients"? If we don't have enough time for a meal or bathroom break, are we being pompous in claiming that our relationship with this clientele is primarily educational or "clinical" rather than mercantile?

Some PharmD's insist that they be referred to as "Doctor." If you don't have time to go to the bathroom, do you feel like a "Doctor"? If your employer has utter disdain for the PharmD degree (preferring, instead, BS pharmacists or techs or robotics), are you being honest with yourself in insisting that people address you as "Doctor"? If your primary relationship with your clientele is mercantile, should you be called "Doctor"? Similarly, if you work at the pharmacy version of McDonald's (complete with a drive-thru window), do you "practice" pharmacy, or do you "practice" fast food? For many pharmacists who feel they work at the pharmacy equivalent of McDonald's, the term "pharmacy practice" is laughable.

Pharmacy chains, like many other businesses, have elevated the titles of employees without necessarily elevating the pay. For example, employees who were formerly called "clerks" may enjoy the fact that their corporate bosses now refer to them as "sales associates." I refer to this as "job title inflation" in lieu of a pay increase.

Which term is more honest for our clientele in the real world of chain pharmacy today: "customers" or "patients"? Do you feel that the term "patient" implies a passive/subservient/dependent recipient of medical care, rather than someone who is fully engaged in the decision-making process?

Patients?

Customers?

Which term is more honest for chain drugstore clientele?

45

The McDonald's-ization of pharmacy

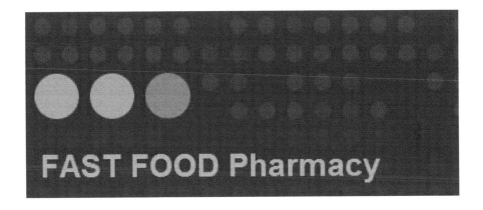

FAST FOOD Pharmacy

Speed may be the core concept that describes chain pharmacy today, just as speed is the core concept that describes fast food franchises like McDonald's, Burger King and Wendy's. Chain pharmacy is based on high volume. High volume and understaffing dictate that employees work at breakneck pace.

Countless times throughout my career, I've worked with pharmacists in their sixties or early seventies and I've felt sad that, after a long career, these pharmacists are still forced to run around the pharmacy like young graduates still in their physical prime. I'm sad when I see these older pharmacists racing back and forth between the pharmacy shelves, then back to the computer, then over to the cash register, then back to answer the phone, then over to the drive-thru window, then back to the register to counsel a customer, then up to the manager's office to get change for the register, then back to check an Rx filled by a tech, then over to a corner of the pharmacy to take a quick bite of a sandwich without customers watching. Many of these steps are repeated 100 to 200 times a day.

It is very sad to see a pharmacist at any age engaging in race-track pharmacy, but it is extra sad to see pharmacists in their sixties or early seventies being forced to run around the pharmacy with the same speed and stamina as a pharmacist 40 years younger. I feel it is demeaning to these older pharmacists. Countless times I ask myself if that's what I want my life to look like when I'm that age.

Unlike many professions in which mastery of the pertinent skills makes one's job easier each year, the pharmacist's job actually becomes more grinding and exhausting as he gets older. That is because the pharmacist's job today primarily utilizes his hands and feet rather than his drug knowledge.

Recent graduates are very happy to be out of school and they're very happy to be earning a nice paycheck, so they're usually quite willing to put up with this pace. After a few years, many of them begin to question how much longer they can maintain that pace. That's why many pharmacists question whether there was indeed ever a true shortage of pharmacists in America, or simply a shortage of pharmacists willing to work at full throttle all day, every day, under meat-grinder conditions. The big chains have been notorious for squeezing blood out of young naive pharmacists, burning them out, and then claiming there was a shortage of pharmacists, for which the big chains had only themselves to blame.

I'd like to ask pharmacists: How long will you be able to maintain your current pace before you find yourself totally burned out? Or is it actually possible that you will find fulfillment in your career by aspiring to enter the ranks of the fastest pharmacists in America? Did you major in pharmacy so that you can prove to the world that you have what it takes to be a fast pharmacist? When you describe your job to your spouse or parents, do you say that speed is the most important factor in your job?

There are possibly three characteristics that are most commonly used to describe pharmacists:

1. The pharmacist has a good rapport with customers and co-workers.
2. The pharmacist is knowledgeable about drugs.
3. The pharmacist fills prescriptions quickly.

From my experience, of these three traits, the big chains unquestionably place the highest value on the third quality: *fills prescriptions quickly*.

In pharmacy school, I felt that my drug knowledge would surely be my biggest asset in my career. In the real world, I discovered that, far more important than my drug knowledge is the speed with which I fill prescriptions. Fast pharmacists are held in high esteem by co-workers, supervisors, and customers. Supervisors ridicule slow pharmacists behind their back. Pharmacists who spend too much time counseling customers, obsessing over drug interactions, and double-checking prescriptions are held in especially low esteem by management. Pharmacists are viewed by management like production workers at a General Motors assembly plant.

One pharmacist wrote a letter to *Drug Topics* describing how some chains monitor pharmacists' speed (Kern Stafford, "Racing the red light," *Drug Topics*, Sept. 1, 2003, p. 16):

...the pharmacist must check literally hundreds of prescriptions on each shift. To slow down will mean, in some chains, a red light showing on the computer screen signifying a pharmacist is behind in checking. This red light affects his bonus and invariably brings the area managers and district managers down on him. If a student really wants to go to pharmacy school for eight years, get that Pharm.D. degree, and then stand in one spot racing the red light with hundreds of prescriptions coming off the conveyor belt, good for him. The money is good, $85,000 and more in some places. But what about the health of the consumer, the drug interactions that are ignored, all in the name of speed?....

The big chains carry out "time and motion" studies to make the pharmacy run more efficiently. The big chains regret that they are not able to re-engineer the genome of pharmacists to make us faster, more accurate, and more efficient like a machine. The suits at the big chains lose sleep over the terrifying thought that a pharmacist somewhere in the chain is actually caught up. If a pharmacist is caught up, that is a sign tech staffing needs to be cut, yet again.

Pharmacists complain that the speed with which we're forced to fill prescriptions endangers the safety of our customers. Our supervisors tell us that more errors occur when the pharmacy is slow because our attention wanders. That is like saying speeding on an icy road is good because the inherent danger forces us to pay attention.

New technology is supposed to make the pharmacist's job easier but it seems that the pace in the pharmacy worsens every year. Pharmacy technology has indeed made the pharmacist's job easier in some ways. Counting machines (pill counters) make the counting of pills less onerous and time consuming. Pharmacy computers are great for "filling and billing" functions. Computerized automatic replenishment of drugs means the pharmacist doesn't have to spend an hour or two each week eyeballing every product on his shelves for the weekly warehouse order. Another innovation is the automatic calculation of the hours that techs and clerks work. Pharmacists no longer have to add up, with a calculator, the hours on each employee's time card at the end of the week. There are many examples of labor-saving and time-saving technology in the pharmacy. The logical question is "Why doesn't the introduction of new technology in the pharmacy make the pharmacy a more relaxed place?" The answer: With each new labor-saving technology, staffing is cut proportionately to the amount of labor that the innovation saves.

Compounding the problem of speed in the drugstore is the widespread expectation among customers for a quick fix for every ill. Customers are not interested in significant discussions about ways they can prevent their condition, nor do pharmacists have the time (or, in many cases, the desire) to engage in such conversations. With the commodification of health in this country, customers have come to believe that the solution to whatever ails them is simply a matter of finding the "right" product. If pharmacies are simply about the distribution of products, can we blame our customers for placing so much importance on the speed with which we provide those products? In this view of pharmacy, prescription drugs are a commodity just like toothpaste, shampoo, and deodorant. In reality, prescription drugs are powerful substances that can cause serious problems if not used carefully.

It is no longer possible to become a pharmacist with a bachelor's degree in pharmacy (B. S. Pharm). All the pharmacy schools now require a doctorate (Pharm. D.) to become a pharmacist. This illustrates the absurdity in pharmacy today. The people who are graduating from pharmacy schools now are armed with more education than pharmacists in the past. But the movement in this country is away from face-to-face contact with pharmacists. Even though all the newly-graduating pharmacists now have doctorates, the big drugstore chains don't like the idea of pharmacists spending time talking to customers because it slows down production. And the big insurance companies are pushing people to have prescriptions filled at distant mail order facilities where the only contact with a pharmacist is via a toll-free phone number. The pharmacy schools are promoting the idea of the pharmacist as drug advisor. The marketplace, however, has not embraced this role for pharmacists. The marketplace is forcing pharmacy and pharmacists into the fast food model which views the pharmacist's advice as unnecessary or a luxury that the system can't afford.

A few years back, Merriam-Webster added the term "McJob" to one of its dictionary revisions. I recall reading a news story that noted McDonald's wasn't too happy with this addition. Many pharmacists refer to our workplace as McPharmacy. One pharmacist sent me an e-mail in response to one of my *Drug Topics* editorials. He wrote simply: "Pharmacist for 38 years: 13 in hospital pharmacy, 14 as store owner, 11 in chain pharmacy. Our profession in the chain pharmacy setting has deteriorated to what I refer to as 'McPharmacy.' Need I write more?"

A third-year pharmacy student wrote to me:

It's so funny that you are comparing pharmacy to fast food. Maybe I'm a little out of the loop here, and maybe this comparison has been made by others but I haven't heard it yet. I thought I was the only one who saw such a similarity between the two. Last week, I went inside the local In & Out. It was the first time I had been in a fast food joint in a long time. While I was waiting for my order, I watched the workers do their thing and I started to get a bit of anxiety, as it seemed all too familiar, despite the fact that I had never ever worked fast-food before. And then of course it hit me. It reminds me of work at the pharmacy. The fast pace, the long lines, the hierarchy, the audience watching and waiting for their order, the drive through!!! I went home and told my mom that I'm nothing but a glorified fast food clerk. Sometimes I'm even the cook (we do compounding at our pharmacy and the standards we use really suck, just like at a fast food place). You are so right about the fast food model and I'm so glad someone with your experience and background sees it that way too. I thought I was going nuts. I feel better now.

Even though the comparison to McDonald's is made constantly in the retail setting, some of our colleagues are angered by this analogy. This analogy often seems to be strongly frowned upon by pharmacists who don't actually toil on the front lines. Among some pharmacists in supervisory, administrative, or executive positions, discussions of working conditions are avoided the way some parents avoid discussing sex with their kids: pretend it doesn't exist. The pharmacy schools, pharmacy boards, and pharmacy associations often consider the McDonald's analogy to be too negative, too cynical, too divisive. Some pharmacists say that the term "McPharmacy" disrespects and trivializes pharmacy. The schools, boards, and associations avoid discussing working conditions because if these groups acknowledged the problem, they would be viewed as wimps for not trying to do something to remedy the situation. These pharmacists with jobs other than dispensing often have a vested interest in downplaying complaints about working conditions voiced by pharmacists on the front lines. These pharmacists do whatever they can to protect their current position so that they can stay away from the hyperstressful environment in drugstores where pharmacists fill prescriptions as fast as their hands and feet will allow. The pharmacists with jobs other than dispensing often seem to have a callous attitude toward their disillusioned colleagues in drugstores, feeling that being positive is more important than being frank: "Stop whining!" "Find another job!" "Don't renew your license!" "Leave the profession!"

Drug Topics occasionally publishes letters from disgruntled pharmacists. The magazine also publishes letters from pharmacists who write something like, "I'm tired of reading letters in *Drug Topics* written by pharmacists who are unhappy! These pharmacists need to do more than complain! They need to find a job with a different employer or leave the profession."

Should pharmacists on the front lines of pharmacy be castigated for using the McDonald's analogy? Should our colleagues who are offended by this analogy bully pharmacy magazine editors into avoiding references to fast food? In my opinion, the pharmacists who would like to prohibit use of the McDonald's analogy prefer a Pollyanna view of pharmacy. They seem to prefer to gloss over the fact that many of our colleagues are genuinely disillusioned with the big drugstore chains. The critics of the fast food analogy strike me as callously unconcerned about their colleagues who, in many cases, are wondering why they ever chose pharmacy.

Despite salaries of close to $100,000 per year directly out of pharmacy school, many young pharmacists are seriously questioning their career choice soon after graduation. Do the pharmacists who are happy with their jobs have a right to silence their disillusioned colleagues? One pharmacist wrote to me, "I cried twice last week. My job is eating me alive." Is it callous for us to suggest that this pharmacist simply discard her years of schooling and leave the profession?

The fast food model makes the practice of pharmacy nothing like the profession pharmacists hoped they were entering. Pharmacists are trained in pharmacy school to be drug experts but the big chains don't want any part of that. Working for the big chains is a production job, just like so many others in the manufacturing sector of our society. Pharmacists are valued for the speed with which we fill prescriptions. In contrast, many pharmacists would like to be evaluated by the quality of advice we give to customers, and how well we are able to help customers achieve a successful outcome with their medications.

The big chains, in adopting the fast food model, want to decrease counseling and decrease circumstances in which a pharmacist's judgment is necessary. Many pharmacists working for the big chains know that their bosses have utter disdain for pharmacists who spend too much time counseling customers.

McDonald's serves fast food. In my opinion, compared to mom's home cookin', McDonald's food isn't really that tasty. It has what can perhaps be referred to as a mass-produced quality and taste. But I suppose McDonald's food can indeed be loosely defined as "food." Similarly, drugstores sling out prescriptions at an incredible pace. Yes, we get the right drug to the right customer most of the time. But few pharmacists would say that we have the time to perform our job in a superior manner. We don't have enough time to counsel our customers adequately or to give adequate attention to potential drug interactions. Sometimes we're forced to take educated guesses when confronted with doctors' poor handwriting or questionable doses.

For many years, pharmacists were tired of hearing the big chains complain about a pharmacist shortage. Most pharmacists felt it was more accurate to say that there was a shortage of pharmacists willing to work in a sweatshop environment that values speed and production only. Quantity is valued much more highly than quality. Churning out prescriptions is valued much more highly than educating our customers about proper use of their medications.

Among the pharmacists I know, most of them remain only a few years, at most, with one chain and then switch to another chain in hopes that surely conditions can't be this bad throughout the industry. Many pharmacists can name several of their colleagues who have left the profession, gone part-time, or happily placed their dispensing career on hold to raise a family.

Many pharmacists resent the fact that the fast food industry doesn't seem to have a problem in providing adequate staffing for the dispensing of hamburgers, while many of the big drugstore chains are clearly unable or unwilling to provide adequate staffing for the dispensing of a far more critical product: prescription drugs.

Perhaps we can trace many of the current problems in pharmacy to the time when the fast food model was first applied to the drugstore.

In response to one of my editorials in *Drug Topics* in which I complained about the speed with which pharmacists are forced to fill prescriptions, the wife of a pharmacist wrote to me saying her husband is a "fast fill pharmacist." (I assume he must be an independent pharmacist. I don't know many spouses of chain pharmacists who would find fault with my criticism of understaffing in chains.) How can the label "fast fill pharmacist" be a description pharmacists aspire to? Does being a "fast fill pharmacist" lead to a fulfilling career? Did we enter pharmacy because we all yearn to "fill 'em faster"? Should pharmacists be proud that "speed" is one of the most important criteria used in judging us?

Pharmacy customers have two primary concerns: How much will it cost and how long will it take. Yet for each prescription that pharmacists fill, we have to check at least five absolutely critical things:

1. the right drug is being dispensed
2. the directions are correct
3. the dosage is reasonable
4. there are no drug interactions
5. the prescription is being filled under the correct customer's name.

If a pharmacist fills 200 prescriptions on his shift, he has to check at least one thousand things (200 X 5 = 1,000), an error in any of which can be disastrous.

It is true that McDonald's clerks, like pharmacists, need to be careful in filling orders, but clearly the consequences of a misfill at the drugstore are potentially a lot more serious than misfilling an order at McDonald's. If McDonald's gives someone a Big Mac instead of a cheeseburger, the customer is unlikely to sue or go to the hospital. At McDonald's, the worst thing that will probably happen is that the customer will be very rude to the clerk who made the mistake. At the drugstore, the worst thing that can happen is that our mistake kills the customer.

McDonald's is sued for ridiculous reasons like failing to warn a customer that the coffee is hot. (That was an actual lawsuit several years ago.) Pharmacists are sued for failing to warn customers about uncommon side effects of drugs, like the anti-depressant trazodone causing priapism—an unusually prolonged erection. (*Drug Topics*, May 6, 2002, p. 42).

McDonald's clerks don't have to learn strange lingo like *hs* (at bedtime), *qid* (four times a day), *pc* (after meals), *ac* (before meals), and *qd* (daily) as pharmacy technicians do. McDonald's clerks don't have the learn a huge list of long generic names in order to fill customers' orders. McDonald's employees usually find hamburgers, fish sandwiches, and Apple Turnovers nicely arranged on stainless steel shelves near the cash registers. In contrast, pharmacy technicians need to learn a long list of generic names so that they will know that cyclobenzaprine is shelved beside Flexeril, prochlorperazine is beside Compazine, doxazosin is beside Cardura, methocarbamol is beside Robaxin, etc. McDonald's has only a few dozen items on the menu, whereas the average pharmacy may have a couple thousand items in its inventory.

So, for our customers who think that drugstores are just like McDonald's (i.e., orders should be ready in less than two minutes), here is my list of reasons why your local drugstore is *not* McDonald's:

• McDonald's doesn't have to screen each order to make sure there are no duplicate therapies, inappropriate dosages, or drugs interactions.
• McDonald's does not accept insurance cards. McDonald's doesn't have to call insurance companies about rejected insurance claims.
• McDonald's doesn't have to explain to customers the fine details of insurance companies' complex tiered co-pay schedules.
• McDonald's doesn't have to deal with arrogant doctors (and their staff) or their illegible handwriting and incorrect dosages.
• McDonald's doesn't have to call doctors' offices for refill authorizations.

- McDonald's doesn't have to call answering services to track down doctors after office hours.
- McDonald's doesn't have to keep records indicating that they were only able to partially fill an order and, consequently, owe a customer, for example, 14 additional Prevacid 20mg.
- McDonald's doesn't counsel customers.
- McDonald's doesn't have orders coming in via phone, fax, and the Internet.
- McDonald's doesn't have to tell customers what foods or drinks to avoid.
- McDonald's doesn't have to tell customers what to do if a dose is missed.
- McDonald's doesn't have to tell customers about side effects, contraindications, precautions, warnings, and potential drug interactions. McDonald's doesn't have to ask customers if they are allergic to penicillin. McDonald's doesn't have to warn pregnant women about the use of certain products.
- McDonald's doesn't have to show customers how to measure 0.5 ml on a dropper or the proper technique for instilling eye drops.
- Whereas McDonald's can just scoop a bunch of french fries into a cardboard container, pharmacists and techs need to count pills precisely. Each french fry is worth one or two cents; in contrast, pharmacists often handle pills than cost several dollars each.

The chain drugstore environment is certainly not conducive to viewpoints that question pharmaceuticals. The typical chain drugstore is highly regimented and requires strict adherence to corporate rules. The modern drug chain is tightly controlled to the point of being nearly coercive. It is in such an environment that nonconformist ideas are highly frowned upon. Our job is to fill prescriptions as quickly as we can and not to question whether nondrug approaches may be more logical.

I can understand that corporations need conformity, efficiency, discipline, and a willingness by employees to work hard. I'm all in favor of efficiency and hard work and discipline. I realize that corporations need conformity if they are to avoid total chaos. But chain drugstores are run on the McDonald's, Burger King, and

Wendy's models. Time and motion studies are done to maximize productivity. All this may serve to make the drug chain more competitive and allow us to sell drugs at a lower price (independent drugstores do, however, often beat the chains' prices). But the consequence of rigid conformity in procedures is a rigid conformity in ideas.

As the huge insurance companies dictate the nature of our medical system, pharmacists are forced to process more customers in less time. This results in resentment by pharmacists toward the system. Customers are viewed as the problem. More customers means more workload, yet staffing always lags far behind workload.

The system is absolutely draining pharmacists of compassion. If we're running behind all day, each customer who approaches the pharmacy is only making the situation worse. Many pharmacists hope that business will not increase (blasphemous thoughts to the corporation) because an increase means that we will have to do more work with little or no increase in staffing.

As you approach the pharmacy, many pharmacists think: *Here comes another customer to get me even further behind.* Customers become the enemy because they rush us when we're already stressed to the breaking point. Even though there may be only few customers waiting near the pharmacy counter at a given time, this doesn't mean that the pharmacist isn't running an hour or two behind with a backlog of prescriptions that customers will be returning to pick up.

I once saw a sign in a restaurant that reminded me of my job: "Waitresses are like swans—calm and collected on the surface but paddling like hell underneath." We pharmacists paddle like hell to keep up with the prescription flow. The system is absolutely turning pharmacists into automatons. Pharmacy has become an endurance contest to see whether we can make it through the day without getting drowned by the prescription flow and without losing control of our emotions.

Pharmacist Bob Crocker from Farmville, North Carolina, ran for a seat on the North Carolina Board of Pharmacy in June of 1995. I received a postcard from him in the mail seeking support for his candidacy. He made several observations about pharmacists' working conditions. His observations about working conditions are as relevant today as they were in 1995.

Fellow Retail Pharmacist

I called a fellow pharmacist a few weeks ago and asked if he could meet me for lunch. He informed me he didn't get a scheduled lunch break and didn't have enough help to leave the pharmacy for even a few minutes. I thought to myself "even galley slaves get a lunch break." I don't know if this situation is the "exception" or the "norm" – but it should be the EXCEPTION!

I have heard from numerous sources that the [North Carolina Board of Pharmacy] has received several letters complaining of dangerous work conditions and asking for help in remedying the situation. To me it is unconscionable to set legal requirements for a professional and not provide him the ability to control his work environment to meet those requirements.

IT IS TIME FOR A CHANGE. Retail pharmacists need someone on the Board who knows what they face on a daily basis. I can be that person. I am a "working" retail pharmacist with both chain & independent experience.

Here's a typical letter to the editor that pharmacists find routinely in the pharmacy magazines. Sometimes pharmacists are brave enough to sign the letters even though we fear that our employer may see them in the magazines. Obviously the big chains would like to keep descriptions of pathetic and dangerous working conditions out of the pages of national pharmacy magazines. The following letter was published as "Name withheld by request." ("Burned-Out Pharmacist," *American Druggist*, May 1995, p. 8)

If honest want ads were run by discount store chains and chain drug stores, here is how they would read: Our pharmacists must be able to—
1. Work 10 hours a day without a break.
2. Answer the phone in three rings while ringing up sales, helping customers, and filling prescriptions.
3. Fill 150 to 250 prescriptions daily, one every three minutes.

4. Control bodily functions in order to limit bathroom breaks to one or two a day.
5. Deal with young, immature assistants who are jealous of your wages.
6. Take constant abuse from customers, store managers, and associates with a smile.

This mess has come about only in the last 10 years. Bottom lines and store traffic should not obliterate patient care. It's time to speak up for the profession. Everyone must protest these conditions. The companies cannot retaliate against us all.

Upon graduation from pharmacy school, young pharmacists very often suffer severe culture shock when they experience the real world of the chain drugstore. Professors in pharmacy schools prepare students to be highly-trained drug experts but the big chain drugstores don't want drug experts. The big chains want fast food experts. I think the pharmacy schools should practice "truth in advertising" by discussing with students what pharmacy is like in the real world. Over the years, I have heard several pharmacists suggest that a class-action lawsuit should be initiated against pharmacy schools for grossly misrepresenting the real world.

What kinds of pharmacists are most likely to have long-term survival in the chain environment? I have concluded that pharmacists with an "attitude" and a thick skin are the ones who are best able to tolerate their jobs. If you are too compassionate, you will soon be run over by rude and impatient customers. A warm and caring pharmacist in a busy chain drug store will soon be mowed down by a clientele that is too often arrogant, aggressive, and abusive.

The fast food model is the only one that works in a typical understaffed pharmacy. Pharmacists often refer to our job as "herding the masses." The education-prevention-caring-listening model simply doesn't work at McPharmacy. If we pharmacists spend too much time giving advice to customers, we're causing the herd to bottleneck. Rudeness increases the speed of herding customers. The friendlier I am to customers, the more they want to tell me their life story or at least their medical history. Countless times people tell me that their spouse is recovering from a heart attack or from bypass surgery or from cancer and all I have time to do is simulate a facial expression that I care. In reality, the speed of the prescription assembly line has drummed out most of my compassion. If I have customers making faces at me all day implying that I'm too slow, how much compassion do you think I have left to sympathize with their health problems? I think many of my colleagues would agree that chain pharmacy can destroy a pharmacist's empathy.

I once spoke with a pharmacist who had just graduated from pharmacy school and was licensed for only about a week. Not surprisingly, he was having trouble entering cardholder information into the pharmacy computer for customers with various prescription insurance plans. Many insurance companies have some unique little quirk with cardholder information that makes pharmacists' lives miserable. This pharmacist told me that he had just made an observation about crowd control. He said that there can be several customers waiting calmly and patiently for their prescriptions. Then, all of a sudden, one customer makes some jackass comment about having to wait too long. Hearing this rude comment, all the other customers collectively become agitated and seem to adopt a herd mentality such as: "Yeah! You pharmacist son-of-a-bitch who is part of the price-gouging drug conspiracy in America. HOW MUCH LONGER IS IT GOING TO BE!!!???" He told me that one of his classmates had experienced the same feeling and that this classmate announced to those waiting at that store, "Now wait just a minute! This isn't Burger King! You'll get your prescription when it's ready!" Throughout this book, it may appear that I repeat the hamburger and fast-food metaphor excessively, but that is only because pharmacists routinely use it to describe our very stressful jobs.

I need to have an attitude if I want to be able to herd customers efficiently and if I want to avoid being run over by an impatient public. It is a fact that the friendlier I am with customers, the more likely that they are to want to talk. And the more likely they are to ask me a question for which I don't know the answer. So then I'd have to take more time to consult reference material. If I'm just barely cordial and very business-like, customers are less likely to set me back with long, involved questions.

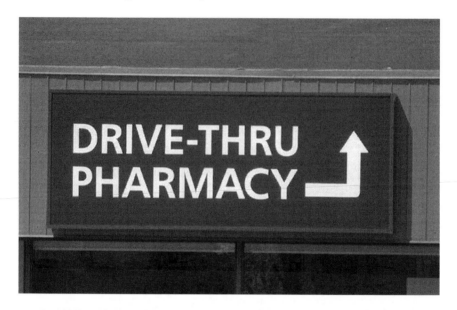

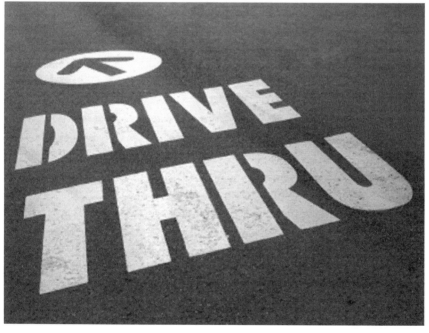

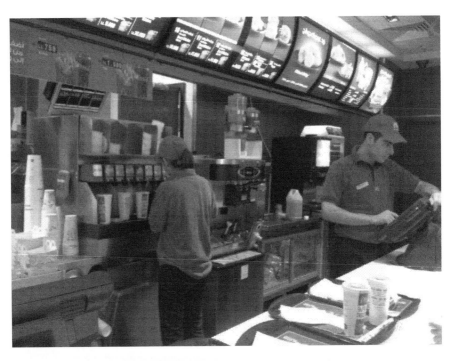

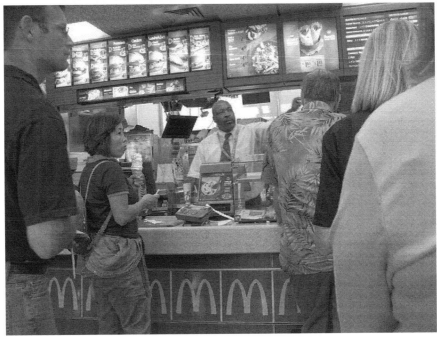

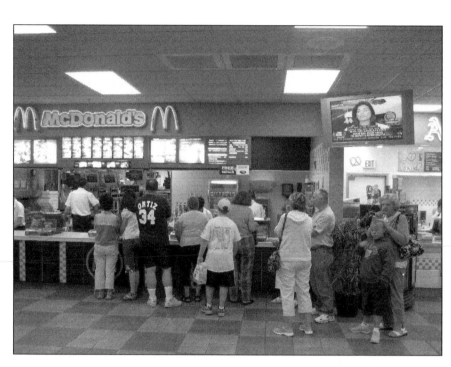

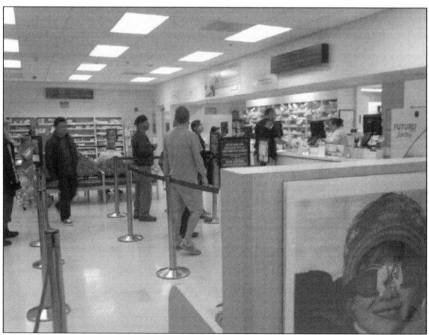

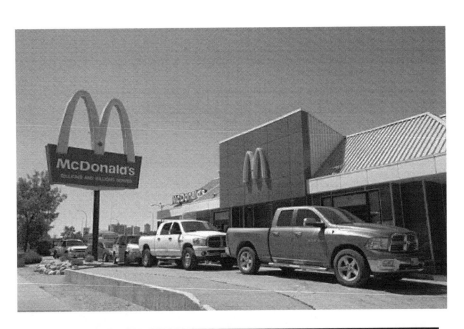

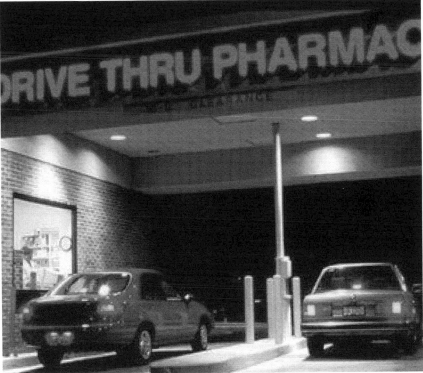

46

Why chain pharmacists hate drive-thru windows

The profession has itself to blame, at least partly, for the culture of speed at the drugstore. With the widespread use of drive-thru windows at pharmacies, we have convinced our customers that prescription drugs are like hamburgers, i.e., the final product should be ready within a couple of minutes. Not surprisingly, the number one question that customers ask us is "How long will it take?" Customers wonder why it should take more than a couple of minutes to fill a prescription for birth control pills since the pills are already in the packet, or a prescription for a skin condition since the cream is already in the tube.

Most chain pharmacists feel passionately about the subject of pharmacy drive-thru windows. In my experience, nearly all chain pharmacists hate the drive-thru since we don't have nearly enough staffing to handle it. People drive up and ask the pharmacist to get them a pack of cigarettes or a roll of film while we've got five to ten people inside staring at us, waiting for us to fill their prescriptions. In total disgust, one pharmacist said to me, "I'm going to start asking them if they want fries, too!" When she was finally transferred to a store without a drive-thru window, she said to me, "You wouldn't believe how happy I was to lock that drive-thru window the night of my last day at that store."

One day I asked a floater pharmacist whom I've known for several years whether he had ever worked in one of the newer stand-alone stores. (A floater pharmacist is one who does not have an as-signed store. He fills in wherever he's needed for vacations, sick days, etc.) These stand-alone stores are not part of a strip shopping center as are most of the stores in the chain I work for. He said that he had no desire to do that because he doesn't like "working at Har-dee's." (Hardee's is a fast-food chain specializing in roast beef sand-wiches.) He said that all these new stand-alone stores have drive-thru windows and that he absolutely hates drive-thru windows.

All the pharmacists I know who have worked at a store with a drive-thru window feel that they're absurd because they increase the already present danger of a mistake in a hyperstressful work en-vironment. Most pharmacists also seem to feel that drive-thru win-dows are demeaning to pharmacy because the drive-thru windows imply that prescriptions are analogous to fast food. The drive-thru window reinforces customers' views that lightning-quick prescrip-tion service is reasonable.

Pharmacists today are trying to convince the public that we do far more than simply dispense drugs. We are available to answer your questions and to advise you on the optimal use of your medi-cations. Pharmacists are very worried about the rapid growth of mail order pharmacy facilities. Pharmacists fear that customers will be satisfied receiving medications from a mail order facility located in some distant part of the country. Pharmacists are afraid that mail order pharmacy will replace community pharmacy. Thus pharmacists are very concerned about job security and the profit-ability of the community pharmacy. The extreme popularity of drive-thru windows at drugstores tells our customers that prescrip-tion drugs are no different from any consumer product that can ar-rive in the mail, like books from Amazon.com. So far, pharmacists have not been very successful in convincing the public that there is value in face-to-face contact with pharmacists.

As we lean our head out the drive-thru window and shout a few words above the traffic noise ("Be sure to take this antibiotic until it's all gone," for example), the parallel to the McDonald's drive-thru window becomes inescapable. McDonald's dispenses fast food. Pharmacists today dispense fast prescriptions and "quick-fix" remedies. Discussions of things like what's actually causing someone's disorder are not even considered important. Our medical system no longer has time to examine causes. There's only time for the prescribing of pills. In my opinion, this can only be described as a cold and impersonal health care system.

Drive-thru windows may be great for burgers, banks, and dry cleaners, but they can be disastrous for prescriptions. After one mix-up at our pharmacy drive-thru, my partner said to me, "This really scares me. Customers need to realize that these aren't cheeseburgers that we're dispensing!"

The pharmacists I know agree that pharmacy drive-thrus are demeaning to pharmacy and represent a decline in professionalism. The drive-thru implies that prescriptions are analogous to fast food and that lightning-quick service is reasonable. Contrast the professionalism instilled in students while in pharmacy school with the real world of McPharmacy.

The public seems to feel that pharmacists do little more than dispense products. Pharmacists are trying to convince the public that we dispense critical drug information to go along with that product. The growing popularity of drive-thru windows creates the impression that it is indeed simply products that we dispense.

I don't know a single pharmacist who enjoys working in stores with drive-thru windows. I heard that one local pharmacist went to work for a competitor when he heard that his employer was replacing his store (in a strip mall) with a freestanding version with a drive-thru.

Customers have the perception that drive-thru windows can provide the pharmacy equivalent of McDonald's with scripts filled instantaneously, no waiting involved. Even repeat customers have a hard time understanding that prescriptions are different from burgers.

Some pharmacists refuse to allow customers to wait at the drive-thru. Yet some customers protest that they've got a sick child or elderly parent at home and that they need to return with the medication right away. Some pharmacists will go ahead and put these prescriptions ahead of others in line. Other pharmacists refuse to give special treatment to drive-thru customers.

Some of the drive-thru windows are bullet-resistant, creating a barricade-like setting complete with pneumatic tubes. The interaction with the pharmacist is as mechanical and sterile as a bank drive-thru. Is this the most conducive environment in which to educate customers about their medications, i.e., through microphones, speakers, with the engine roaring, and the car stereo blasting? You've never really experienced pharmacy until you've attempted to answer customers' questions at a drive-thru window without pneumatic tubes, where car exhaust fumes drift into the open pharmacy window.

Drive-thru windows may be good if we want to change the name of our store to something like Drugs-R-Us or Speedy-Rx or Drug-In-A-Box. And when customers ask for a two-month supply of their meds (rather than their usual one-month supply), maybe we should begin saying that the customer wants to SUPER SIZE his Rx order.

As if we didn't already have enough problems in the pharmacy, now we've got to endure the absurdity of people honking their horn at the drive-thru window, wondering why their prescriptions haven't been filled in two minutes. I once witnessed the second-in-line customer at our drive-thru honking his horn at the customer in front of him for being at the window too long. Or was he honking his horn at us (the pharmacy staff) for failing to move traffic through the window as quickly as McDonald's?

In one store, I was told that a customer at the drive-thru got the wrong medications as follows. The tech went to the window and asked for the patient's name. The tech misunderstood the patient's name and picked up the Rx bag for a customer with a similar-sounding name. The tech then read the name on the Rx bag to the customer at the drive-thru. Apparently the noise of the engine interfered with clear communication. The customer nodded in agreement when the tech read the name on the Rx bag. The customer went to the local emergency room when he discovered the error (after he had taken some of the wrong medication). There was no harm to the customer but I am told that he did indeed sue. I did not hear the final outcome of the lawsuit. Probably my employer quietly agreed to a small settlement. In my opinion, this type of error would be less likely to occur if the customer had picked up the medication inside the store rather than at the drive-thru window. I make the following observation only half-jokingly: It seems that the customer was guilty of *contributory negligence*. The customer contributed to the error by choosing to pick up his medications at the drive-thru window. Pharmacy customers need to realize that communication at the drive-thru window can be difficult and that drive-thru windows increase the chances of an error at the drugstore.

On days that we're severely understaffed, the pharmacist on duty may decide to close the drive-thru window for a few hours. In my experience, this always irritates the non-pharmacist store manager because he (the non-pharmacist store manager), like our customers, thinks drugstores dispense burgers. I've seen many non-pharmacist store managers who sit comfortably in their office (resting, eating, talking on the phone, etc.) for periods of time that pharmacists can only dream of. Yet these same non-pharmacist store managers call our district manager when the pharmacist closes the drive-thru window in response to dangerous understaffing.

I worked in one store in which the drive-thru window is located an insanely long distance from the rest of the pharmacy. One pharmacist there said that the architect who designed the layout of that store deserves to be hanged from a rafter in the ceiling. The technicians at this store were engaged in an ongoing grudge match with each other. Each tech criticized the other techs for not taking their fair share of the long walks to assist customers waiting at the drive-thru window.

There was one pharmacist at this store who was an absolute stickler for following rules. But he followed only those rules he agreed with. He was, of course, well aware of the pharmacy board's counseling requirement but he felt that the insanely long walk to the drive-thru window released him from his duty to counsel customers at the drive-thru.

The boards of pharmacy are good at mandating lots of things that pharmacists view as non-critical. For example, the boards enforce regulations specifying that we have on hand certain reference books or compounding equipment that we never use. But where are the boards when we need them to do something useful like outlawing drive-thru windows as a threat to the public safety?

Pharmacists who have been out of school for only a few months very often begin comparing our jobs to McDonald's or Burger King. It doesn't take long for these young graduates to become disillusioned. In my experience, the McDonald's analogy is possibly the single most frequently used description of our workplace by pharmacists on the front lines of chain pharmacy. The only difference of opinion among pharmacists as regards the fast food analogy seems to be which specific burger outlet pharmacists cite in comparison. For example, one pharmacist posted a message on the Internet discussion group sci.med.pharmacy: "The drive-thru has really cheapened the image of the pharmacist as a professional. Drive-thru windows have given people the impression that going to the drugstore is like going to Burger King or the bank."

The message sent to the public by drive thru windows is directly opposite the message that most pharmacists hope to send to the public. The public logically asks, "If drugstores aren't associated with speed, why do they have drive thru windows?" Our message should be that pharmacy is about advice on using medications for maximum benefit. The drive thru window convinces the public that pharmacy is simply about products, not advice. Pharmacists have inadvertently given the public the impression that pharmacy is simply about the speedy dispensing of products, that the pharmacist's relationship with customers is mainly mercantile, not cognitive.

In my experience, in contrast to chain pharmacists, independent pharmacists seem to love the drive thru window. Independent pharmacists would probably characterize the drive thru as being about convenience, not speed. The difference is that independent pharmacy owners can increase staffing sufficiently to handle the drive thru, whereas chain pharmacists don't even have enough staffing for stores without a drive thru. Staffing levels at chain drugstores are tightly controlled by the corporate office based on numbers of prescriptions filled. For example, chain pharmacists can usually determine technician scheduling, but not the number of technicians we can hire or the 'budget hours' for technicians.

Both drugstores and fast food outlets have to contend with drive-thru windows and impatient customers. Unless the pharmacy has the latest pneumatic tubes, pharmacists (like McDonald's clerks) have the pleasure of inhaling car exhaust fumes as we lean our head out the window to hand our customers their orders. Drugstores and fast food outlets both have high school girls who work part-time and who are more interested in jabbering about their boyfriends than filling orders correctly.

Sheryl Szeinbach and colleagues at The Ohio State University College of Pharmacy co-authored a study examining whether pharmacy drive-thrus contribute to errors. They concluded that this is indeed the case. (Emily Caldwell, *OSU Research News*, "Pharmacists Believe Drive-Through Windows Contribute to Delays, Errors."
http://www.pharmacy.ohio-state.edu/news/med_errors.cfm):

Consumers who pick up their prescription medications at a pharmacy drive-through window might be jeopardizing their own safety in the name of convenience.

A new study indicates that pharmacists who work at locations with drive-through windows believe the extra distractions associated with window service contribute to processing delays, reduced efficiency and even dispensing errors.

The surveyed pharmacists reported that the design and layout of their workplace has an impact on dispensing accuracy, especially the presence of drive-through window pick-up services.

The study suggests pharmacy design should emphasize minimal workflow interruptions but it also offers a caution to consumers to check their prescription medications, especially those obtained from a pharmacy's drive-through window, said Sheryl Szeinbach, the study's lead author and a professor of pharmacy practice and administration at Ohio State University.

"Maybe we ought to stop and consider: 'Am I likely to get the same level of service from the drive-through as I am actually interacting face-to-face with a health-care professional?'" Szeinbach said.

With the number of prescriptions dispensed annually in the United States nearing the 4 billion mark, Szeinbach said the public is best served by pharmacists with the fewest possible distractions. Even with stringent internal quality controls, pharmacists nationally make an estimated 5.7 errors per 10,000 prescriptions processed, according to the study, which translates to more than 2.2 million dispensing errors each year.

Responding pharmacists attributed about 80 percent of dispensing errors to cognitive problems that Szeinbach said could be associated with various disruptions that interfere with their work.

The survey results were published in a recent issue of the *International Journal for Quality in Health Care.*

Szeinbach and colleagues surveyed 429 U.S. pharmacists working at pharmacies located within mass merchant retailers, traditional chain drugstores or independently owned shops. The questionnaire sought pharmacists' perceptions of how their practice was affected by the pharmacy layout and design, the presence of a drive-through window and the availability of an automated dispensing system. Specifically, they were asked whether those factors had a positive or negative influence on errors in dispensing, communication between staff and pharmacists, prescription processing time, efficiency and physical mobility in the practice setting.

Participating pharmacists were asked to respond to questions using a scale from 1 to 5, with 1 indicating pharmacists strongly disagreed with suggestions that their practice was affected by these factors and 5 meaning they strongly agree.

While the responding pharmacists agreed that the layout and design of their workplace could contribute to errors and reduce efficiency, the presence of a drive-through window elicited a much more definitive response, Szeinbach said.

"The drive-through window, overall, poses a huge problem with respect to causing dispensing errors, contributing to communication errors, delaying processing and forcing staff to take more steps," Szeinbach said. "Think about it – that window has to be in an area that's convenient for the patient driving up to the window, yet may not – and obviously is not –

convenient to the pharmacist and the staff. The link between drive-through and dispensing errors alone should be a concern to the public."

She said the findings suggest that consumers should always check the prescription medications they pick up at a pharmacy to confirm they received the right medicine.

According to the survey, pharmacists perceive that the drive-through window has the biggest impact on causing pharmacists and their staff to take extra steps (average agreement response of 3.7 on a 5-point scale); reducing efficiency (average response of 3.8); and causing delays in prescription processing (average response of 3.7). The respondents also attributed dispensing errors (average response of 3.2) and communication errors (average response of 3.3) to the presence of a drive-through window.

Szeinbach suggested the addition of a drive-through to a pharmacy has the potential to place unreasonable multitasking demands on professionals whose job includes counseling patients about medication use, not simply dispensing the drugs.

"A pharmacist or staff member could be responsible for four or five tasks, and serving people at the drive-through window is just one of them," she said. "Some people seeking the convenience of the drive-through window don't care about getting information. They just want the medication, and they want it as fast as possible. They should probably think about that and at least look at the medication and make sure it's OK. And if they have questions, it may behoove them to come into the pharmacy."

She noted that an additional study comparing actual error rates at pharmacies with and without drive-through windows is needed to verify her results.

"There's a potential bias that could exist against drive-through windows," she said. "But since the responding pharmacists pointed out the drawbacks of both drive-through windows and the entire layout and design, and their responses are fairly consistent, it leads me to believe their perceptions are probably accurate."

Szeinbach co-authored the study with Enrique Seoane-Vazquez and graduate students Ashish Parekh and Michelle Herderick, all of Ohio State's College of Pharmacy.

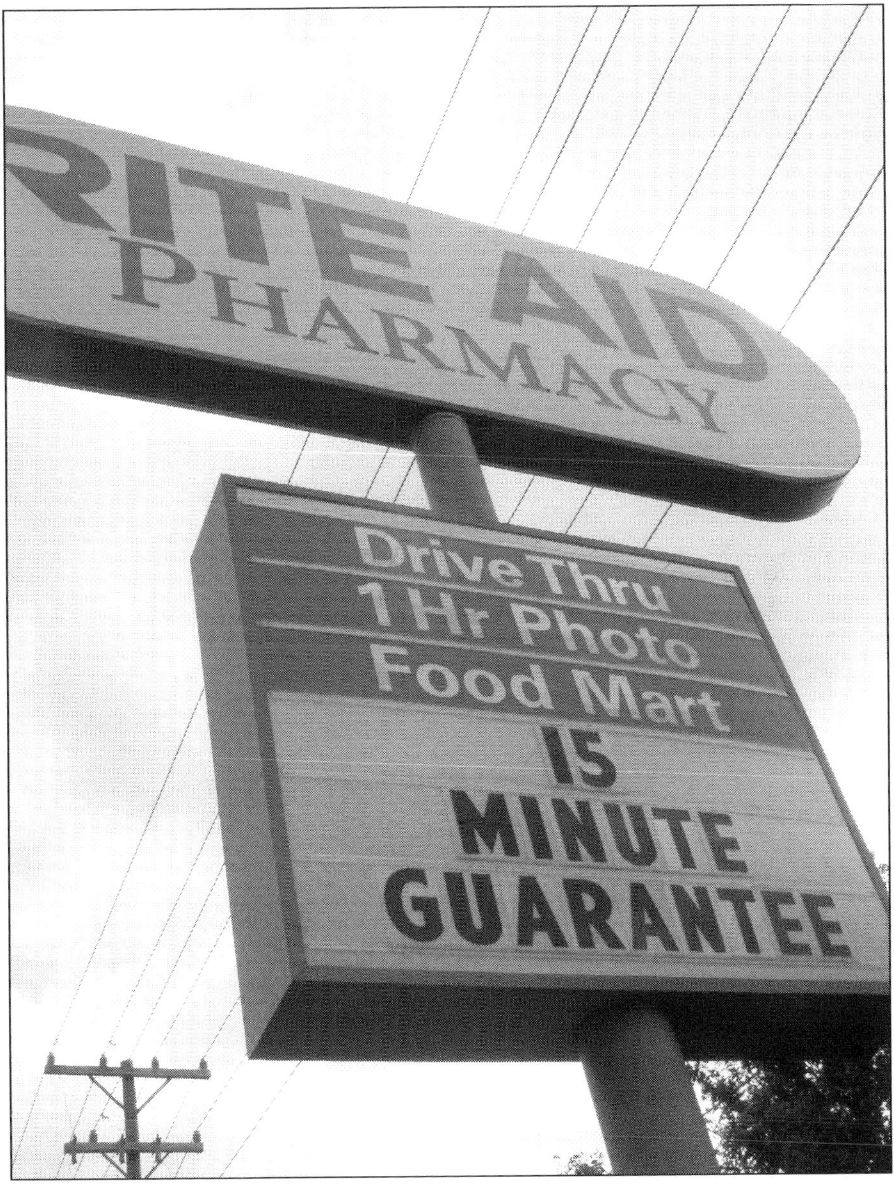
RITE AID
PHARMACY
Drive Thru
1 Hr Photo
Food Mart
15
MINUTE
GUARANTEE

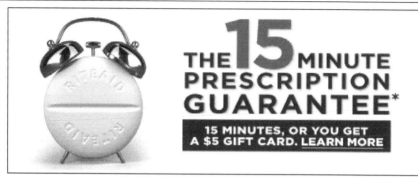

THE 15 MINUTE PRESCRIPTION GUARANTEE*

15 MINUTES, OR YOU GET A $5 GIFT CARD. LEARN MORE

Let us fill your prescription in 15 minutes. Guaranteed.

Bring your prescriptions in to Rite Aid today and we'll fill them in 15 minutes guaranteed – or you get a $5 Rite Aid Gift Card.*

After all, we care about your health and wellness. Helping you achieve your goals is what we're all about.

We also care about your time. Just bring your prescriptions in today and you can get well – Sooner.

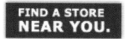

FIND A STORE NEAR YOU.

* **Not available in NY.** Guarantee applies to prescriptions dropped off in-store and at drive-through only. Offer is limited to one gift card per order of 3 prescriptions maximum. Certain exclusions apply including services, or prescriptions requiring ordering, prescriber contact, third party assistance, professional services, or prescriptions presented immediately before or during Pharmacist lunch break.

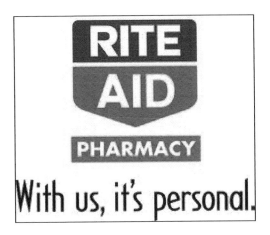

With us, it's personal.

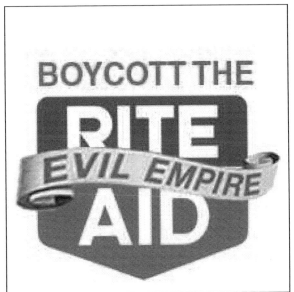

http://www.bridesburg.net/Rite_aid_sucks/rite_aid_sucks.htm

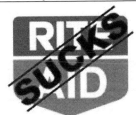

With us, it's personal too.

Rite-AidSucks.blogspot.com

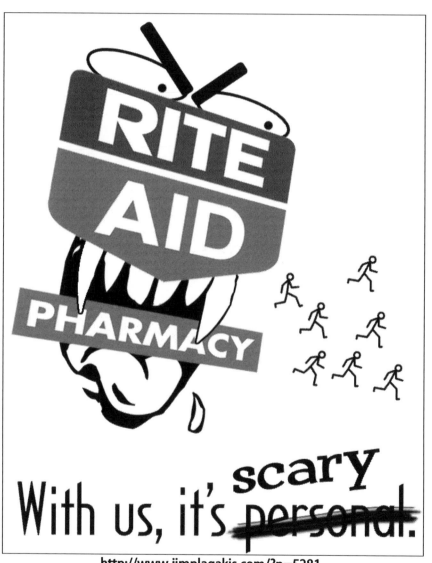

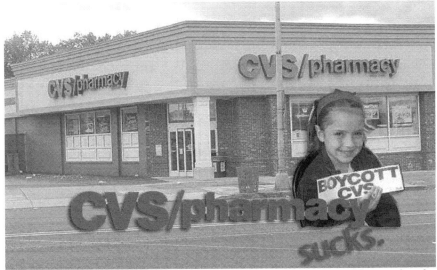

http://cvssucks.blogspot.com/2005/10/welcome-to-anti-cvs-blog-yo.html

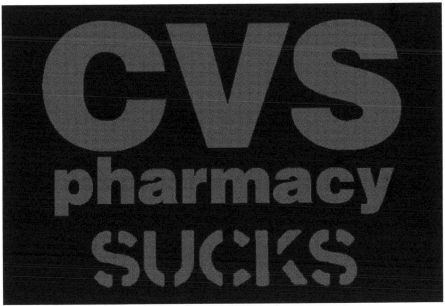

http://sullivan1985.deviantart.com/art/CVS-Sucks-39307559

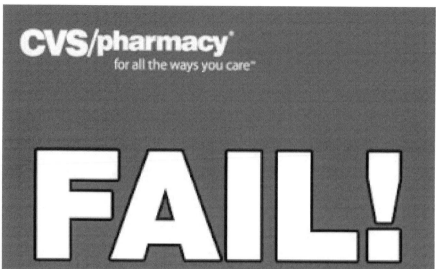

"CVS Pharmacy sucks! I had to go a bit insane last night to finally get my meds! It was not pretty, but I do kind of wish I had some pics to share the moment! Little boy 'Josh' working the drive-thru ended the ordeal with a sarcastic 'you have a marvelous night now Mrs. H.' I seriously wanted to punch him in the face!"
http://www.bitchyrunners.com/2011_01_01_archive.html

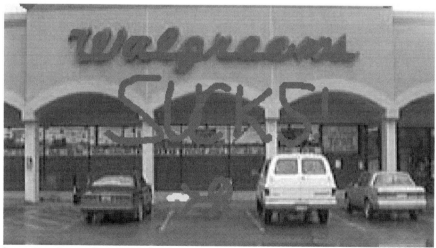

http://walgreenhater.synthasite.com/

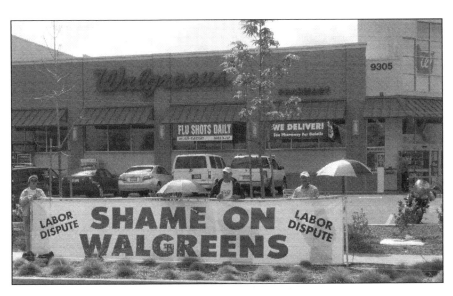

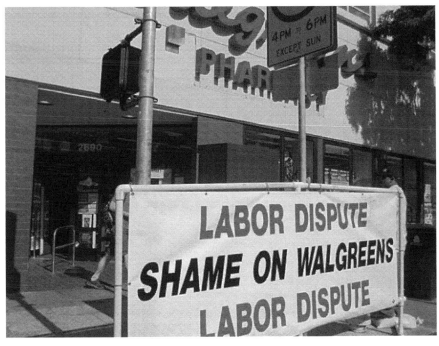

47

Are chain drugstores a threat to the public safety?

Do chain drugstores have a higher error rate per 1,000 prescriptions compared to locally-owned, independent, "mom and pop" drugstores?

Do the big chain drugstores have a higher error rate (per thousand prescriptions filled) in comparison to the error rate (per thousand prescriptions) at locally-owned, independent, "mom and pop" drugstores? I don't believe I've ever seen a study that attempted to answer this question directly. But a survey of Oregon pharmacists by the Oregon Board of Pharmacy in July 2011 strongly suggests that working conditions at chain drugstores are inferior to working conditions at locally-owned independent drugstores. Most pharmacists feel that there is a direct relationship between working conditions and pharmacy mistakes. The survey found that only 25.9 percent of *chain store* pharmacists agreed working conditions promoted safe and effective patient care—compared to 76 percent of pharmacists at *independent* pharmacies. (Oregon Board of Pharmacy, "Working Conditions Survey," July 2011 http://www.oregon.gov/pharmacy/Imports/OBOP-Pharmacy_Working_Conditions_Survey_Results11.11.pdf?ga=t)

If it is true that chain drugstores have a higher error rate per thousand prescriptions in comparison to locally-owned independent drugstores, what could explain this? Here is my theory.

If I were a pharmacist who owned the drugstore in which I worked, I would be extremely afraid of making an error in filling prescriptions because I would worry that a serious error in a small community could damage my reputation in that community and severely hurt my business. Do chain pharmacists care any less about making mistakes than pharmacists who own the drugstore in which they work? In my opinion, it depends on several factors.

I've worked for three large chains in my 25-year career. I worked for a small independent for only a few months during a summer in which I was in pharmacy school. All three of the chains I worked for had at least a thousand drugstores, divided into local districts usually consisting of fifteen to twenty drugstores. At each chain, I had a "district manager" who was in charge of these fifteen to twenty stores.

With a large turnover in chain pharmacists during most of my career, my district supervisor (or his secretary) would fill openings with any of the thirty to forty pharmacists in the local district. Thus, for example, it was quite common for the district secretary to call me and ask if I would be willing to work at a nearby store on my day off. "Nearby" could mean anything from a store that was two or three miles away to one that was thirty miles away. Most of the stores within the district were within an hour's drive of each other.

During times of pharmacist shortages or pharmacists' vacations or sick days, a large number of pharmacists could end up filling in at given stores. It would not be uncommon, for example, to have a different pharmacist on duty at a particular store each day of the week. For example, Pharmacist A worked there on Monday, Pharmacist B worked there on Tuesday, Pharmacist C worked there on Wednesday, Pharmacist D worked there on Thursday, etc. No continuity at all.

What are the consequences of having so many pharmacists filling in at a store, as opposed to having one or two pharmacists who have worked at that store regularly for many years? The most likely consequences are 1) chaos, 2) bad morale, 3) rudeness toward customers, 4) rudeness toward the doctors and nurses who phone in prescriptions, 5) "lost" prescriptions (for example, a customer dropped off a prescription on Tuesday and returned on Wednesday only to find that the pharmacy staff can find no trace of that prescription—it happens more often than you think!).

"Fill-in" or "floater" pharmacists often have a bad attitude because they hate to arrive at a drugstore and find poorly-trained techs or no techs at all. This can be a prescription for disaster, i.e., the combination of poorly-trained techs (or no techs), high prescription volume, and a pissed-off pharmacist filling in at an understaffed store with which he is unfamiliar.

My point is that small, locally-owned, independent drugstores often have a totally different culture from that at the chain drugstores. With the pharmacist/owner present most of the time, there is a stability at independent mom-and-pop drugstores that is very often lacking at chain drugstores. The pharmacist/owner has the power to keep good technicians and he has the power to hire an adequate number of technicians.

In contrast, a chain pharmacist filling in at any of the fifteen to twenty stores in the local district is in an utterly different situation. That fill-in chain pharmacist has no control over the number of techs who happen to show up for work that day or the training level of those techs. That fill-in chain pharmacist has no incentive to nurture long-term relationships with local customers or with the doctors and nurse-receptionists who phone prescriptions to that drugstore.

Many fill-in chain pharmacists feel that they parachute into one drugstore in the district for one or two days and then they may never work in that drugstore again for many months, if at all. So why give a damn about that store? If these fill-in pharmacists arrive at that drugstore and find poorly trained techs (or no techs) and that fill-in pharmacist is "slammed" with a deluge of prescriptions, that fill-in pharmacist's attitude is very often, "Screw this company!" Such an attitude can lead to carelessness and mistakes.

Only pharmacists understand the sky-high stress levels, disgust, and sometimes rage that often results from working for a huge corporation that routinely places us in positions that jeopardize our license and make errors inevitable. Our attitude is often, "If this chain doesn't give me enough trained staffing for the safe filling of prescriptions, why should I give a damn about this chain and this store?"

The subject of "working conditions" is possibly the number one topic (hassles with customers' insurance may be number two) of pharmacists who write letters to the editor at pharmacy magazines like *Drug Topics*. The majority of these letters complain bitterly about our working conditions. But there are always a few pharmacists who write "I love my job" or "If you're unhappy, find another job." It is a fact that chain pharmacists are the largest single category of pharmacists, exceeding the numbers of pharmacists who work at independents or hospitals. So the alternatives for employment outside chain drugstores are not always great.

To be fair, there are very many chain pharmacists who are extremely concerned about mistakes, and who are extremely concerned about maintaining good relationships with customers, doctors, and nurses in the local community. Thus it is a generalization to say that pharmacists at chain drugstores have a higher error rate per store than pharmacists at small, locally-owned, independent drugstores.

Nevertheless, in my opinion, real-world conditions mean that the morale at the average independent drugstore is likely to be better than at the average chain drugstore, and that attitudes toward customers and doctors at independent drugstores are likely to be better than at the average chain drugstore. Chain pharmacists very often have a feeling of overwhelming powerlessness as we experience daily the reality of having no control over factors (like staffing levels) that can lead to serious errors. You do not want a pharmacist filling your prescriptions who feels utterly overwhelmed, panicked, and powerless. In addition, many pharmacists feel a sense of rage against the chain for such work environments.

Some chain pharmacists have worked at the same location for many years and they are very happy in their jobs. I don't personally know many of these happy pharmacists, but I see from pharmacy magazines and the pharmacy blogosphere that they do exist. Some of them are recent graduates who love their paycheck and have not yet realized (or have suppressed the fact) that their daily high-speed, high-stress, high-stakes reality is not conducive to their long-term career satisfaction and their physical and mental health.

Some pharmacists have suggested that young female pharmacists (who make up an increasing percentage of graduates from pharmacy schools) are more likely to accept bad work environments without complaint, in comparison to males, or in comparison to pharmacists who have worked for chains for more than a year or two.

The chain drugstore model seems to mean burning pharmacists out and then replacing them with recent graduates who are too naïve or docile to question things. After six or more years of college, it often takes a year or two for pharmacists to realize (or accept) that the real world is nothing like what they learned in pharmacy school. This leaves a huge number of pharmacists with a feeling of disgust toward their alma maters for misrepresenting the fact that the real world of chain drugstores is nothing like the model of pharmacist-as-drug-expert that they were taught in pharmacy school.

The Oregon Board of Pharmacy survey of pharmacists' working conditions (July 2011) was covered by both *The Oregonian* and by *Oregon Public Broadcasting.* See the following two chapters for excerpts from both of those websites regarding this survey.

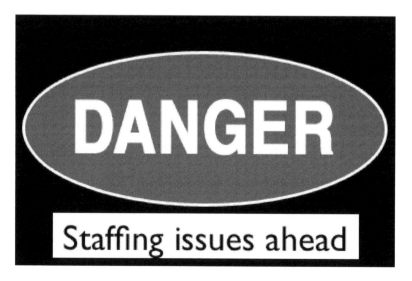

48

Pharmacists' working conditions—*The Oregonian*

Nick Budnick, "Workloads, chain stores add to safety risks, Oregon pharmacist survey says," *The Oregonian*, OregonLive.com, Feb. 12, 2012 http://blog.oregonlive.com/health_impact/print.html?entry=/2012/02/workloads_chain_stores_add_to.html)

A retired Paisley minister experiences sudden Parkinson's disease symptoms, so severe he believes death is imminent—only to learn it's due to the wrong medication.

A pharmacy technician in Hillsboro sells an Ativan prescription to the wrong man, who gets pulled over for driving erratically.

An Astoria woman suffers a cardiac arrest, and later learns her pharmacy for months had overdosed her with thyroid medication.

These are among the estimated hundreds of pharmacy errors reported in the last few years, either to state agencies or in lawsuits. And some pharmacists say errors are happening more than ever.

A recent survey by the Oregon Board of Pharmacy reported that more than 350 chain pharmacists—more than half of those responding—said their working conditions don't promote safe and effective patient care.

Many complained it is getting worse. "I feel that we are operating on the edge of disaster," wrote one. "It is a danger zone for us and our patients."

Last summer, the state board hosted an online survey for roughly 5,700 licensed pharmacists licensed in Oregon. The results were gratifying and disturbing, says board member Ann Zweber. She hadn't expected so many to respond—more than 1,300; unfortunately, many responded by reporting safety concerns.

"People had a lot to say," she says. "It concerns me greatly."

The survey results describe a profession in transition. Independent pharmacies, which once dominated Oregon, now number just 214 out of about 750 retail pharmacies, according to state records. As independents give way to large chains and mail-order operations, increased competition is inserting a bottom-line mentality into the way people get their pills.

Only 25.9 percent of chain store pharmacists agreed working conditions promoted safe and effective patient care—compared to 76 percent of pharmacists at independent pharmacies.

Not only that, more than 200 hundred chain pharmacists commented about workload and safety.

The survey data isn't perfect. It's anonymous and pharmacists were allowed to self-report their type of workplace. But the board believes the survey is credible, Zweber said.

Many complained of having to fill more prescriptions each day with fewer staff; of 12-hour shifts with scant breaks; and constant distractions, such as administering immunization shots to augment profits.

One reported quitting a chain job because of feeling "like I'm going to jeopardize the patients every time I stepped into that pharmacy." Another said because of lack of staff, "we have seen a huge increase in errors. We used to have a couple per month, now we have a couple per week and sometimes more than one in a day!"

Blake Rice, a pharmacist who used to sit on the state board, thinks many errors are caught internally by improved safety procedures. But he agrees chain stores don't protect the public, giving drugs "the same lack of oversight as the sale of bread and milk or canned beans."

There is no data to definitively show more pharmacy errors are occurring, or that they happen more often in chains. Pharmacies do not have to report errors to any public agency. The pharmacy board considers roughly 80 cases a year involving reporting errors. The Oregon Patient Safety Commission encourages voluntary reporting, but only 94 pharmacies have signed up.

The Institute for Safe Medication Practices solicits confidential reports of pharmacy errors from consumers and pharmacists. The group is seeing a steady increase in such reports nationwide, said Michael Cohen, a pharmacist who heads the group.

He said the group is sending its own survey. "It's hard for the pharmacists who work at these chains to complain too loudly to their manager or go public because they work there and they don't want to undergo any type of job issue," Cohen said.

Joseph Lassiter, a Pacific University pharmacy professor who sits on the Oregon Patient Safety Commission, said the Oregon survey results are disturbing. "This survey is a signal for us that there's something going on."

The board of pharmacy is considering rules to keep an eye on working conditions. The rules do not set strict workload levels, but allows the board to fine or suspend a pharmacy license over safety issues.

Patrick Bowman, owner of Tualatin Pharmacy, says he's not surprised at the survey. He founded his business 11 months ago after working in chains. "I don't have headaches anymore. I don't have trouble sleeping anymore," he said. "People come to me because they're not a number."

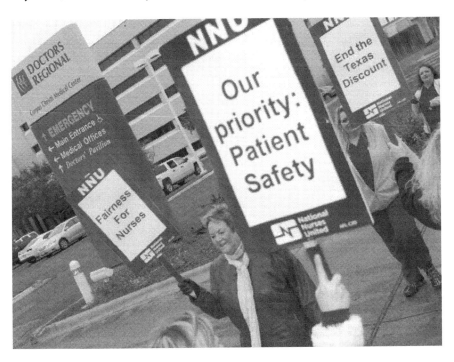

49
Pharmacists' working conditions –Oregon Public Broadcasting

"Preventing Pharmacy Errors," Oregon Public Broadcasting, AIR DATE: Wednesday, February 22nd 2012
http://www.opb.org/thinkoutloud/shows/preventing-pharmacy-errors/

When you get a prescription filled, you assume that the pills in the bottle are the ones that your doctor prescribed. But if there's a mistake, the consequences could be serious. The Oregon Board of Pharmacy sent out a survey to about six thousand licensed pharmacists, trying to get a better idea about the state of the industry and pharmacists' working conditions. About 20 percent responded. The results of the non-scientific study were surprising. About 75 percent of pharmacists working for chain stores said they felt working conditions did not promote patient safety. About 25 percent of those working in independent pharmacies said the same. Board member Ann Zweber told the Oregonian that the results concerned her greatly.

GUESTS:
—Ann Zweber: Member of the Oregon Board of Pharmacy, instructor of pharmacy at Oregon State University, part-time pharmacist at Bi-Mart

—Joseph Lassiter: Pharmacy Professor at Pacific University, member of the Oregon Patient Safety Commission

Comments posted by Oregon pharmacists on the *Oregon Public Broadcasting* website

I'm a practicing retail pharmacist who took part in this survey last year. I would have been surprised had the results of this survey NOT shown that most pharmacists feel as though their working conditions were not safe on the whole. We work very long hours (12-hour or more) and get very few breaks since most of us, if not all, are salaried and not expected to adhere to hourly labor laws. I am very disturbed when we find a mistake and we take it very seriously at my workplace. While we have put many procedures in place to prevent such mistakes and thus many procedures to deal with mistakes, they are inevitable, we are human. It seems as though the state of retail pharmacy has gotten to a point where people expect their prescriptions filled as fast as they expect a cheeseburger and french fries at a fast food chain. It is no wonder with drive-thrus in pharmacies and commercials promising 15-min wait times that people have developed ridiculous expectations of pharmacists. Also, it seems as though most pharmacies are always cutting how many hours we get for technicians and auxiliary help. We need more people in place to prevent more mistakes. **–Oregon pharmacist #1**

I'm a retail pharmacist in the Portland metro area who graduated within the past 5 years. I have been with my current company since I started school as an intern and then hired on as a pharmacist. In the years that I have been with the company, I have seen drastic decreases in the amount of technician hours a store is allowed with subsequent increases in job expectations. When I started I remember being thrilled with the profession and being able to talk to people and help them, and as much as corporate pharmacy would like you to believe that they are there to do this, we as pharmacists are stretched to the limit with our workloads. It absolutely kills me when someone comes in who really needs medical help, or needs advice on an OTC product, and I have to give them a very short/abrupt answer just so I can get back to spitting out prescriptions. As for errors in the pharmacy, they are on the rise. Pharmacists are forced to rush through verifying prescriptions. I consider myself very accurate at data verifying, but very rarely actually get the chance to think about the whole patient profile. I often catch myself thinking of things to look at after I hit enter, instead of having an extra two or three minutes to actually evaluate the patient profile. I also don't take breaks ever, and when I go to the bathroom (God forbid), I can almost count on being paged back to the pharmacy in ten seconds time. **–Oregon pharmacist #2**

I have professionally advised pharmacists caught in management squeezes in large chain store settings. Many times a pharmacist has to supervise pharmacy techs who actually answer to non-pharmacist managers in the larger retail setting of a supermarket or large chain pharmacy. Pharmacists actually have little supervisory clout within the organization and are subject to constant demands to speed up service and provide whatever the customers want. This results in mistakes, stressful personnel conflicts and a lack of accountability for the pharmacy function. I would not go to a large chain pharmacy because of the safety concerns in that environment. **–Oregon pharmacist #3**

I thought I would be working till 65 and then part time after that since I enjoyed my job as a pharmacist. Things changed as the independent stores fell to the chains and their main focus is on SPEED! It has become McPharmacy, few patients want to listen to counseling, sit in their car at the drive up texting away. Speed is most important to the patient however many (most) of them refuse to provide the pharmacy with their current insurance information. More time is spent dinking around trying to find out who we are supposed to bill than actually filling the prescription. I miss the days when I actually had time to talk to the patients who seek advice, current time pressures do not allow in-depth discussions.

Long hours, no lunch, no breaks...many a day I worked 8 hours without a bathroom break. Technicians' hours have been slashed, so more and more the pharmacist is like a plate spinner, hoping to heaven that no plates drop and break. Corporate pharmacy would like nothing better than to have NO pharmacists on the payroll and as soon as they get a machine to replace us.

In the meantime they keep increasing the workload, adding vaccines, blood pressure checks, Medicare part D counseling, and cutting tech hours. Installing monitors on computers to track speed of rx filling.

I am a dinosaur from the days when pharmacists knew their patients and had time to talk to them and help with their healthcare decisions. Back in the old days when patients sometimes called you "Doc" and not while they were on their cell phone. I used to enjoy going to work. When it got to the point of shifts ending in tears of frustration, I had to quit. – **Oregon pharmacist #4**

I am a relatively new retail pharmacist (licensed less than three years) practicing in the Portland area. I completely agree with "Portland Pharmacist" but would like to emphasize the topic of "cutting hours" for ancillary staff as well as pharmacist hours and how it relates to safety in the pharmacy. Just a few years ago in a pharmacy that averaged around 1000 prescriptions per week, most pharmacies would have two pharmacists working together (overlapping with 2-3 technicians and a clerk) for at least 4-6 hours per day on busier days (Mon/Tues) and maybe 2-4 hours on less busy weekdays. It was possible to take a lunch, breaks and finish all of the prescriptions, daily filing, inventory control, ordering, re-stocking, cleaning etc.

Then, as the economy started taking a turn, and Wal-Mart's "$4.00 List" came out, our company decided that the current "labor model" wasn't working. They started basing the number of [staffing] hours they would give each pharmacy to operate with on the previous years' prescription volume, assuming no growth, and they decided to keep the pharmacies open later each night. Oh… and they implemented an "auto-fill" service that added to our prescription volume initially, but in many cases, we end up filling the same prescription 2-3 times because patients (still) don't pick up their prescriptions within the time allotted. So, they cut several hours out of every pharmacy's labor budget/schedule and eliminated several positions while asking us to work longer hours and duplicate work/fill additional prescriptions unnecessarily and significantly increase our vaccination services. This eliminated almost all pharmacist overlap and forced pharmacists to start working alone on weekends and evenings with no ancillary staff help and marginal help during the busier times during the week.

Pharmacists went from focusing on whether the prescriptions they were filling were clinically appropriate, correct, and that their patients were benefiting from their therapy with minimal or no side effects, providing thorough counseling (Medication Therapy Management-MTM) to just trying to get the right pills in the bottle before the end of their shift. Pharmacists are doing all of the ancillary work that used to be covered by technicians and clerks on top of all the added responsibilities of providing professional health services, immunizations, and final verification that all prescriptions in the pharmacy are correctly filled during their shift.

I saw a steady decline in morale and our work environment made many people see patients as the enemy because when they call or come to the counter they are interrupting our ability to get the work done. This is exactly the opposite reason why we became pharmacists. We wanted to promote patient safety and educate patients about the safe use of medications as well as prevent prescribing errors, but there isn't time for that in the average retail pharmacy anymore. We are overeducated pharmacy clerks (with doctorate degrees) answering the phone, running the cash register, ringing up donuts and dish soap while juggling 10 or more drug related issues per minute with our one technician yelling "Override!"

I have found and fixed many errors made by other pharmacists and admittedly I do not always report them because I don't have time. I have reported the serious errors and I have reported myself when I've made an error because I wanted to believe it would make a difference if the conditions of the pharmacy environment at the time of the mistake would be a reason for the company to give us our labor hours back. It doesn't matter and I have never been spoken to about any mistakes that I have made or reported.

I have worked several 12-13.5 hour shifts (not including travel time) with no pharmacist overlap where my ancillary staff is either untrained or not intelligent enough to occupy the position they are in. Training of pharmacy technicians and the hiring process for them are separate topics we could discuss as it pertains to patient safety. Most mistakes start with the technician typing a prescription incorrectly. This happens several times per day in most pharmacies unless you are working with an experienced, conscientious, fastidious technician. They are very rare and if you have one, it makes all the difference. The most egregious errors I have witnessed were made solely by pharmacists working alone or in under-staffed busy pharmacies. The errors occurred due to not looking at the pills in the bottle that they were labeling (that had been counted by a machine or technician) or by not actually reading the stock bottle that they were putting a label on, resulting in the patients receiving the wrong medication and having serious side effects. The side effects could have been life threatening and/or deadly.

Whether you are salaried or hourly, it is impossible for pharmacists to have a 30-minute uninterrupted lunch break if there is no pharmacist overlap. It is unlawful for any prescription to be sold if it is labeled as "New" (even if it is not new) without having a pharmacist consult with the patient. This happens on all highly controlled (C-2) medications and many refills that have been newly authorized by a physician ("reassigns" labeled as new). Whenever there is a question about an over-the-counter medication, the pharmacist has to be interrupted. If a patient has a question about a refill, the clerk or technician must interrupt the pharmacist to answer the question before the medication is sold. If a patient comes in and wants to get a flu, shingles, or travel vaccination, we are supposed to be readily available to provide this service, so once again, our break or lunch is cut short, postponed, or interrupted.

Many pharmacies are finding themselves getting one, two, even three days behind on filling prescriptions. It is disheartening when every person that comes to the pharmacy expecting their prescriptions to be ready finds they are not ready and the pharmacist has to stop what they are doing and fill that script on the spot. This constant interruption is a set-up for mistakes. Not to mention the pharmacy is understaffed on top of having the extra burden of being behind. It is a downward spiral only alleviated by the salaried managers staying late every night or coming in early to "clean-up." The managers in most cases are working 50-60 hours per week (but getting paid for 40) but would never in a million years complain to "corporate" for fear of appearing weak or incompetent. It is very sad. We used to get paid for every hour we had to stay over and we were allowed to work as long as it took to get the work done. Now that they have eliminated most of the "slow" or "weakest links" in the pool of pharmacists, with little or no regard for the quality or supply of technician help, we are all saying "Something's Gotta Give." Currently it is our health (the pharmacist's physical and mental health), our attention to "customer service," patient safety, and our career satisfaction. Does someone have to die before they realize the new labor model is not working?

All pharmacists that graduated after 2003 receive a doctorate degree. Most of us have 8 or more years of college education. We have a great responsibility to provide safe, professional healthcare services to the public. If we work for a corporation, we have little control over the tools we are given to provide the professional services we are licensed and highly educated for. We have unlicensed, unprofessional, middle management, high school dropouts micro-managing labor hours (likely because their bonuses are affected by it) and ultimately affecting safety outcomes for patients.

In school they say, "If you don't like retail then go do something else." Why does it have to be that way? Why not change retail pharmacy so it provides a professional environment for pharmacists to provide safe, professional healthcare services as well as have career satisfaction and feel like we don't have to kill ourselves attempting to make sure patients get the correct medications in a timely manner? Is it too much to ask that we close for an hour for lunch, and actually have a clean, quiet place to eat that lunch? Is it too much to ask that we not be shamed into standing for 12 hours for fear of appearing lazy or weak if we sit on a stool (if the pharmacy even has one)? I know of several pharmacists that have had deep vein thrombosis (blood clots in the legs), strokes, or are heavily medicated themselves on antidepressants, anti-anxiety, and pain meds. These issues are undoubtedly related to working conditions and stress levels. We joke around saying things like "corporate would prefer that we wear a catheter or a diaper so we don't have to leave for a bathroom break." It's just pitiful. We all have hope that somehow things will change because we enjoy the direct patient contact that retail provides and so we hang in there, but really, does someone have to die, patient or pharmacist, before retail pharmacy provides a safe, professional environment for everyone involved? **–Oregon pharmacist #5**

I have been a pharmacist in a retail setting for 20 years. I agree with every word you've said. And I'll bet you work for Safeway, just as I do. I complain often to my district manager about our unsafe working conditions, as they relate to the health and safety of all of us working in retail pharmacies (I guess I can speak only for Safeway pharmacists) AND as they relate then to patient safety. I have been in contact with the Board of Pharmacy a couple of times in the past month begging them to DO SOMETHING about the very unsafe state of retail pharmacy in Oregon today. I, like you, know that the only thing that will prompt some legal/regulatory changes is for patient deaths to occur. I am furious and sad and just plain exhausted. I am a pharmacy manager and I can't wait to get out of this business. **–Oregon pharmacist #6**

You guessed it. I do work for Safeway. It is very sad indeed. I hope the Board of Pharmacy will do something that corporate can't maneuver around with some clever policy change like our laughable meal and rest period policy. It looks great on paper but try actually implementing it in an understaffed pharmacy. It just doesn't happen. I'm hopeful that something good will come out of all the negative attention pharmacy is getting. If nothing changes, I will be looking at other options. **–Oregon pharmacist #5—Part 2**

Insurance-mandated mail order prescriptions play a major role in the erosion of patient care. As an independent pharmacist I find myself bailing out the mail order system when a prescription is not delivered on time. The cost of filling these prescriptions usually is far greater than the reimbursements. The mail order system saves the insurance provider money by shifting the cost of delivery errors to the local pharmacy. We recently filled a prescription that had a total reimbursement of 36 cents. This Rx took no less than 1 and 1/2 hours of phone time with the doctor, the insurance company, the mail order company. We often spend a great deal of time helping mail order subscribers pick out appropriate over the counter medicines. If we are lucky the patient brings in their list of current medicines, otherwise they have to go from memory of the medications and health conditions. Your corner pharmacist has always been trusted to give out free advice. I hope we can survive the mail order and loss leader chains. **–Oregon pharmacist #7**

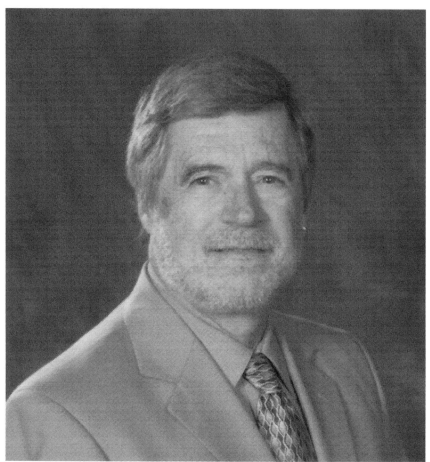

Gary Schnabel, RPh, Executive Director of the Oregon State Board of Pharmacy: "A pharmacy is a professional environment. It is not the deli counter."

50

Pharmacists' own words about working conditions

This chapter consists of two parts:
1. "Letters-to-the-editor" from various pharmacists published in major pharmacy magazines
2. Comments posted by pharmacists on two Internet pharmacy discussion groups (pharmacyweek.com and sci.med.pharmacy)

1. Letters-to-the-editor at various pharmacy magazines regarding pharmacists' working conditions

Letters-to-the-editor #1

[This pharmacist writes in response to an article in Drug Topics (March 18, 2002, p. 21) describing a pharmacy disaster in Southington, Connecticut in which a customer died as a result of a pharmacist mistakenly dispensing opium tincture instead of paregoric.]

I have quite a bit to say about your March 18 article "Lawsuit alleges fatal paregoric mix-up," but I'll try to keep it short. I used to be a pharmacist for CVS in Connecticut and would "float" through most of the stores in the area where the misfill occurred, including the Southington store. I also went to pharmacy school with the pharmacist whose name was on the prescription and worked with her several times at her store.

Your article left out many important facts. First of all, with the switch to Pharm. D. at the state's only pharmacy school, we were left with a crippling shortage of pharmacists at CVS. Many of the stores were closed several times a week for lack of a pharmacist. Imagine coming into a store that has a two-day backlog of prescriptions, not to mention angry, screaming customers. Also, in some stores with two pharmacists per shift due to heavy prescription volume, the second pharmacist was "pulled" to keep another store from closing. This happened in the store in question many times to my knowledge. Having one pharmacist to fill 500+ prescriptions in 12 hours (plus answer phones, tend the drive-in window, check Rxs, and monitor technicians) leaves little choice for us to "take our time when filling a prescription ... and not rush from one script to the next." This is, in my opinion, a very naive statement to make, especially coming from a lawyer who I'm sure knows nothing about working the bench.

Why are we, as pharmacists, not defending each other? Why are we agreeing to work in those potentially dangerous situations? The pharmacist in question may not remember me, but I certainly remember her. She is conscientious, intelligent, and hardworking in an impossible situation. This mistake could have happened to any one of us. The victim, and the pharmacist, are the result of a corporate push to open new stores on every corner with no thought of who will staff them. I have been in this same situation many times. I was labeled as a "troublemaker" by my district manager because I began to refuse to work in stores where I felt there was not enough help and too much room for error.

No job is worth making a mistake you can't undo. Please, I'm begging all pharmacists, let's stick together and start demanding better working conditions, for our sake, and our patients' sake.

–Heather Fontaine, R.Ph., Atlanta, GA, Letters: "Demand Better Conditions," *Drug Topics*, May 6, 2002, pp. 12, 14

Letters-to-the-editor #2

I cannot believe that working 12- and 13-hours days or 50- to 70-hour weeks is conducive to good, safe pharmacy practice. ...I have yet to work in an independent retail practice that has placed upon it the same extraordinary demands found in a busy chain store, both in terms of prescription volume and the need for personal counseling by the pharmacist.

I am appalled that any chain would allow a pharmacist to work 60, 70, even 80 hours a week, which happens regularly. Were I an attorney representing a client who suffered an injury related to a dispensing error, my first question to the pharmacist (and his employer) would be, "How many hours had you worked in the five days immediately preceding the error?"

It is my belief that pharmacist fatigue is a bigger contributor to dispensing errors than workload. Pilots and truck drivers are limited by law as to how many hours they may work without mandated idle time, thus helping to ensure the public safety; why do we expect more from ourselves?

–Mitch Fields, R.Ph., Royal Oak, Michigan, "Is this safe pharmacy?", *Drug Topics*, April 7, 1997, p. 12.

Letters-to-the-editor #3

It is incredible that pharmacy corporate officials, academics, and state boards do not simply observe the pharmacist during a normal workday and realize immediately the legion of reasons that contribute to dispensing errors. They are almost ridiculously obvious to even the most casual observer. Most of us are so stressed by many of the issues discussed in the poll that it is miraculous that there are not more errors.

When are retail pharmacy corporate officials, academics, and state boards going to come down to earth and address the real issues facing the practicing pharmacist? What person in the performance of such a critical service is regularly required to work 12-hour shifts without meal breaks and with limited comfort breaks, while attempting to be a switchboard operator, receptionist, insurance billing clerk, and cashier, as well as performing critical professional duties, all at breakneck speed?

It is time for retail corporate officials, academics, and state boards to get the stars out of their eyes and stop spewing their idealistic rhetoric long enough to look and listen. They must see the reality of how the pharmacist is actually required to perform, and hear what the pharmacist is trying to tell them regarding these conditions. Then and only then can the subject of dispensing errors begin to be positively addressed. The recent rash of bad press about pharmacists should be a loud wake-up call to more groups than pharmacists.

It is time that pharmacists stand up for themselves and say, "Enough!" Our patients deserve better, and our profession deserves better, and we as individual pharmacists deserve better.

Since my employer sees any views, comments, or ideas such as those expressed above as an "attitude problem" rather than legitimate feedback about an alarming situation, I hesitate to sign my name, but I hope that fact does not preclude the use of my letter.

–Name withheld by request, "Wake up to reality," *Pharmacy Today*, Jan. 15, 1997, p. 5.

Letters-to-the-editor #4

Why is it that pharmacists are expected to work 8-13 hours straight in one day without a break, lunch, or just some time to relax? There is a trend in this country that doctors have adopted by closing their office for lunch approximately one hour per day. In this time nothing takes place and all the phones are turned off. They still have patients! I don't know of one doctor who went out of business because he slowed down for one hour a day, and yet pharmacy management feels that this would cause such a hardship for the customers.

I have also heard the argument that it would not be cost-effective to give a pharmacist an uninterrupted lunch and break. I just wonder how cost-effective a multi-million-dollar lawsuit would be when a mistake that was made by an exhausted pharmacist was determined to be due to the unreasonable schedule that the pharmacist was forced to work.

This is not an isolated problem, it is widespread over the entire country. Wake up pharmacy leaders! People have not worked like this since the days of the sweatshop....

I don't care about all of this political stuff that is in *Pharmacy Times*. I don't care about insurance reimbursement. Let's concern ourselves about the unprofessional workload first and get pharmacists feeling professional again, then we can think about the other issues.

–Stephen D. Davis, R.Ph., "Unprofessional Workload," *Pharmacy Times*, March 1997, pp. 17-18.

Letters-to-the-editor #5

I have noticed that a number of Walgreen's stores are popping up with drive-through service. Now this may be great for the patient/customer, but I see it as another headache for the pharmacist who is already overworked with walk-ins and telephone orders. When will pharmacy stop being viewed and treated like McDonald's, and respected as a profession with a professional who is an expert on medications? ...

Pharmacists are professionals who know and understand medications. We should be there to counsel and advise patients on medical needs. We are not robots designed to churn out 350 scripts in a day, we are definitely not insurance agents who know about copays and deductibles, and finally we are human beings, not supermen from the planet Krypton. If pharmacy is going to continue to be like McDonald's, then let us have the support hours McDonald's has. After all, if a person accidentally gets a pickle when they didn't want it, is it going to kill them?

–Elas Dray, R.Ph., "Future of Pharmacy," *Pharmacy Times*, September 1996, p. 14.

Letters-to-the-editor #6

I am going to tell you what is wrong with retail pharmacy today. It has nothing to do with managed care, i.e., drug formularies, OBRA '90, declining margins on third party prescriptions. It's about greed, selfishness and non-loyalty to employees. ...

The simple truth is that retail chain pharmacy has nothing to do with patient care; the only thing the big boys give a hoot about is money, money and more money. The pharmacist's job is to fill customers' prescriptions at the speed of light (the faster you fill, the more money they make), explain their drugs only so the chain doesn't get fined for noncompliance with OBRA, and get them out as soon as you can.

–Lawrence Barusch, R.Ph., Clifton Park, New York, "Revco: A Friend for Life?" *American Druggist*, March 1997, p. 8.

Letters-to-the-editor #7

After reading many articles and editorials expressing pharmacists' plight for fewer interruptions, more technician help, much-needed and deserved lunch, dinner and bathroom breaks, and the need for a more "professional" environment, I've come to a conclusion.

On one particularly busy day, one of our regular customers could tell we were swamped and wanted to do something nice for us. She offered to bring us lunch. She asked, "Have you had your lunch break yet?" It was all we could do to not burst out laughing at such a silly question. I begrudgingly told her we did not get lunch breaks. Nor any kind of break for that matter, but I kept that to myself. The woman was extremely surprised and somewhat taken aback upon hearing my response. She couldn't believe that pharmacists don't get breaks, and, needless to say, she didn't bring us lunch.

Which brings me to my point. These articles and editorials that describe pharmacists' working conditions are only in pharmacy journals and are not likely to be read by average citizens. If our plight was more publicized, people might take notice. They may well be concerned that their prescriptions are being filled often by worn-out, food-deprived, urinary-challenged pharmacists who would function much better if they had better working conditions and got to sit down and detach the phone from their heads occasionally.

–Angela Stadler, R. Ph., Charlotte, North Carolina, "Give Us a Break," *American Druggist*, April 1997, p. 8.

Letters-to-the-editor #8

In pharmacy, most of us have at one time or another been the victim of a corporate policy that doesn't allow pharmacists to act professionally. No time for meals, no time to use the restrooms, no time to legally comply with OBRA regulations, no time to consult with patients, no time to adequately ensure that prescriptions are filled correctly. You know the story. We all know the story.

We can wait for the pharmacy boards to change the business by mandating tech-to-pharmacist ratios or pharmacist workload limits. But the dollar power of Big Business will stall any bills considered in the legislature. We can wait for Big Business to change the profession (through massive layoffs due to technology and outrageous use of technicians to perform pharmacist functions).

Or we can demand protection and change in our business by unionizing. Few pharmacists have considered unionizing but we need the strength that a union could provide.

Standing alone we have no bargaining power. We are at the mercy of our employers to adequately staff the pharmacies.

–Name withheld by request, "Time to Unionize," *American Druggist*, April 1997, p. 17.

Letters-to-the-editor #9

...In what other profession do you have to worry about finding time to take a bathroom break? In what other profession do you constantly feel guilty for trying to take 30 minutes to eat a meal, relax, and regroup to work the next few hours? Is it any wonder colleagues are leaving the profession and new pharmacists quickly become disillusioned with it?

These working conditions affect the safety of the public. It is only logical that a pharmacist working under these conditions day in and day out has a greater chance of making an error than someone who works under more humane conditons. Boards of pharmacy are charged with the protection of the public safety. Unfortunately, most boards have chosen to ignore working conditions in the mistaken belief that working conditions of pharmacists are a business issue rather than a public safety issue. Personally, I do believe boards should be setting some standards. ...

–Stanley L. Tetenman R.Ph., Auburn, Maine. "The Enemy Is Us," *Drug Topics*, April 16, 2001

Letters-to-the-editor #10

Regarding the article "Pharmacy boards of two minds about R.Ph. breaks," which appeared in *Drug Topics,* Feb. 19 issue, I lasted nine months as a retail pharmacist. The job, if done right, is grueling as well as emotionally and physically costly. I cannot believe that breaks are even an issue. What other profession or nonprofession works employees for 12 hours without scheduled breaks? I lost 15 pounds from a 100-pound frame in the nine months I worked in retail. My partner would get so nervous about coming to work that she would regularly vomit from the anxiety.

We are an educated group of professionals, and we are treated like slave labor. The current conditions are deplorable and need to change. I would never encourage a young person to pursue a career in pharmacy. Pharmacists have such a huge responsibility and workload but are not given the support they need to perform the job even marginally.

I have spent the last nine years as a hospital pharmacist and, because of the working conditions of that environment, would never even consider going back into retail.

–E. Stewart, R. Ph. (Etstewart5@aol.com)
"Retail work is grueling," *Drug Topics,* April 16, 2001

Letters-to-the-editor #11

...No one knows what we go through in a day but us. The closest people to understanding us are our techs, because it is they who see us being abused, disrespected, overworked, and walked on daily.

Just yesterday, during the worst part of the dinner rush, my two techs were stuck at the counter, leaving me to process, fill, check, and try to get the phone. Needless to say, I began ignoring the phone. As more and more lines were ringing, the assistant store manager started answering the phone and paging me to get the lines on hold. It took all of my willpower to keep my mouth shut and not blow up on him. You would think that someone who works in the same building as we do would have some idea what we go through. I guess that's too much to ask.

Hard as we try, we can't even fully make our families understand. I've told my wife, who is a teacher, everything imaginable about pharmacy. But she still is shocked when I tell her I don't have time to chat when she calls me in the middle of the day. "Why are you so hungry?" she'll ask. "Because I've worked all day and eaten only a Kudos bar and two packs of Smarties." They just don't get it. ...

–Jason Martinazzi
dr_of_rx@hotmail.com
"We're misunderstood," *Drug Topics*, Dec. 8, 2003, p. 22

Letters-to-the-editor #12

...The chain pharmacy retail sector lags considerably behind in examining profiles for drug interactions due to the fact that the pharmacist must check literally hundreds of prescriptions on each shift. To slow down will mean, in some chains, a red light showing on the computer screen signifying a pharmacist is behind in checking. This red light affects his bonus and invariably brings the area managers and district managers down on him. If a student really wants to go to pharmacy school for eight years, get that Pharm.D. degree, and then stand in one spot racing the red light with hundreds of prescriptions coming off the conveyor belt, good for him. The money is good, $85,000 and more in some places. But what about the health of the consumer, the drug interactions that are ignored, all in the name of speed.?....

–Kern Stafford, "Racing the red light," *Drug Topics*, Sept. 1, 2003, p. 16

Letters-to-the-editor #13

...I managed to stick out 4 years at CVS before the night of January 2, the Monday after New Year's and the busiest day of the year, when I worked a 14-hour shift with one 10-hour technician, filled 240 prescriptions, fell asleep driving home, and ended up crashing my car into the median. As soon as I woke up, I gave notice. Now I work at a grocery pharmacy for the same money, with much better hours and 10 times less stress.

CVS is an extreme case among retailers. Its new hires are almost always either recent grads or people who have bounced around the pharmacy world so often that they have nowhere left to go.

When are we pharmacists going to rise up and say that this treatment is completely unacceptable?

–Conchetta Lesser, PharmD, Phoenix, Ariz. "Wake-up call," *Drug Topics*, December 2011, pp. 8-9.

Letters-to-the-editor #14

...I spent my career at a drug company, retired 10 years ago, and returned to retail. The R.Ph. [registered pharmacist] works more than half the time without any [technician or clerk] help. I feel like a grocery clerk ringing up milk, soup, bread, etc., the way I did as a 16-year-old cashier in a supermarket. Some profession. We are nothing more than "high-priced clerks," who spend too much time with insurance problems, waiting on obnoxious, rude, impatient people who consider us as clerks; and work in high-pressure jobs that don't pay what we are worth. Pharmacy is no longer a profession. It's no wonder the young pharmacy students want no part of retail, as it is underpaid, understaffed, and overworked.

–Paul D. Rowe, "Associations are wanting," *Drug Topics*, April 19, 2004, p. 16

Letters-to-the-editor #15

Having read *Drug Topics* for years, I am increasingly glad I decided upon hospital pharmacy over the retail setting.

I have worked in the same hosoptial for 17 years, and I can honestly say I like my job. I have great co-workers, plenty of quality technician help, time for lunch and breaks, respect from management, involvement in many clinical activities, and I never have to deal with insurance problems—all in a safe and secure setting.

Almost every Letter to the Editor and many articles in *Drug Topics* are about how terrible retail pharmacy is, of which I am well aware.

Considering a pharmacist I know recently had to tackle and disarm a gunman (gunwoman actually), and that my other retail pharmacist friends hate their jobs, it would take a very significant pay increase or something like 10 weeks of vacation (which obviously will never happen) to ever persuade me to work in the retail setting.

–Jennifer Prazenica, R.Ph., Kittanning, Pennsylvania. "Job Satisfaction," *Drug Topics*, April 2012, p. 21

---

2. Comments posted by pharmacists on two pharmacy discussion groups (pharmacyweek.com and sci.med.pharmacy) regarding pharmacists' working conditions

Pharmacy discussion group post #1
Internet discussion group: Pharmacyweek.com
Author: emmyjay (3/23/2006)
Subject: RE: retail setting vs. hospital setting

Oh my God, where do I start???? I would HIGHLY recommend that you spend some time in a retail pharmacy. See if a local big chain will let you job-shadow a few days (especially a Monday at the beginning of the month). You will soon see what a nightmare it is.

1. Rarely do you have enough competent tech help

2. When you come in first thing in the morning, your voice-mail is already full of refill requests, so you are running behind right off the bat

3. Customers are rude, demanding, nasty, impatient, and give you no respect

4. You are bombarded by phone calls from doctor's offices, patients, people who AREN'T your patient but want to get your opinion of what their regular RPh told them, people who get their drugs mail-order but still want you to spend time answering their questions, and people who just need someone to yak at

5. INSURANCE HASSLES!! Non-formulary drugs, drugs that need prior authorization, refill-too-soon rejects, requests for early fills, etc. Every phone call takes forever and you get that much more behind in your rx filling

6. Patients who expect you to know every insurance company, plan, copay, and deductible amount off the top of your head. "I don't have my card with me—just bill Blue Cross"...

7. People who come in at 5pm with no refills on their controlled substance rx but expect you to fill it anyway.

8. Drug-seekers and narc abusers who bullshit you with stupid stories (my dog ate my Vicodin) that insult your intelligence.

9. People who think just because there's nobody waiting at the counter, you're not busy. They don't see the 40 rxs lined up back behind the counter, not to mention the dozen on voice mail and the other dozen called in by the docs!

10. Medicaid patients who bitch about $1 copay, then go up front and buy cigarettes & beer.

11. People who pay no attention to the letters their insurance company sends them, then yell at you because you're charging them a $10 copay instead of $5.

12. Working at a furious pace for 8-12 hours with (maybe) 1 potty break, no meal break, and praying you don't make a mistake and hurt or kill somebody!

There is a reason they pay so much to retail pharmacists. Nobody wants to do it. They lure new grads with the big bucks, but most quit within a couple of years. It will wear you down and make you a nasty person. Don't take our word for it—go and witness it yourself. Talk to some pharmacists who work in retail and see what they have to say.

Hospital can be very hectic as well, depending upon the staffing situation, but it's nowhere near as bad as retail. In my area, hospital pays about $5/hr less than retail but my mental health is worth the pay difference!

http://www.pharmacyweek.com/job_seeker/discussions/thread.asp ?board_id=2&conference_id=18&post_id=22699&thread_id=5500&p aging_CurPage=2 (Accessed 4-26-06)

Pharmacy discussion group post #2
Internet discussion group: Pharmacyweek.com

Got out of retail long ago, but still remember the pain. My relatives don't understand when I try to explain what a hellhole retail is. They always say, "it doesn't look busy" just cuz there's nobody standing at the counter. They don't see the 40 rxs [prescriptions] in line & all 7 phone lines blinking, plus the computer screen saying "prior auth required" or "non-formulary", etc. AAARRRGGGHHH!

I wish Oprah or 20/20 would do a show about it. Film a busy retail store on a Monday at the beginning of the month that only has 1 RPh [pharmacist] and a couple of techs. SHOW people that all the insurance crap is NOT OUR FAULT!!! And that for every rx [prescription] that is brought to the counter, there are 5 more off the voice mail & from doctor's offices. And show people what NOT to do: don't make us call your doc for refills; don't park at the drive-thru; don't ask for 5 other things along with your rx at the drive-thru; pay attention to changes in your insurance; I could go on and on.

I don't know how you retail dogs stay sane and not kill anyone..............
Emmajay 7-19-05

http://www.pharmacyweek.com/job_seeker/discussions/thread.asp?board_id=2&conference_id=18&post_id=21376&thread_id=5126" \l "pid21376"

Pharmacy discussion group post #3
Internet discussion group: Pharmacyweek.com
Author: SlaveRPh (2/15/2005)
Subject: RE: New pharmacists getting a dose of reality

Well golly gee. Isn't this what I have been talking about for a long time? The big lie about pharmacy. You see most jobs are nothing more than assembly line functions. I'm surprised someone has not filed legal action against the schools for misrepresenting what pharmacy really has to offer. It's very sad that people who are so intelligent end up doing nothing with their knowledge. And its not going to change in the near future. Heck this clinical stuff was being pushed 30 years ago. It's gone nowhere. Why? Because it doesn't fit the system. I have found maybe 3 pharmacists over the last 40 years who were happy. They both owned their pharmacy. How could anyone with a 6 year degree be happy with the environment found in most pharmacy jobs? My god 6 years and you work at the local grocery store or mass merchandiser. Those are the places you think about when you think about a professional and rewarding career in pharmacy? And more time is spent fighting PBM's and the ignorant public just to fill a script than is ever spent on professional functions. I hope more articles like this [John Strahinich, "Bitter pill: New pharmacists getting a dose of reality," *Boston Herald*, February 13, 2005] get printed and all students read them. It's not too late to get out of pharmacy if you're a student. A doctor and you can't even get a potty break or lunch break. Absolutely ridiculous.

http://www.pharmacyweek.com/discussions/thread.asp?board_id=2&conference_id=18&post_id=20291&thread_id=4831&paging_Cur-Page=3#pid20291

Pharmacy discussion group post #4
Internet discussion group: sci.med.pharmacy
12-21-2003

...because physicians are spending less time with patients, the pharmacist is receiving more and more calls with medical questions. Why don't they call their doctors? I don't know why you were prescribed Neurontin. Shouldn't you know? I mean you went to the doctor for SOMETHING. I would be glad to discuss the various off label uses of Neurontin plus its plethora of side effects, but you are going to send the script off to mail order anyway!

This past week was hellish. I finally decided to tell everyone it would be a 2 hour wait (with the exception of mothers with children or adults with elderly parents). I couldn't help but notice that most customers don't extend the favor of calling refills in a day in advance, or keeping up with their own insurance plans. Why should I convenience someone who is making my job that much harder?

I WILL take bathroom breaks and eat lunch. Being busy does not equate to working faster. My mistakes can kill you or get me sued. If you want to be part of the problem, you are encouraged to go to another store. I tried consulting for several years but grew weary of the hotel stays. Tried hospital and am now waiting for an opening to go back.

skipperdogs.
skipperdogs@whatever.com

Pharmacy discussion group post #5

Internet discussion group: sci.med.pharmacy
12-21-2003

...I don't have any statistics, but from conversations with young pharmacists in my state, there is quite a large number that are disenfranchised with pharmacy, particularly retail and hospital. When asked my opinion on the future of our profession, the best I can offer is usually a shrug and "If only" RPhs took back the profession, were allowed to practice what they learn, and make a living by that practice. I find it increasingly difficult to recommend an intelligent young person choose pharmacy for a career....

Glenn Gilbreath Jr., Registered Pharmacist
Wizard57M@SurfBest.net

Pharmacy discussion group post #6

Internet discussion group: Sci.med.pharmacy
From: Ftino (FSCIORTINO@worldnet.att.net)
Subject: Re: pharmacist shortage
Date: 2003-10-17

There is no pharmacist shortage. There are a lot of "vacant job positions" because working conditions are terrible. Many pharmacists won't work more hours or have cut back hours because they hate the job. CVS lost over a dozen pharmacists in my area. Not because they died or retired but because they QUIT. Now they are "short". That's not a shortage.

Pharmacy discussion group post #7
Internet discussion group: Sci.med.pharmacy
From: skipperdogs (skipperdogs@whatever.com)
Subject: Re: Worked to Death
Date: 2003-04-22

I and my two technicians/cashiers did 119 scripts from 9 am to 12 noon today. That's 40 per hour. I had a customer "jesus christ"ing and "goddamn"ing at the register because he thought I was taking too long on his refill which he failed to call ahead with. I guess he wanted me to up it to 50 per hour. I am going to have to write a legal disclaimer for those types of customers to sign whereby I am not responsible for any errors/deaths resulting from their fastfood pharmacy excursion. No. I did not rush him through nor put him ahead of anyone else in line. I know full well he would be the first person to sue me if something was done incorrectly.

Pharmacy discussion group post #8
Internet discussion group: Sci.med.pharmacy
From: Dazed&Confused (nate@nowhere.net)
Subject: Oh, what to do... Any rural US pharmacists read this newsgroup?
Date: 2001-04-19

Hello all. ***WARNING—Whining Ahead***
I am just finishing my first year of a Pharm.D. program and am wandering what the &*## I'm doing here. I'm from a small town and plan on returning to a small town (pop. <10K) after graduation.
For some masochistic reason, I work as an intern for one of the major chains, and I absolutely hate it. I think I thought that if I could stand working there, I could work anywhere. Now I know I couldn't stand it if I were to have to work there full-time. It's one of the busiest (if not the busiest) of their stores in this town (pop

~600K), and it's what I'd expect working at a McDonald's in hell at noon hour would be like. Not a day goes by that at least one of the female pharmacists or techs aren't in tears. (It may sound sexist, but its a fact.) I usually get by OK, as insults, etc. don't bother me much. I'm pretty thick-skinned at my ripe old age, but I have absolutely no skills in consoling people, and it does bother me to see my coworkers so upset all of the time (bit of a softie deep down I guess). That statement itself kinda scares me, as it sounds like it's an "us against them" situation, and that's not the way it should be. Getting jaded and cynical before my first year is even over is a bad sign. Granted, the vast majority of our customers are civil and understanding, but we're busy enough that the small percentage of true buttheads adds up to substantial numbers.

I guess I'm just looking for pity, or a shoulder to cry on, because I am so close to quitting. It's not something I want to do, as I'm kinda an old fart already, and I've had to bust my butt to get to where I am now, like working 7 days a week during most of my undergrad. But yet, the old proverb about throwing good money after bad keeps coming to mind.

So, if any small-town pharmacists happen to read this newsgroup, I'd love to hear some positive comments on your personal situation. (Are there any?) I plan on being a floater for a few years after graduation, eventually taking over a pharmacy of my own as someone retires. (Pipe dream?) If anyone has done something similar, I'd like to hear about that too.

Well, thanks for letting me babble on. –Nate

Pharmacy discussion group post #9
Internet discussion group: Sci.med.pharmacy
From: Name withheld (kmcl@zianet.com)
Subject: Wal-mart customers
Date: 2000/04/01

I just got home from another overwhelming day at Wal-Mart. I find it hard to continue day in, day out being insulted, harassed, pressured, accused of not doing theirs fast enough, etc., by customers. We often fill a little less than one prescription per minute. That's not fast enough for most customers, who arrive with 25 people ahead of them, and expect a 5 minute wait. Sure, they're in a hurry to go home to their soap operas, but we are hurrying as fast as we can up to 12 hours straight. If they want it fast, at least they could call it in a few hours in advance. I have been tempted to just lock the door and walk out. Does this ever end?

Pharmacy discussion group post #10
Internet discussion group: Sci.med.pharmacy
From: Liza57 (liza57@aol.com)
Subject: Re: Wal-mart customers
Date: 2000/04/05

Nope! It doesn't ever end—not in a retail pharmacy. But there are some things you can do for yourself. First, SLOW DOWN !!!! As was said before, you are setting yourself up for Rx errors that could cause a serious problem with your customer/patient and will ultimately affect you and the Board of Pharmacy when the mistake gets reported to the Board. No obnoxious customer should force you into feeling that you have to move faster to feel competent in your profession.

Second, realize that there is no way you can please every customer. Don't try to please everyone. Just do the best you can and when someone bitches about the how long it takes you to fill their prescription, ask them quietly and nicely whether they would care to have you fill it or would they care to take the Rx somewhere else and pay a higher price, which IS their prerogative. If they say yes, go back to work. If they say no...well...you certainly have enough to do already, right?

Third, take a really deep breath when you start to feel this frazzled. Step OUT of the pharmacy for a few minutes and take a few more deep breaths and keep repeating that you are doing your best and that faster doesn't mean better/safer for your customers and that NO ONE (customers included) should have this amount of power over you—to make you SO STRESSED OUT! I know this one takes practice. I've been doing this for 20 years and it still gets to me, too, but I'm getting better at it.

Pharmacy discussion group post #11

Internet discussion group: Sci.med.pharmacy
From: Liza57 (liza57@aol.com)
Subject: Re: public health issue.
Date: 2000/03/23
Re: What public health issue is most important to the profession of pharmacy? Why?

I believe the most important public health issue involving the profession of pharmacy involves prescription errors and the impact those errors have on the health of those involved in such incidents. I believe the error rate has risen due to a decline in the amount of ancillary help within the pharmacy thanks to low reimbursement rates from third party providers. I believe that corporations (both hospital and retail ~ independent or chain) were wrong to accept such low reimbursement in the first place and I don't feel that a pharmacist's ability to practice pharmacy in a competent manner should be jeopardized because of poor business choices. I also believe that it's time to step back and re-evaluate things like drive-through windows in pharmacies for convenience that can lead to yet more problems with drug therapy thanks to a lack of counseling. I think that this issue is by far the most critical issue facing pharmacy AND public health.

Pharmacy discussion group post #12

Internet discussion group: Sci.med.pharmacy
From: Paul (arghhspam@ctel.net)
Subject: Re: Pharmacy working conditions - New laws, N.C.
Date: 1998/12/25

I would probably bet that a break or two during the day would let all of us pharmacists live a little longer. Still, I don't know how I would ever be able to be caught up enough to take a 15-30 minute break. It might make it worse upon returning and attempting to catch up. My two techs have worked thru most of their lunch breaks (unpaid) for a long time just to try and keep up. What do you do about the truly sick patient or the one who has driven an hour (I live and work in the boonies) to get their meds? Do you make them wait? Would they get upset and go elsewhere? I don't know how you could make the system work. I think that all the pharmacies would have to close at the same time and for the same amount of time, just to be fair and consistent. In response to the original thread of this post, the profession is not fun, rewarding, stimulating or respected. It's just a job, as well as a few other adjectives that shall not be stated here, and I don't care where you work or who you work for, the grass isn't any greener. It's the same no matter where you are, it just plain stinks. On the bright side however, the money is pretty good and it does pay the bills. –Paul

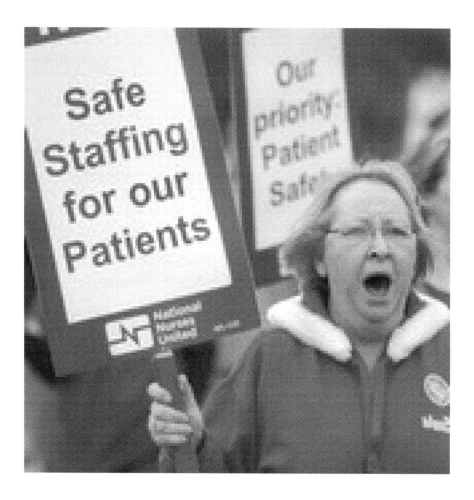

51

Pharmacist considers suicide because of working conditons

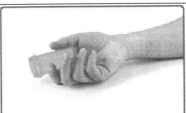

I work under very stressful conditions every day. I literally never eat or drink anything while I'm at work, been doing this for 1.5 years. Just recently, I had a misfill because I was the only one typing, dispensing and verifying all while the phones are ringing and long lines at drive-thru and drop off and pick up. I was rushing and glanced at the prescription and pulled the bottle and typed the rx and filled it because this person wanted her prescription done in 15 mins and it was dropped off over 10 mins ago and the rx still hasn't been typed because we had a long line. I did have a tech with me, but she is one of the most incompetent techs I have ever worked with. I just let her check people out when I work with her and there's a line. Thank God, I didn't dispense something that would seriously harm the patient. The patient ended up taking 2 doses before I caught the mistake. That day had to come one day considering the conditions I'm working under....

I'm seriously tired of having to work understaffed and with incompetent and slow technicians. I find myself getting so frustrated with them that I'm always getting upset with them and telling them that they make my job so stressful and that I will end up in the mental institution or on anti-psychotics because of them. I don't have a partner (other partner left because she couldn't take it anymore), but this one pharmacist who's been filling in at my store said she dreads coming to my store and sometimes wants to kill herself or wishes she was dead so she didn't have to come to my store. I myself have once thought about committing suicide because of work, I actually Googled ways to die painlessly.

If I knew I was gonna end up with a job like this, I would have never done pharmacy... How can the boards of pharmacies allow us to work under these conditions? They should make it a law that no pharmacist should work alone without a technician and that we should have sufficient help because we are dealing with people's lives here and working under these conditions just increases our chances of making mistakes.
http://forums.studentdoctor.net/showthread.php?t=891478
Last edited by rx2010; 03-05-2012.

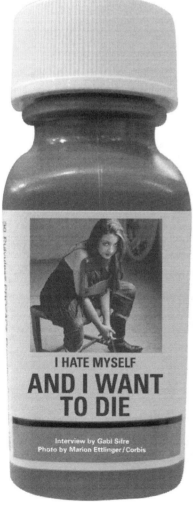

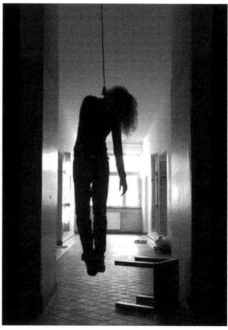

52

Pharmacist says he's "had enough" and "will no longer practice pharmacy"

I am writing to you as a pharmacist who as of today will no longer practice pharmacy. My feelings and thoughts about the profession are so strong that I wanted to compile them in a letter that you might want to publish for other pharmacists and the industry, to possibly stimulate change.

It's change that has been needed for a long time. OBRA is a tremendous spark plug, but the real changes will occur in the coming months and years as pharmacists like me finally say, "I've had enough!"

There's a passiveness that has allowed pharmacists to put up with all the injustices dealt them in their practice settings. My experience has been in chain retail, where the abuses have always been at the ridiculous level. I perceived that the level of what was expected of me was so high in terms of quality, professional duties, and non-pharmacy job responsibilities that I could not personally meet it. This has led to a building frustration, a lack of job satisfaction, and a stress that has pushed me out of the practice. The battle of "pharmacy as *fast food*" versus "pharmacy as true profession" makes it impossible to fulfill what's expected of us by the public and the profession. The OBRA counseling requirements just may be "the straw that broke the camel's back"!

I'm a very strong advocate of quality communication and of teaching every customer (patient) anything that will improve his or her health. This desire for a decent quality practice of the profession has to go out the window when the scripts pile up and 90% of the incoming phone calls are for the single pharmacist on duty who has to ring the register, answer OTC questions, get change to the front register, [all] without a technician or anyone in the store who has been properly trained to dive in and get that level of "quality" back to where it should be!...

It has also been my experience, in 12 years of pharmacy practice, that pharmacists have always been grossly overworked—expected to be salesmen, bookkeepers, and "nice guys"...at all times, despite any and all stressful circumstances....

The pharmacist gets little appreciation, little sense of having actually helped anyone, the stress of knowing he cannot possibly do what's expected of him, and the frustration of knowing his existence and value to society in the first place are constantly questioned! In talking to my pharmacist partner, we decided that it was necessary to have an "attitude" just to get us through our workday, because our working situation was so stressfully bad. Where is pharmacy taking its pharmacists?

The "professional puppet"—the pharmacist—may rear back and fight when finally, after years and years of punishment, he wakes up and demands decent treatment....

[Right now] it's a spineless, voiceless, robotic type of pharmacist I observe around me. With this as a profile of the profession, I don't see any significant changes occurring anytime soon. What I probably will see are a lot of pharmacists going to stress-management programs and the profession being possibly "gobbled up" by other, stronger interests and powers. We'll see. But as for me. . . I'm outta there!

—Mark W. Tillack, R. Ph., Charlotte, N. C., "Enough's enough," Letters to the Editor, *Drug Topics* (Feb. 7, 1994, pp. 12, 14).

53

Pharmacist describes pharmacy as "a horrible profession"

I graduated from St. John's University College of Pharmacy, Jamaica, NY, in 1995 in hopes of having a fulfilling career as a pharmacist. I have yet to find such a position. I worked at a hospital where the conditions were terrible and then at a chain pharmacy on Long Island for three months. In search of better working conditions, I moved to Florida where I currently work at a chain drug store. I have to say, "I hate my job!" Pharmacy working conditions are the same everywhere: Horrible!

A typical day starts with scripts and problems left from the day before and people waiting for the store to open. My pharmacy has six phone lines, two fax lines, a drop off/pickup window and a drive-through. Usually there is one pharmacist to deal with all these possible incoming problems. Today my tech called in sick and I have a register person who has never worked in the pharmacy before. By the way, my tech didn't graduate high school, can hardly count to 100 without help and gets paid less than a register person at Burger King. So much for tech training.

After just five minutes at work I feel the pressure. All six phones are ringing and people at the drop-off window are already complaining. Someone is yelling in the drive-through to speak to the manager because he's been sitting in his car too long. My store manager is not a pharmacist. He is 23 years old and can fire me for poor customer service. I go home hating the world, my job and my life.

What a reward for five years of education! I have been told that I get paid too much money. Plus, if I make a mistake filling one of the 400 scripts in my typical day, with basically no help, I can get sued for everything and feel terrible that I hurt someone. But the pharmacy would remain open and someone else would take my place. Employers don't care. I have been told that if I don't like it, leave. How can we still call pharmacy a profession? ...

According to the Gallup poll we are the most respected profession, yet I have had people curse at me, spit on me and throw stuff at me, usually due to an insurance problem or having to wait for their prescription. I consider myself an excellent pharmacist with the knowledge to provide information to people, but in reality it doesn't happen.

I would like to stand up for my dignity and personal sanity. But if I do, I will lose my job. Pharmacy is a small world and your name will get around if you are seen as a troublemaker.

Pharmacy is a horrible profession and I see no end in sight. The associations have not done anything to help our cause nor do I expect they will in the near future. We need studies conducted in every state on how many pharmacists actually enjoy their jobs. Please help us by continuing to publish articles on the poor work environment. It gives us some hope that maybe in the distant future we will be able to do what we were taught to do: provide care and information to our patients in a caring environment. The public needs to be educated and maybe they would have some patience with us. All we want is to be able to do our jobs well and we can't do that without proper help. Thanks.

—A young, frustrated pharmacist licensed in New York and Florida
Letters, "Pharmacy: A 'Horrible' Profession," *American Druggist*, January 1999, p. 10.

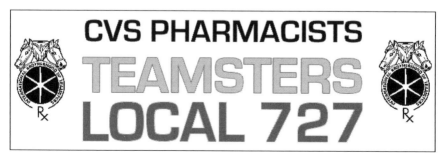

CVS PHARMACISTS TEAMSTERS LOCAL 727

54

Pharmacist asks, "Should I leave the profession?"

As I read your editorial in the November issue, "Stand Up for Pharmacy," tears rolled down my face. I had just finished working a full weekend at my retail store, Saturday and Sunday, 12-hour shifts, alone.

I came home complaining to my husband how much I dislike my job now. I feel like a robot. Customers demand faster service while waiting times are increased due to insurance rejections, etc. I have never felt so stressed, not to mention the lack of breaks. I have three children ages five, two and six months and I need to keep my focus and maintain a positive attitude at home. It's becoming an impossible task but I can't afford to stop working.

I have been contemplating returning to graduate school to earn a Pharm. D. because I love the patient counseling aspect of pharmacy practice but I must find a way to leave the frustrations of the retail-bench setting. I wonder if the time and money spent on graduate school will be worth the sacrifice. Or should I leave the profession all together? My only hope is that pharmacists will stand up for our profession and changes will be made. I hope all the other states will conduct a survey like New York did, but more important, I pray that everyone involved will open their eyes and realize how devastating and disastrous things will become if nothing changes. I'm ready to take a stand. What can I do?

—Pharmacist in Massachusetts
Letters, "Where To Turn?", *American Druggist*, January 1999, pp. 10-11.

55

Pharmacist says chain drugstore understaffing is a "cancer" destroying the profession

The following is, in my opinion, one of the best editorials published in Drug Topics in the last ten years. (Charles L. Duhon, Viewpoint: "Is pharmacy a profession or a trade?", Drug Topics, Oct. 23, 2006, p. 52)

I've been in the retail practice environment for more than 30 years and have realized that at the very heart of our profession lies a cancer that's been eating away at its core for decades. The cancer is called inadequate staffing, and it has caused myriad ills to befall the profession. I'm convinced that one of the primary contributors to the pharmacist shortage today is the disillusionment factor caused by stress brought on by inadequate staffing. I've known many R.Ph.s who early in their careers chose to pursue other career paths because of work environment issues. I've seen many female R.Ph.s, who are often secondary breadwinners, opt out of their profession because of intolerable stress levels due to inadequate staffing.

It should be obvious there is a problem when one of the most profitable drug chains in the nation, which offers high sign-on incentives and salaries cannot keep pharmacists. The chain is quick to blame the pharmacist shortage. What it, like most retail chains, fails to acknowledge is that the shortage has been created to a great extent by the working conditions behind the counter.

One national chain has added a new high-tech innovation to the practice of pharmacy. If you are filling scripts fast enough, a green light appears on the computer screen. If you fall behind, a red light appears. Records are kept and the red-light R.Ph.s are deemed incompetent because they are too slow. It is amazing to realize that, after six years of college taking such courses as biochemistry, pharmacognosy, physiology, and physics, your competency level is judged solely based on the number of Rxs you can fill per hour.

When are we going to realize that this is an albatross around the neck of our profession? The sheer fact that several state boards have attempted to address this issue gives it legitimacy. North Carolina and West Virginia are two that have passed legislation addressing this ongoing problem. In Oklahoma, I formed a committee to come up with a solution. We formulated a plan whereby any pharmacist who felt he did not have sufficient staffing could document it on a state-provided form. The board would investigate each incident, thus encouraging all employers to be competently staffed at all times. We formulated legislation that was passed, only to be blocked by the legal departments of a number of large chains.

I firmly believe that it is in the best interest of the state board and the people we serve each day, and more significantly in the best interest of the profession, that we be adequately staffed at all times. How can we project a professional image and be taken seriously by other healthcare providers as long as we keep trying to provide pharmaceutical care at the same time we are ringing up purchases, fighting with insurance carriers, entering data into the computer, and manning the drive-up window?

The pharmacy schools have been telling us for years that pharmacy should expand from providing products to providing services. But we will never get there until we are willing to recognize that we have a major problem with inadequate staffing and we are willing to come together as a profession to figure out how to fix it. We must be willing to surgically remove the tumor at all cost so that the patient might survive.

My tenure in this profession is almost over, and when I look back over the years I've invested in this great profession, I have mixed emotions. I know that I've helped many people physically, emotionally, spiritually, and sometimes financially. I know I made a difference when it came to helping people, but what have I done for the profession? In that regard I have failed miserably—primarily because I, like most other pharmacists, have allowed the cancer to grow and done very little to stop it.

I felt the pain 30 years ago when, right after graduating, I was sent to a high-volume store that filled more than 300 Rxs a day and had only one cashier. I saw the pain on the faces of my colleagues as they changed jobs over and over again trying to find a better work environment. I knew about the cancer and for years did little to correct it. If you ignore the pain long enough, the ailment that causes the pain will consume you. We've ignored the pain for too long, and the ailment has begun to consume us.

Ask yourself, "What have I done to change what is happening?" If your answer is "nothing," then you have only yourself to blame.

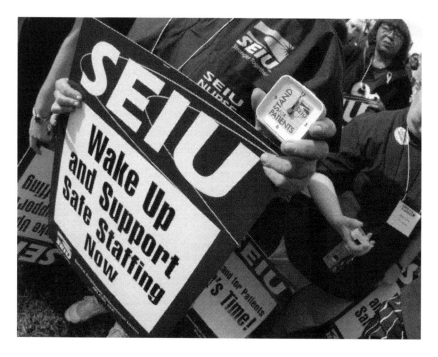

56

Severely disillusioned hospital pharmacist says errors are "too numerous to count"

PharmacyGal.com

I did it again!

Posted on August 19, 2013

Well, I did it again. I just returned from a state association-sponsored seminar. I made new friends, learned new skills, and got excited about pharmacy again. My enthusiasm lasted for about a minute once I returned to work. Obviously the job is the problem. I still have a passion for practicing pharmacy.

I maintain that it is impossible to expect a highly-trained professional to sit in a chair 8-12 hours a day verifying orders as fast as they can day-after-day from an endless queue and expect them to have job satisfaction. Better yet, some days we do nothing but walk back and forth on a concrete floor initialing labels and transferring medications from a paper envelope to a plastic bag. (Dumping the medications out of big envelopes into little plastic baggies is absolutely my favorite!) Hospital pharmacy is just a glorified assembly line. The pharmacists go home each night praying they didn't miss anything important…praying they didn't hurt anyone. There is no possible way to give every order an appropriate amount of review when you are expected to process orders for complicated hospitalized patients at a rate of one order every 1.5 minutes. Sometimes it takes two minutes just to get by all of the worthless pop-up warning screens! Actually, it is a great day if you can even get your computer to boot up in less than 20 minutes. Every order is a rush order. Meal breaks are permitted but you pay dearly for them. When you return from break there will be an even larger mountain of orders stacked up in the queue. The pharmacist left to cover the break will be completely stressed out by the time you return. It is almost not worth going.

This is the insanity pharmacists on the front lines face on a daily basis. The fact is: there are not enough "clinical" jobs to go around. Front line pharmacists work like dogs but are significantly under-utilized for the skills they have learned. When will hospital administrators realize the talent they have under their roofs? When will patients benefit from pharmacy services rather than be put at risk by pharmacy volume, fatigue, and over-load? Until that day, newly trained pharmacists will be disappointed in their career choice. Experienced pharmacists will continue to battle job burn-out.

I will continue to go to seminars. I owe it to my patients to be as current and knowledgeable as I can be. But the post-seminar let-down is getting harder and harder to face. It may be easier to not love pharmacy. I guess I did it again.

Searching for Pharmacy Excellence
Posted on August 1, 2013
Yesterday was a particularly trying day at the hospital pharmacy. Unfortunately, difficult shifts are becoming more and more the rule rather than the exception. Once again I refused to "bless" several intravenous products that had visible cores in them. Even worse, a nurse administered a chemotherapy drug I had prepared to a different patient than for which it was labeled. She had contaminated the medication made for the first patient of the day and upon comparing the labels determined that the 2nd patient was receiving the same drug. It was just a quick little label switch except pharmacy was totally out of the loop. What do our nurses do when the package or label doesn't scan? They document on paper. Then they call pharmacy. Expediency is always the rule. Get the job done how-

ever you have to do it. Policies and procedures were made to be broken. Processes developed to keep patients safe take a back seat to throughput. We are constantly expected to go faster and faster…

Most troubling of all was a young colleague who exclaimed, "That is just the way health care is today. It is like this everywhere." I really don't want to believe that. Call me "old school" but back in the day pharmacists checked labels 3 times and took every precaution to get the right medication to the right patient. Errors were abhorred. Now they are accepted as a "cost" of doing business. Our young pharmacists are very focused on pumping the orders out as fast as they can-making their numbers look good. Who taught them this? We are dealing with patient's lives; not making widgets here.

Controlling quality in a service business takes hard work. It takes time and effort to develop good employees into great employees. You can't do it by staring at a spreadsheet on your computer or giving a single power-point presentation at a staff meeting. You cannot expect excellence when only quantity and speed are rewarded. It is going to take individual pharmacists to stand up for their patients and the MBA masters of the bottom line to step out from behind their desks. Our patients expect quality. Our professional futures depend on it.

Dear God
Posted on June 27, 2013

Am I where I should be? I entered the profession of pharmacy to help people. Why do I feel so helpless and abandoned? Why do pharmacists accept mediocrity now instead of excellence? Why can't things be different? We used to do everything we could to prevent errors. Now they are too numerous to even count. We used to care about people. Now we care mostly about the bottom line. I used to be proud of my profession. Now it is just a JOB. What happened? Where did we go wrong? Please answer. I am listening.

The 70%

Posted on June 19, 2013

According to a recent Gallup survey, most workers are either not engaged or actively disengaged at work. In fact, only 30% of workers are enthusiastic about their jobs! Think about it. Seventy percent of our full-time workforce is unhappy at work! This is costing American companies a lot of money in terms of lost productivity. In my opinion, I would add this must also be costing employers a tremendous amount of money for healthcare benefits due to stress-related illness.

Gallup broke down the numbers into three categories.

30% of workers are actively engaged or enthusiastic about their work

50% of workers are "disengaged" from work. They only go through the motions when on the job.

20% of workers are "actively disengaged" from work. They hate their jobs and undermine their employer.

This pharmacist is desperately trying to stay among the enthusiastic and engaged 30% of workers. It is getting harder and harder. Several of my colleagues are now just putting in their time. You can see it in their eyes and feel it in their attitude at work. They are just trying to survive. Are you in the 30% or the 70%?

http://www.mercurynews.com/business/ci_23479060/most-workers-hate-their-jobs-or-have-checked?source=rss

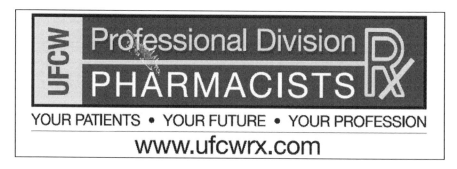

57

Should pharmacists admit fault for errors caused by working conditions?

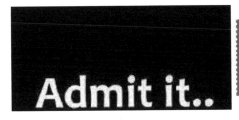

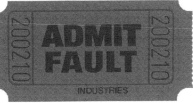

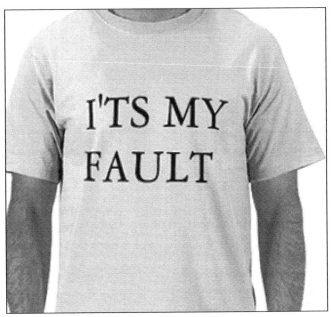

Many of our pharmacy leaders tell us that we should immediately fess up after a mistake. Let me make the case why I don't think the issue is quite that simple.

I happened to be visiting my mother and stepfather when my stepfather noticed that half the pills in one of his Rx bottles looked strange. It turns out that a national chain mistakenly dispensed Glucophage (for type 2 diabetes) to my stepfather instead of Toprol XL (for blood pressure). My stepfather has never had diabetes. I told my stepfather that I would like to accompany him when he asked the pharmacist what happened. During my stepfather's conversation with the pharmacist, I never identified myself as a pharmacist nor did I say a single word. I've witnessed similar scenarios too often in my career. The pharmacist who made the mistake was not on duty but the pharmacist-in-charge spoke carefully. He told my stepfather, "I'm sorry for the inconvenience." He did not say "I'm sorry for the error." I confess that I probably would have handled the situation similarly.

The issue of whether pharmacists should admit an error and apologize to the customer is one of considerable controversy to pharmacists in the trenches. Several years ago at a day-long meeting of about two dozen of the chain's pharmacists in my local district, our supervisor and his boss said that we should admit errors to customers and apologize. There was a great deal of discussion of this point. I have come to the conclusion that it was indeed a corporate decision that the pharmacist responsible for the error should apologize to the customer.

During our lunch break that day, the half-dozen pharmacists sitting around my table discussed this idea of admitting our error and apologizing to the customer. A couple of older pharmacists said they had never done it that way before and they didn't want to start now. The implied best way to handle errors was to try to obfuscate the whole thing by claiming, for example, that the drug is a generic. If the customer may be in danger, obviously we have to take more direct action. We always correct the error by saying something like "It's made by a different company but we'll give you the one you had before."

One of these older pharmacists said that most auto insurers recommend that policyholders not admit fault. I went home and checked my State Farm car insurance policy and, sure enough, on the back of my wallet card are these exact words: "Do not admit fault. Do not discuss the accident with anyone except State Farm or Police."

So why would my employer (one of the largest drug chains in the country) suggest that we admit fault to the customer and apologize? At our table, we concluded that the corporation was trying to protect itself by isolating us on a limb and then, if necessary, cutting off that limb. We figured that the chain would endeavor to get rid of us through various means or transfer us to a different town if the dispensing error were so serious that it received widespread publicity in our community. As a result, most of the pharmacists I know are not eager to admit fault and apologize to customers.

I wouldn't necessarily mind apologizing in the following manner: "On behalf of (Walgreens, CVS, Wal-Mart, Rite Aid, etc.), I apologize for the error." But this is precisely the opposite of what our employer wants. Our employer wants us to blame ourselves as individual pharmacists rather than blame the corporation for the understaffing that guarantees errors. The corporation wants to divert attention from its own negligence and responsibility to provide conditions in which accuracy is more than a matter of being lucky.

Why should all the blame be directed at the pharmacist when he is often simply the victim of a dangerously understaffed pharmacy? Are you to blame when the store you're working in (for example, for a pharmacist who is sick or on vacation) has poorly-trained techs, or no tech, or a tech who is off sick, or a tech who is on vacation? Are you to blame for the fact that your employer intentionally understaffs pharmacies to increase profitability? Are you a victim of the system just as much as the customer who received the wrong drug?

I simply have a hard time admitting fault for an error in which there are factors beyond my control. Little did I know in pharmacy school that the most difficult problem in my career would be having adequate staffing. It is shameful that pharmacists are not given enough staffing for the safe filling of prescriptions. Pharmacy school professors tell us we are professionals. In the real world, we quickly realize that we are piece-workers on a fast food assembly line.

If you are an independent owner and you dispensed the wrong medication, perhaps you have a greater responsibility to admit fault. After all, you have the power to determine staffing levels in the pharmacy. In contrast, employee pharmacists who work for the big chains are powerless to set tech staffing levels.

By admitting fault, will we increase the likelihood of the customer initiating a lawsuit? Are we essentially telling the customer that he has legitimate grounds for legal action? After one error that my partner made, he mentioned to me that he didn't know whether he should call the customer at home and apologize. My partner did decide to call the customer. My partner said the customer appreciated the apology. But it turns out that the customer sued my partner and our employer anyway. I never learned the outcome of the lawsuit. I felt it was too sensitive to discuss.

As regards the incident involving my stepfather, I was not angry at the pharmacist who was responsible. I know that the McDonald's model of pharmacy makes errors like this inevitable. Nevertheless, we all know pharmacists who are an accident waiting to happen. If the pharmacist responsible for the error in my stepfather's Rx was simply reckless and careless, a forgiving attitude would probably not be warranted.

In my opinion, there are two types of pharmacists: The first type tries very hard to prevent errors. These pharmacists lose sleep worrying about the possibility of errors. The second type of pharmacist slings out prescriptions all day long seemingly unaware of the tremendous liability riding on each prescription and without a clear understanding that the legal profession is salivating over the chance to take a big bite out of our posterior.

A shorter version of this discussion was published as an editorial in *Drug Topics* ("Should you admit fault after a dispensing error?" June 16, 2008, p. 60). With each of my editorials in *Drug Topics*, I include my e-mail address in case pharmacists care to comment. Here are three of the e-mails I received following my editorial:

E-mail from pharmacist #1

Dennis,

I just finished 7 straight days totaling 80 hours (6 X 12 hr. days and one 8 hour Sunday), working with one 24hr/week experienced tech, the other 5 techs are inexperienced, and they all do data entry. Not an envious situation. They learn from their mistakes as I point them out and correct them. And brother are they ever doing a lot of learning.
[Anonymous pharmacist]

E-mail from pharmacist #2

Hi. Thanks for your excellent article on pharmacists and apologies. I could not agree with you more.

Several years ago, I was working for a grocery chain pharmacy. I had a technician who was incompetent, insubordinate, and mentally unstable. I had tried to fire this tech for over a year, but Safeway pharmacy management would not let me do this, despite the fact that I was the pharmacy manager—and supposedly was responsible for staffing the pharmacy.

One day, a regular customer returned to the pharmacy with the complaint that she had received a prescription intended for another patient. She had taken two doses of the medication and had suffered no ill effects from it, but was understandably angry. We were still keeping manual signature logs at that time, and when I looked to see who had given the wrong Rx to this patient, it was that technician!

The patient had refused counseling, so I never saw what was actually given to her. The patient asked for a written apology from Safeway, and my store manager and pharmacy district manager tried to persuade me to write a personal letter of apology to her. I refused, as I saw a great deal of personal liability in doing this. Certainly, the technician was under my supervision at the time that this error occurred, but I had no realistic way of preventing it, short of watching over each prescription she passed to the customers, and this store was way too busy and understaffed to allow this. And if I had been allowed to terminate this employee as I had tried to several times before, this event would not have occurred.

The patient brought suit against Safeway, not me, and they ended up making a five-figure settlement to her. This event was not tied to me or my license in any way. I did feel horrible for the patient as she was a good customer, and also a good person. But I refused to make the pharmacy's staffing problem my own personal problem.

There was a huge teachable lesson for corporate pharmacy managers in all of this, but they never got the message, as the tech in question is still working for the chain. Fortunately, I am not, having left to pursue a very happy career in biopharmaceutical manufacturing operations for Amgen.

Have a good day!

[Pharmacist R. H.]

E-mail from pharmacist #3

Hi Dennis,

I read with interest your editorial in *Drug Topics* about pharmacists admitting to errors as they happen. I am a retail pharmacist and appreciate your opening dialogue on a topic that needs serious attention—the state of current pharmacy. You hint at many sad and dangerous trends in our business—understaffing, increasing errors, strained relationship between corporation and pharmacist, lawsuits, liability, and lying. Each of these can and should be discussed by all pharmacists. But I had read years ago that pharmacists tend to be an introverted group, so it's not surprising that we have been led like sheep to the "job" each day.

...Errors do happen, and part of our job is education. One of the myths out there is that pharmacies don't make mistakes. Think of how many times someone has come in and whispered "I am bringing my prescriptions over here because they made a mistake at CVS," or some other pharmacy. I always let them know at that moment that mistakes are made in EVERY pharmacy, as we are all staffed by human beings. I encourage them to call if ever anything looks different, and that in this day of hectic doctor visits and busy pharmacies you (the customer) need to look out for yourself and ask questions.

Several years ago our local paper (*Portland Press Herald*) had a lead story titled something like: "Pharmacy Errors—All Pharmacies Make Mistakes But Why does Rite Aid Get Sued More?" This was actually an eye-opening article. The writer had done his research and checked the number of errors/complaints that were brought to the attention of the Maine Board of Pharmacy, and sure enough the numbers were similar for most chains. But the number going to trial (at that time) was much higher for Rite Aid. The conclusion of the article was that how a patient is treated at the time of the incident is critical. If you are arrogant or callous in your approach, you are more likely to get sued. Since reading this article I have made it a point to develop good relationships with customers from the start. When the shit hits the fan, I want that angry customer to be a friend. If you have been an arrogant pharmacist (and there are plenty out there), then you are writing your own legal prescription. Keep that personal liability insurance handy.

...I will also say that I keep memos of correspondence between myself and the corporation when it comes to staffing. If I ended up in court I would present papers and emails to show that I tried to warn the corporation that we were dangerously understaffed. I won't go down alone; I'll drag as many of my supervisors into court as possible. Sad that this is how I look at my job, but this is my liability insurance.

Your article, hopefully, will be another push toward galvanizing pharmacists to be a more cohesive group. We are the only ones that can change this. Think about it—what if pharmacists walked off the job like the air traffic controllers did back in the 70's? Hopefully that would never happen but my point is that we need to ALL work toward change. The corporations have no interest in that. Keep up the dialogue.

[Pharmacist B. Y.]

58

Who is to blame for pharmacy mistakes?

The issue of pharmacy mistakes is possibly the most serious issue facing our profession. Why have we been unable to solve this problem? I blame the following:

1. State boards of pharmacy

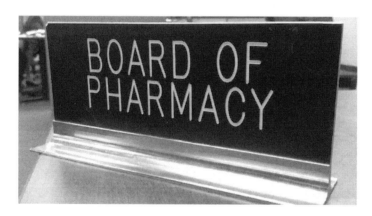

In my opinion, the state boards need to have the authority to levy hefty fines against those employers who don't provide adequate staffing for the safe filling of prescriptions. The fines need to be more than a slap on the wrist. As it is now, the big employers find it less expensive to pay customers harmed by pharmacy mistakes, rather than hire adequate staffing. The state boards need the muscle and willpower to aggressively go after the big employers, rather than slap them with a fine that means nothing to these multi-billion-dollar corporations. The fines need to be big enough so that the big employers conclude that understaffing and the inevitable pharmacy mistakes are simply not a profitable business model.

2. National Association of Boards of Pharmacy (NABP)

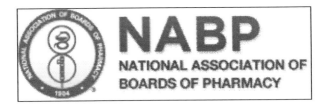

According to its website, NABP is "the impartial professional organization that supports the state boards of pharmacy in protecting public health." In my opinion, this places NABP in a unique position to make a difference with the issue of pharmacy mistakes. I would like to see NABP take its role seriously in protecting public health by making a forceful presentation to Congress that safe staffing in pharmacies must be assured. Surely NABP could do more in this regard than it is now, i.e., nothing.

3. American Pharmacists Association (APhA)

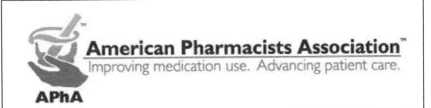

Many pharmacists harbor a tremendous amount of contempt for APhA for not focusing on those working conditions (primarily staffing levels) that make errors inevitable. The American Medical Association seems to be far more effective in addressing working conditions for doctors than APhA is for pharmacists. Many pharmacists are incredulous that APhA appears to be too timid to fight for pharmacists' working conditions. Many pharmacists feel that APhA's timidity in addressing this issue is more than enough reason to refuse to join that organization.

4. State legislatures

The anti-regulatory ideology that predominates in America to-day (even after the near-collapse of our financial system) holds that the market should be left to its own devices to fix every problem, and that no governmental agency should intervene in the private sector. Accordingly, workplace issues such as understaffing are conveniently viewed by state legislatures as employer-employee is-sues rather than public safety issues. But state legislatures have a duty (like state boards) to protect the public safety. Fear of being labeled by state legislatures as anti-business causes leaders of pharmacy boards, NABP, and APhA to avoid focusing on under-staffing. Unfortunately, state legislatures have tremendous power to overturn helpful workplace regulations that any pro-employee state board dares to pass. I would like to see some head of a state pharmacy board put his job on the line by standing up to the big chains even at the risk of being labeled by that state legislature as anti-business. We need courageous leaders who put this issue above their own job security. It seems that our leaders prefer to bask in the prestige that accompanies their positions, rather than use their visibility to make a real difference for pharmacists in the trenches.

5. Employers

I know many pharmacists who privately welcome the huge multi-million dollar jury awards against the big employers as a re-sult of serious and/or fatal mistakes. Many pharmacists hope that these huge jury awards will embarrass and shame the big employers into providing adequate staffing so that pharmacy mistakes are a rarity. As it is, pharmacy mistakes are a predictable consequence of this business model based on slinging out prescriptions as fast as McDonald's slings out burgers. Many pharmacists are disgusted that McDonald's seems to be far more capable of providing ade-quate staffing for the preparation of hamburgers, whereas the huge drugstore chains seem to be incapable or unwilling to provide adequate staffing for the preparation of a far more critical product: prescription drugs.

6. Pharmacists

Every pharmacist knows that many of our colleagues are an accident waiting to happen. These pharmacists would make errors regardless of prescription volume and regardless of staffing levels. Some pharmacists seem to have no clue about how high the stakes are with each prescription we fill. They seem to be completely oblivious to the fact that lawyers are salivating over the possibility of taking a huge bite out of our posterior.

7. Cultural factors

Our quick-fix, pill for every ill culture has commodified health. When health is seen simply as the result of the consumption of commodities, it is not surprising that the rapid distribution of those commodities is seen as paramount. Mistakes are inevitable when pharmacy is seen primarily as a distributive activity rather than a cognitive activity.

8. Pharmacy schools

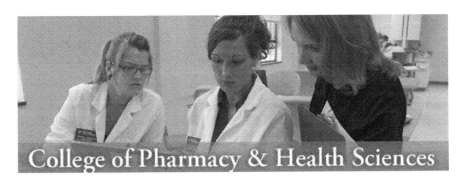

Pharmacy schools inculcate in students a view of pharmacy that is at profound odds with the real world of chain drugstores. Pharmacy schools tell students that they are drug experts whereas the big drug chains absolutely don't want drug experts. The big chains want fast food experts. Failure to be frank with pharmacy students about the real world ill-prepares students for the lightning quick pace with which they will be expected to fill prescriptions. Pharmacy schools are afraid that students will question their career choice if they are told that they'll be evaluated by chain drugstores primarily on how fast they fill prescriptions. Failure to understand these realities sets up freshly-minted pharmacists for culture shock, disorientation, disillusionment, disgust, rage, powerlessness, feelings of being overwhelmed, etc. These feelings increase the likelihood of pharmacy mistakes.

9. Pharmacy customers

Our customers deserve a big chunk of the blame for pharmacy errors because they—like our employers—seem to judge pharmacists solely by how fast we fill prescriptions. Unfortunately, drive-thru windows send an unmistakable message to customers that prescriptions are no different from burgers.

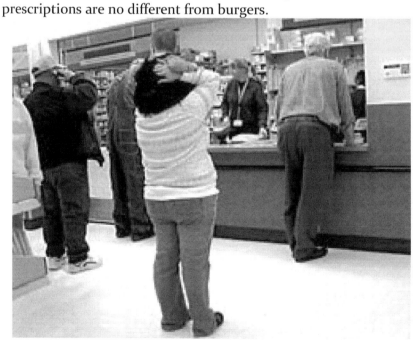

PART X

STATE BOARDS OF PHARMACY

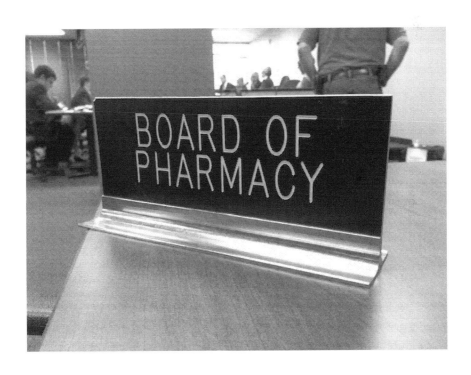

59

State boards of pharmacy disciplinary actions

DISCIPLINARY ACTIONS

The purpose of the board of pharmacy in each state is to protect the public. The state boards do things like licensing pharmacists to ensure that those pharmacists are competent. The boards try to prevent pharmacists from breaking laws pertaining to drugs. The most common disciplinary actions taken by state boards of pharmacy are usually for one of the following three reasons: (1) the pharmacist abuses drugs and/or alcohol, (2) the pharmacist is involved in illegally selling or distributing drugs, or (3) the pharmacist makes an error in dispensing drugs (for example, giving a patient the wrong drug, wrong dose, wrong directions, etc.).

Most of my career as a pharmacist was spent in North Carolina. How common are pharmacy errors in North Carolina? In my opinion, they are probably just as common as in most other states, despite some well-intentioned workload regulations that were passed by the state board of pharmacy. During the years I worked in North Carolina, most of these workload regulations were ignored by employers unless or until, for example, the board got involved in investigating an error that was reported to the board of pharmacy. In my experience, only a tiny fraction of errors are ever reported to state boards of pharmacy, mainly because pharmacy customers do not know they have that option, or because they do not perceive the error as having been serious, or because they shrug it off by telling themselves, "Errors happen. Pharmacists are human."

The NewsChannel 36 investigative team at television station WCNC in Charlotte, North Carolina analyzed a spread sheet with five years worth of errors that were reported to the North Carolina board of pharmacy from 2006 through 2010. The WCNC-TV investigative team found that the most common error was the substitution of the wrong drug, which happened 226 times in that five year period, accounting for more than half the documented errors. Other errors included wrong dosage, wrong directions, wrong patient (one patient's drugs given to a different patient), and the wrong count or number of pills or tablets in the bottle. (Stuart Watson, NewsChannel 36, Charlotte, North Carolina, "Pharmacy board documents hundreds of pharmacist errors," Posted on WCNC.com on May 3, 2011.
http://www.wcnc.com/news/iteam/NC-Pharmacy-board-documents-hundreds-of-pharmacist-errors-121189759.html#)

Errors reported to North Carolina Board of Pharmacy: 2006 -2010
(Analysis by WCNC-TV in Charlotte, North Carolina, May 3, 2011)
Wrong medication: 226
Wrong dose: 80
Wrong directions: 77
Wrong patient: 24
Wrong count: 12

Here is a sample of disciplinary actions taken by the North Carolina Board of Pharmacy for pharmacy mistakes that were reported to that board. Most of these mistakes involve the wrong drug being dispensed, or the right drug was dispensed but in the wrong dose, or the wrong directions were typed on the patient's label. These disciplinary actions are from the January 2002 and October 2001 issues of the *Newsletter* published by the North Carolina Board of Pharmacy (www.ncbop.org). Starting with the April 2002 issue, the North Carolina Board of Pharmacy stopped providing detailed descriptions in that *Newsletter* of disciplinary actions, so I am unable to provide more recent examples that are as detailed as those below. A notice in the April 2002 issue of the *Newsletter* states, "The format for "Disciplinary Actions" will change with this *Newsletter*. In this and all future *Newsletters*, there will be information listing a general summary of actions taken by the North Carolina Board of Pharmacy." From my perspective, there is no reason to assume that the incidence of pharmacy errors has decreased in the interim. (Please note: Brand name drugs are capitalized. Generic names are in lower case.)

DISCIPLINARY ACTIONS—JANUARY 2002

Clonidine dispensed instead of Premarin

[Pharmacist J. Z.] was the subject of a Prehearing Conference held April 9, 2001 with Mr. Watts regarding the dispensing of clonidine on a prescription which called for Premarin 0.3 mg and the patient ingesting one dosage unit of clonidine before discovering the error. Recommendation: Letter of Warning and directed to be more careful in the dispensing of drugs in the future and comply with statutes and regulations governing the practice of pharmacy and the distribution of drugs. Accepted by: [Pharmacist J. Z.] 6/28/01; the Board 7/17/01.

Tussionex dispensed instead of prednisolone

[Pharmacist V. F.] was the subject of a Prehearing Conference held May 21, 2001 with Mr. Overman regarding the dispensing of Tussionex on an order for prednisolone. The Tussionex was also labeled prednisolone. Recommendation: Caution and within 90 days of Board's acceptance of this order he shall submit a written proposal to the Board for the lawful and accurate dispensing of multi-orders of liquid prescription drugs to the same patient and that for 12 months from the date of the Board's acceptance of the order the respondent shall notify the Board's director of investigations of any error committed by him if the patient leaves the store with the prescription. Accepted by [Pharmacist V. F.] 6/23/01.

Amoxicillin dispensed instead of naproxen

[Pharmacist J. M.] was the subject of a Prehearing Conference held June 20, 2001 with Mr. Haywood regarding the dispensing of amoxicillin on an order for naproxen with the patient ingesting the incorrect product for three days before the error was discovered. Recommendation: Warning to exercise greater care in his dispensing practices in the future; review his practice environment and make any changes necessary to prevent the occurrence of dispensing errors; not violate any law or regulation governing the practice of pharmacy. Accepted by [Pharmacist J. M.] 7/10/01.

Incorrect directions on Cefzil label

[Pharmacist A. C.] was the subject of a Prehearing Conference held April 26, 2001 with Mr. Rogers regarding the dispensing of Cefzil to a patient with incorrect directions on the label and also indicating no refills when refills were left on the prescription. Recommendation: Letter of Caution for his actions in this matter and cautioned to be more careful in the dispensing of drugs in the future and to comply with statutes and regulations governing the practice of pharmacy and the distribution of drugs. Accepted by [Pharmacist A. C.] 6/26/01.

Wrong strength of Tapazole dispensed

[Pharmacist S. S.] and The Medicine Shoppe were the subject of a Prehearing Conference held May 21, 2001 with Mr. Overman regarding the dispensing of Tapazole 100 mg. on an order for Tapazole 5 mg.; failure to conduct Drug Utilization Reviews on prescription drug orders; failure to make and keep an accurate record of prescription drugs compounded in the pharmacy; failure to make and keep records regarding patient's refusals to accept counseling on new drugs. Recommendation: For the actions in committing an error in the dispensing of a prescription drug the license is suspended for a period of 3 days, stayed 1 year with specific conditions. Accepted by [Pharmacist S. S.] 7/13/01; accepted by [Pharmacist S. S.] on behalf of The Medicine Shoppe 7/13/01.

DISCIPLINARY ACTIONS—OCTOBER 2001

Zoloft dispensed instead of metronidazole
[Pharmacist C. B.] Dispensed Zoloft on a prescription for metronidazole; no patient counseling offered; the patient ingested the wrong medication for a period of four days before the error was discovered. Official Board Warning.

Incorrect directions on Dilantin
[Pharmacist J. H.] Heard by Board Member Crocker. Filled an order for Dilantin suspension with incorrect directions for administration on the vial resulting in the patient being hospitalized for approximately eight days. Recommendation: License suspended seven days, stayed two years with active three-day suspension of the license and other conditions. Accepted by [Pharmacist J. H.] March 19, 2001; the Board April 17, 2001.

Incorrect directions on Histinex DM
[Pharmacist D. H.] Heard by Board Member Watts. Dispensed Histinex DM Syrup to a patient with incorrect directions on the vial. Recommendation: Letter of Concern. Accepted by: [Pharmacist D. H.] March 13, 2001; the Board April 17, 2001.

Synthroid dispensed instead of Maxzide
[Pharmacist R. R.] Heard by Board Member Nelson. Dispensed Synthroid on a prescription for Maxzide with the patient ingesting the wrong medication for approximately seven days before the error was discovered. Recommendation: License suspended five days, stayed three years with active suspension of one day and other conditions. Accepted by: [Pharmacist R. R.] April 10, 2001; the Board April 17, 2001.

Incorrect directions on Dilantin
Indian Trail Pharmacy. Heard by Board Member Overman. A pharmacist working at that facility dispensed Dilantin liquid with incorrect directions on the bottle with the patient receiving nine administrations of the product before the error was discovered. Recommenda-

tion: Permit suspended one day, stayed two years with conditions. Accepted by: [C. S.] on behalf of Indian Trail Pharmacy March 20, 2001; by the Board April 17, 2001.

Zyrtec and Lipitor dispensed in same vial

Eckerd Drugs, 945 N Harrison Ave, Cary. Heard by Board Member Crocker. Pharmacist dispensed Zyrtec 10 mg with both Zyrtec and Lipitor 10 mg dispensed in same vial. The error resulted from Zyrtec and Lipitor being placed in a "Baker Cell" without the knowledge of the pharmacist. The patient ingested at least four dosage units of Lipitor as a result of the error. Recommendation: Letter of Warning with the pharmacy to implement an effective Policy and Procedure for automatic devices used in the dispensing of prescription drugs. Accepted by: [J. C.] on behalf of Eckerd Drugs March 27, 2001; by the Board April 17, 2001.

Wrong strength of isosorbide dispensed

[Pharmacist R. B.] Heard by Board Member Haywood. Dispensing isosorbide 60 mg on a prescription for isosorbide 30 mg. The patient did not ingest any of the incorrect medication. Recommendation: Reprimand and violate no laws governing the practice of pharmacy or the distribution of drugs. Accepted by: [Pharmacist R. B.] April 17, 2001; the Board May 15, 2001.

Hydralazine dispensed instead of hydroxyzine

[Pharmacist K. S.] Heard by Board Member Nelson. Dispensing of hydralazine on a prescription for hydroxyzine 25 mg with the order being refilled several times from the original dispensing date, resulting in the patient ingesting the incorrect product. Recommendation: License suspended five days, stayed three years with active one-day suspension of the license and other conditions. Accepted by: [Pharmacist K. S.] May 2, 2001; the Board May 15, 2001.

Fiorinal dispensed instead of Florinef

[Pharmacist O. O.] Heard by Board Member Nelson regarding the dispensing of Fiorinal on an order calling for Florinef with the patient ingesting three dosage units before the error was discovered. Recommendation: License suspended five days, stayed three years with active one day suspension and other specific conditions. Accepted by: [Pharmacist O. O.] April 23, 2001; the Board May 15, 2001.

Vibramycin dispensed instead of vitamins

[Pharmacist L. R.] Heard by Board Member Watts. Dispensing Vibramycin 100 mg on a prescription for vitamins with the patient ingesting the incorrect medication for approximately 34 days before discovery of the error. Recommendation: Warning to exercise greater care in his dispensing practices in the future. Accepted by: [Pharmacist L. R.] May 10, 2001; the Board May 15, 2001.

Sulfasalazine dispensed instead of sulfadiazine

[Pharmacist H. M.] Heard by Board Member Rogers. Dispensing sulfasalazine 500 mg to a patient on a prescription order for sulfadiazine 500 mg. Recommendation: Letter of Warning for his actions in this matter. Accepted by: [Pharmacist H. M.] May 30, 2001; the Board June 26, 2001.

Prednisone dispensed instead of glipizide

[Pharmacist M. D.] Heard by Board Member Rogers. Dispensing prednisone 5 mg to a patient who was to receive glipizide. Recommendation: Letter of Warning for her actions in this matter. Accepted by [Pharmacist M. D.] May 30, 2001; the Board June 26, 2001.

Verapamil dispensed instead of Zantac

[Pharmacist T. L.] Heard by Board Member Watts. Dispensing verapamil to a patient on a prescription calling for Zantac with the patient ingesting two dosage units of the incorrect medication before the error was discovered. Recommendation: Letter of Warning for his actions in this matter. Accepted by: [Pharmacist T. L.] May 23, 2001; the Board June 26, 2001.

Pharmacist committed seven errors in six months

[Pharmacist W. F.] Heard by Board Member Watts. Embezzlement or otherwise diversion to his own use of approximately 900 dosage units of hydrocodone; during the first six months of the year 2000 committing seven errors in the dispensing of prescription drugs to patients; history of alcohol and controlled substance abuse for approximately 25 years. Recommendation: License suspended indefinitely, stayed five years with specific conditions. Accepted by: [Pharmacist W. F.] May 15, 2001; the Board June 26, 2001.

Propylthiouracil dispensed instead of Purinthol

[Pharmacist D. M.] Heard by Board Member Watts. Dispensing propylthiouracil to a two-year-old patient on a prescription calling for Purinethol with the patient ingesting the wrong medication from January 10 until June 20, 2000, when the error was discovered. Recommendation: License suspended 30 days, stayed three years with an active suspension of seven days to begin no later than June 30, 2001, and other conditions. Accepted by [Pharmacist D. M.] May 17, 2001; the Board June 26, 2001.

Morphine dispensed instead of Roxicodone

[Pharmacist A. A.] Heard by Board Member Watts. Dispensing morphine 15 mg on a prescription calling for Roxicodone 5 mg with the patient ingesting 81 morphine 15 mg dosage units before the error was discovered. Recommendation: Letter of Warning for her actions in this matter. Accepted by: [Pharmacist A. A.] May 17, 2001; the Board June 26, 2001.

Wrong dose of doxepin dispensed

[Pharmacist P. H.] Heard by Board Member Overman. Dispensing of doxepin 10 mg to a patient on an order calling for doxepin 100 mg. Recommendation: Warning to exercise greater care in his dispensing practices. Accepted by: [Pharmacist P. H.] June 15, 2001; the Board June 26, 2001.

60

State boards of pharmacy are intimidated by the political and legal clout of chain drugstores

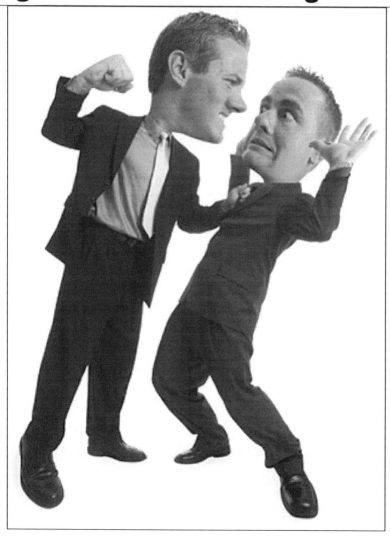

I have very mixed feelings about the state boards of pharmacy publishing (in their newsletters and/or websites) disciplinary actions taken against pharmacists. For those pharmacists who try very hard to avoid mistakes, but occasionally make them anyway, I have the greatest sympathy. If these pharmacists make an error because of inadequate staffing in the pharmacy, I consider it unfair to blame the pharmacist rather than the employer. Employers benefit from understaffing because it forces everyone to work harder, thereby increasing the productivity and profitability of the pharmacy. But understaffing also increases the chance of pharmacy mistakes.

There are a very large number of mitigating and aggravating factors that, in my opinion, should be considered before pharmacists are disciplined by state boards of pharmacy. Here are just a few:

• If a pharmacist makes a mistake because he was working overtime due to, for example, another pharmacist's vacation or illness, I find it hard to blame the pharmacist for being exhausted. However, if the pharmacist made the mistake because he asked to work those extra hours (and there were other pharmacists available), then blaming that pharmacist may be more reasonable if he claims the mistake was due to the fact that he was exhausted from the long hours on his feet.

• If a pharmacist makes a mistake because he was up all night with a sick child, then I have a hard time blaming the pharmacist.

• If a pharmacist makes a mistake because he was unfocused due to the fact that he just had an unavoidable fight with his spouse, children, or boss, I have a hard time blaming the pharmacist.

On the other hand,

• If a pharmacist makes a mistake because he was simply careless (for example, he was more interested in chatting with one of his young female techs or clerks) and there was adequate staffing in the pharmacy, it is probably more reasonable to blame the pharmacist.

Fear is a powerful motivator causing pharmacists to be careful. These fears include: 1) the fear of being sued and ending up in court, 2) the fear of harming one of our customers as a result of a mistake, 3) the fear of being disciplined by the state board of pharmacy, and 4) the fear of having our name listed in the board of pharmacy newsletter.

For those pharmacists who are extremely careful yet occasionally make errors, I feel it is unfair to publicize their names in the board of pharmacy newsletter. For those many pharmacists who are an accident waiting to happen, publicizing their names in the board newsletter may be one of the biggest things that can give these careless pharmacists a wake up call.

Potentially the most serious mistake I made in my 25-year career was when I did not catch a doctor's error on a prescription. In this case, a local doctor wrote a prescription for the sleeping pill Halcion with directions, "Take one tablet 3 times a day." Obviously sleeping pills are usually taken once a day (at bedtime). At that time, Halcion had just come on the market, and, as much as I hate to admit it, I dispensed this drug without knowing what it is used for (i.e., it is sleeping pill). The doctor had clearly made an error in the directions and I did not catch that error. I typed "Take one tablet 3 times a day" on the label just as the doctor specified. If the customer had reported this error to the state board of pharmacy, I would have been very upset but perhaps I would have deserved being disciplined for this error.

As best as I can recall this incident, there were not any exacerbating circumstances that I can blame for my role in this error. I did not make this error because of understaffing. It is true that I was sometimes exhausted at this store. I was routinely working fifty hours a week because this was in a new store and my district supervisor hadn't yet found a second pharmacist to split the eighty hours the store was open each week. "Floater" pharmacists filled in whenever I asked for a day off. I can't remember whether I was fatigued that particular day.

Surely I should never have dispensed Halcion (or any other drug) without knowing what it is used for. But I did and I am lucky that no harm resulted. The customer apparently called his doctor and asked the doctor about the directions. The doctor phoned me and asked, "Why would you put three times a day on a sleeping pill?" I asked the doctor to hold on for a few seconds while I pulled the hard copy of the prescription from our files. What I discovered when I pulled the hard copy from our files was that the doctor had indeed mistakenly specified "three times a day" on his handwritten prescription. I told the doctor, "I have your prescription here in my hand. You wrote "tid" [the Latin abbreviation for three times a day]." I think I then offered to fax him the prescription so he could see that he had made a mistake. He did not ask to see a copy of the prescription so I assume he believed me that he had made the mistake. The doctor's main question was why I had not caught the error. So the doctor and I were basically even. The doctor had screwed up and I did not catch the mistake.

If this customer had indeed taken the pill three times a day and attempted to drive a car, the results could have been disastrous. I assume that the customer realized that the Halcion is indeed a sleeping pill, so I assume he knew enough to question why the label instructed him to "Take one tablet 3 times a day." Many customers are on so many medications that they have a hard time keeping track of what each one is used for. And many pharmacy customers are illiterate or poorly literate or elderly and never question things. This customer had the misfortune of being the recipient of the most serious mistake I made in my career, but I am lucky that he knew enough to question things.

Pharmacy customers need to realize that only a tiny percentage (maybe as few as one in a thousand) of mistakes made by pharmacists are reported to state boards of pharmacy. Why? Most customers do not know that they have this option. Many customers do not realize that pharmacy mistakes can vary in significance from those that are trivial to those that are deadly. Many customers have a hard time believing that pharmacists and techs do indeed make mistakes. Many customers are, thankfully, quite forgiving. When my stepfather was given a drug for Type 2 diabetes (he's never had Type 2 diabetes) by mistake instead of his blood pressure pills at a local WalMart pharmacy, my stepfather said to me "Accidents happen. If it happens again, I'll get mad." Even though I've seen or heard about many mistakes made by pharmacists in the stores I've worked in during my career, I can't specifically recall hearing that a single one of those mistakes was reported to the state board of pharmacy.

The purpose of the state board of pharmacy is to protect the public from harm as it relates to pharmacies. Since pharmacy mistakes can and do cause harm to the public, many pharmacists feel that state boards of pharmacy should be a powerful force in preventing these errors. Pharmacists feel that working conditions (including inadequate staffing) are a primary cause of pharmacy mistakes. Therefore pharmacists feel that boards of pharmacy should take a very aggressive role in prohibiting those working conditions that contribute to pharmacy mistakes. Many pharmacists feel that state boards of pharmacy have been afraid to blame the big drugstore chains for inadequate staffing. Many pharmacists feel that the state boards are afraid to challenge the immense legal and political clout of the big drugstore chains. In a phone conversation, the head of one state board of pharmacy told me that the worst part of his job was dealing with lawyers representing pharmacists and/or the big chains.

In my opinion, another factor that prevents state boards from blaming the big chains is that the boards don't want to be seen as having an anti-business outlook in the eyes of state legislatures if those legislatures indeed have a largely pro-business orientation. In the event of a pharmacy mistake, many pharmacists are disgusted and angered by the fact that many state boards focus aggressively on the weakest player (the individual pharmacist) but appear to be afraid to focus on the strongest player (the big drugstore chains). Pharmacists feel that the big drugstore chains routinely understaff pharmacies to increase profitability and that, therefore, mistakes are inevitable.

Many pharmacists hope that the reporting of mistakes to boards of pharmacy and local newspapers will result in efforts that require adequate staffing for pharmacies. It just doesn't seem to be happening. Unfortunately the public seems to have a hard time believing that the big chains are often reckless in how they staff pharmacies.

Issues of working conditions and public safety are not unique to pharmacists. Many nurses complain that unbearable workloads endanger hospital patients. Medical residents complain that their long work weeks cause fatigue which decreases their level of performance, putting patients at risk. Airline pilots say that pilot fatigue endangers passengers. Are all these examples strictly employer/employee issues between nurses, medical residents, and hospital administrators, or between airlines and pilots? Or are they public safety issues? Long-haul truck drivers who are exhausted from spending too many hours on the highway are clearly a hazard to the public safety.

At what point do employer/employee issues justifiably become public safety issues? Are nurses, pharmacists, medical residents, airline pilots, and long-haul truck drivers simply crybabies in search of cushy jobs? At what point does governmental regulation of the private sector for public safety reasons trump the rights of private corporations to control their workplace? How many deaths must occur before regulators are justified in intervening? Republicans typically favor less regulation of the workplace than Democrats.

The pharmacy boards act as though pharmacists' working conditions are a private matter between employers and employees. Pharmacy boards seem to feel that if pharmacists dislike their working conditions, they are free to change jobs. Indeed, some pharmacists write angry "letters to the editor" telling their disillusioned colleagues: "If you're unhappy, CHANGE JOBS!!"

Is it simply a matter of disgruntled pharmacists changing jobs? Each year the pharmacy workplace shows more resemblance to a factory assembly line. The mail order model of high volume dispensing seems to be the direction in which the profession is headed, to the dismay of many pharmacists. It may be that alternatives for disgruntled pharmacists are diminishing as more employers embrace the fast food model. Even though the schools of pharmacy continue to promote the model of the pharmacist as drug expert, the big chains have shown little enthusiasm for that concept. The schools of pharmacy convince students that they're professionals. So it comes as a powerful shock when these students graduate and begin working as licensed pharmacists and discover that the big chains are only interested in how many widgets (prescriptions) we can produce per hour. When the big chains talk about productivity, what they mean is getting pharmacists, techs, and clerks to do more work with less staffing.

One definition of a dysfunctional family is a family that avoids addressing the most pressing issues facing it. For example, a dysfunctional family avoids discussing a father who is an alcoholic or who abuses his children or beats his wife. In my opinion, pharmacy boards are significantly dysfunctional because they are afraid to openly confront the most crucial issue facing chain pharmacists: working conditions.

The boards of pharmacy say that they can't do anything about pharmacists' working conditions. The boards say that if pharmacists have complaints about working conditions, we need to form a guild or union. Are the pharmacy boards simply passing the buck? Is this a legitimate position for the boards to take? Or is it simply a cop-out? Should employee pharmacists let the boards off the hook so easily? Or should we organize and hold their feet to the fire and force them to address the immediate concerns of employee pharmacists?

In my opinion, the boards of pharmacy are afraid to challenge the immense power of the big chains. What happens when some pharmacy group stands up to the big chains? The big chains or their proxies may take you to court as the North Carolina Board of Pharmacy discovered several years ago when that Board tried to address pharmacists' working conditions.

Even though I admire the North Carolina Board's efforts to pass a regulation requiring a lunch break for pharmacists, I don't see how such a regulation would have a major impact on our workplace. No employer is so stupid as to say we can't take a lunch break. Many pharmacists choose to skip meals for the simple reason that we're so far behind in filling prescriptions that taking a break would put us even further behind.

I don't see how the National Association of Boards of Pharmacy (NABP) can continue to say that pharmacists' working conditions are outside their purview when they see that the North Carolina Board has taken courageous stands in an effort to address this issue.

Employee pharmacists need to collectively put pressure on the leaders of the state boards and NABP. We need to get the dead wood out of the pharmacy boards. The boards of pharmacy tell us that they don't have any power to improve working conditions and that they can only pass regulations that protect the public safety. But surely pharmacies that are dangerously understaffed are a threat to the public safety. Surely a pharmacist who hasn't eaten any food or taken a break in ten hours is a threat to the public safety.

In my opinion, the state boards of pharmacy, as official state regulatory bodies, need to capitalize on their ties to state legislatures in order to address pharmacists' working conditions. Employee pharmacists need to hold the state boards and NABP accountable in their responsibility to protect the public safety. We need to put pressure on the boards to address working conditions the same way that the boards put pressure on us to counsel customers even though, too often, pharmacists don't have enough staffing to allow proper counseling.

Pharmacists are tired of hearing that the state boards' hands are tied by the organizational structure of state governments. The state boards need to stop making excuses and learn to think outside the box. Let the state board members jawbone the state legislators at non-official gatherings if necessary, like at social functions, football games, etc. We need results—not excuses—from state boards.

The Auburn University School of Pharmacy study (Elizabeth Flynn, et. al., "National Observational Study of Prescription Dispensing Accuracy and Safety in 50 Pharmacies," *Journal of the American Pharmacists Association*, March/April 2003, pp. 191-200. (http://www.medscape.com/viewarticle/451962) concludes that "51.5 million errors occur during the filling of 3 billion prescriptions each year." Since most pharmacists feel strongly that there is a direct relationship between understaffing and errors, I think the boards are being less than honest when they claim that they have no role in the pharmacist's workplace. If the state boards and NABP are to properly carry out their role in protecting the public safety, they have a duty to speak out about pharmacists' working conditions.

The boards have credibility with state legislatures because the boards are not seen as promoting the economic interests of pharmacists. The boards need to use their position as watchdogs over public safety to get the attention of the state legislatures. If the main function of the boards of pharmacy is to protect the public safety, then, based on the occurrence of 51.5 million errors each year, the boards are doing a very poor job of protecting the public from this unacceptably high number pharmacy errors.

I have received a large number of e-mails from pharmacists who are fed up with state boards of pharmacy. These pharmacists feel that the state boards are negligent in their duty to protect the public safety by failing to address the threat posed by dangerous dispensing speeds. Pharmacists should realize that, collectively, we have tremendous power to influence the agenda of the state boards. If huge numbers of pharmacists complain to state legislators about the state boards, surely the boards will feel the heat.

We need true leaders at all the state boards, not people who pass the buck to protect their own position. (One state board director told me that "prestige" is a big reason why some people desire to be on state boards of pharmacy.) We need dynamic leadership and people who are willing to take courageous stands in the fight for employee pharmacists. Too many pharmacy boards are wimps on the issue of pharmacists' working conditions. Collectively, pharmacists need to become more forceful and sophisticated in shaping the agenda of pharmacy boards. A major shake-up is long overdue.

David Work, formerly the executive director of the North Carolina Board of Pharmacy, is an attorney and a pharmacist. He is one of the few people with a prominent role in pharmacy who has taken a courageous position in the fight for better working conditions for pharmacists. Pharmacists should encourage him to seek the helm at one of pharmacy's major national organizations or associations. In my opinion, he should be one of the most prominent voices for pharmacy and pharmacists.

Even though I would like to see state boards of pharmacy mandate adequate staffing in pharmacies, I admit that writing such a regulation would be difficult. For example, a regulation might state that, for example, a pharmacy filling 200 prescriptions per day must have "x" number of techs on duty, a pharmacy filling 300 hundred prescriptions per day must have "y" number of techs on duty, and a pharmacy filling 400 prescriptions per day must have "z" number of techs on duty. Wording a regulation in that way fails to take into consideration the quality of each technician. It is important to realize that techs vary in performance from those who are the greenest rookies to those who are absolutely fantastic. The best techs can work circles around the weakest techs. A pharmacy filling, say, 250 prescriptions on a particular day can be bearable with good techs, but it can be an absolute nightmare with weak techs. Mandating certification of techs is not, in my opinion, the answer. Certification of techs does not mean that those techs are fast or smart. I'd rather work with non-certified techs who are fast and smart, rather than work with certified techs who are slow and not very bright. At the very least I would like state boards of pharmacy to make an attempt to mandate adequate staffing, even though I acknowledge writing such a regulation would be difficult. In my dream world, a pharmacist would have the ability to walk out of a pharmacy that he felt was inadequately staffed and a threat to the public safety. In the real world, such a pharmacist would stand the very real risk of being fired.

Many pharmacists have a great deal of anger toward state boards of pharmacy for not standing up to the big chains and requiring conditions and staffing in drugstores so that errors are not inevitable. Pharmacists express these sentiments routinely in private conversations among ourselves and, often, in letters to the editor at pharmacy magazines. The following letter-to-the-editor published in *Drug Topics* is one of many examples (Ann Greene, R.Ph., "A Matter of Time," *Drug Topics*, October, 2010, p. 13). This letter was in response to an article in that magazine about Rajendra Bhat, a former Medco pharmacist who went on a hunger strike to protest production requirements at that huge pharmacy mail order facility. Although most pharmacists would probably agree that a hunger strike is an extreme reaction to workloads, these same pharmacists would probably emphasize that Mr. Bhat's main point is exceedingly important.

Re: "Desperate measures" [*Drug Topics* Viewpoint, Sept. 2010]:
I have been a retail pharmacist for 20 years and have seen the error rates progressively getting worse. I find it appalling that a state board

could turn its back on not only the pharmacists but the patients as well. Rajendra Bhat should be commended for taking a stand while the rest of us cowardly pharmacists trudge on, knowing that patient lives are in danger.

The major chains care only about money; they add more responsibilities, such as immunizations, while providing no additional help. It is only a matter of time before a major tragedy occurs. Shame on Medco, shame on the board, and shame on the retailers who have the same quota systems in place.

--Ann Greene, R.Ph., Nottingham, Penn.

An Ohio grand jury indicted pharmacist Eric Cropp for manslaughter and reckless homicide in the death of a two-year-old child, which resulted from an improperly compounded IV solution. The medical error occurred in 2006 at Rainbow Babies & Children's Hospital where the child, Emily Jerry, was a patient undergoing chemotherapy. According to testimony presented before the Ohio board of pharmacy, the prescription for etoposide with a base solution of 0.9% sodium chloride was instead compounded by a technician with a base solution of 23.4% sodium chloride. Three days after receiving the medication, the child died. The grand jury declined to indict the technician, Katie Dudash. (Reid Paul, "Former pharmacist indicted for manslaughter after med error," *Drug Topics*, Sept. 17, 2007, p. 10. See also the Emily Jerry Foundation emilyjerryfoundation.org and http://emilyjerryfoundation.org/man-seeks-nationwide-law-after-toddlers-death/) This case settled for seven million dollars. Pharmacist Eric Cropp served time in prison for the pharmacy mistake.

Emily Jerry's father blames the Ohio State Pharmacy Board for the death of his daughter. I know this will sound extreme on my part, but I firmly believe that pharmacists across America should publicly ridicule state boards of pharmacy and the National Association of Boards of Pharmacy for being too timid to take meaningful action that actually decreases the occurrence of pharmacy mistakes. Here is the comment from Emily Jerry's father on the website (emilyjerryfoundation.org) he set up to promote the prevention of pharmacy errors.

(http://emilyjerryfoundation.org/discovery-channel-to-air-
%E2%80%9Csurfing-the-healthcare-tsunami-bring-your-best-
board%E2%80%9D-on-april-28th%E2%80%9D-featuring-initial-
interview-between-christopher-jerry-and-eric-cropp/

...I truly believe that the Ohio State Pharmacy Board, at that time, should have really been held culpable in Emily's death. The reason I say this is due to the simple fact that it was determined that a pharmacy technician had actually made the fatal error that had killed Emily. After the incident, the pharmacy technician had mentioned that she never really knew that highly concentrated sodium chloride (salt) could actually kill people. With that in mind, I have always asked myself why the Ohio State Pharmacy Board at that time had absolutely no training requirements, licensing requirements, or oversight of pharmacy technicians in the state of Ohio. To make matters worse, they had to know that pharmacy technicians were being used on a daily basis at all of Ohio's medical facilities to routinely compound IV medications going directly into patient's circulatory systems. With that being said, I believe the Ohio State Pharmacy Board was really not doing their primary job, which was to protect the residents of their state from unsafe pharmacy practices. Bottom line, as Emily's father, had I known that there would have been a very high likelihood, or probability, that a pharmacy technician who had little, to no, training would have been compounding my daughter's IV medications, I never would have allowed it to happen. I would have insisted that only a registered pharmacist, with years and years of training, prepare all of Emily's IV medications during the course of her treatment.

PART XI

PHARMACY SCHOOLS

College of Pharmacy

61

Pharmacy schools aren't frank with students about chain drugstore working conditions

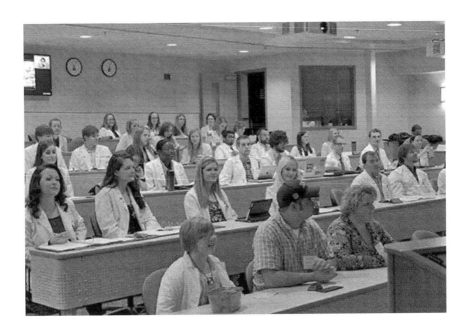

"Clinical pharmacy" is an inside-the-profession term that means a pharmacist utilizing his knowledge about drugs to optimize drug therapy just as a physician uses his "clinical medicine" skills to optimize the diagnosis and treatment of disease.

"Alma mater" is Latin for "nourishing mother" or "fostering mother." We were coddled in pharmacy school by professors who

were protective of us, as if they were our second mother or substitute parents. Sure, we had to study hard to graduate, but once we were accepted into pharmacy school, our professors seemed to feel it was their duty to help us become pharmacists. The big chains have no similar protective view toward pharmacists.

Teachers and professors in all fields are accused of building the self-esteem of students to sky-high levels, almost to the point where high school and college graduates view themselves as the center of the universe. Pharmacy professors convince students that they will be valued for their drug knowledge when, in fact, the big chains are contemptuous of the product of today's pharmacy schools, the Pharm D. The big chains were happy with BS pharmacists, or even techs or robotics. Pharmacy professors don't level with students and tell them that the model they're pushing in pharmacy school is completely unrealistic in the real world of chain drugstores.

Psychologists say that humans replay in our minds the audio recordings that our brains make of our conversations with our parents. Ideally, our parents are our moral compass. From them we learn compassion and right from wrong. We replay those recordings in our brains for the rest of our lives.

Similarly, pharmacy professors imprint in the minds of young, naïve, impressionable students a model of pharmacy that, in reality, reinforces the occupational and intellectual interests of those professors far more than it does the needs of pharmacists in the trenches. I view the switch to the PharmD degree as a turf grab by pharmacy professors concerned about their academic standing among university faculty who wanted to be able to tell medical and dental professors that the pharmacy curriculum is equal because our entry level degree is now a doctorate just like theirs.

For the rest of their careers, pharmacists ask themselves, "Where is the clinical nirvana that I was promised in pharmacy school?" We graduate from pharmacy school and never recover from the fact that our alma mater wasn't honest with us in describing the real world. It is too painful for us to accept that our pharmacy professors sold us a bill of goods about what pharmacy is really like.

Over the course of my career in chain drugstores, I've heard it said many times (only half-jokingly) that pharmacists need to bring a class action lawsuit against the pharmacy schools in America for misrepresenting the real world. In pharmacy school, our young minds are imprinted with a professional model of the pharmacist that simply does not (and, I predict, never will) exist in the chain drugstore setting.

Pharmacy students graduate with a view of themselves as skilled professionals and experience profound culture shock in the real world in which they don't even have time to eat or go to the bathroom. How could our alma mater have misled us so fundamentally during our college years about the nature of pharmacy in the real world?

Pharmacy students graduate with a belief that they're god's gift to the world of health care, that their drug knowledge will be highly valued in our health care system. That naive view puts them at a severe disadvantage when it comes to dealing with our employer. We see ourselves as professionals while our employers see us as disposable wage laborers. The unspoken corporate attitude toward pharmacists seems to be, "Burn 'em out and hire someone younger." So pharmacists are unprepared to fight the big chains with the only thing they understand: power. We tell ourselves, "True professionals don't need unions."

Acknowledging the real world (i.e., that we need a union) is just too painful for precious young graduates who've been led to believe they will be the savior of our health care system. Pharmacists prefer to carry around in our heads a view of ourselves as highly trained professionals. The big chains are happy that we view ourselves as professionals who are above unions. That's because the biggest thing that scares the chains is powerful unions.

Students' brains are filled with a vision of clinical nirvana, a carrot that has been dangled in front of students at least since I graduated in 1975. From the perspective of a chain pharmacist, I would say that the average chain pharmacist is no closer to the clinical model today than when I graduated 35 years ago. Pharmacy professors are afraid to level with students about real world working conditions out of fear that those students will begin wondering whether pharmacy is the right choice. For their own job security, professors fear declining enrollments in pharmacy schools.

The current pharmacy school model stressing a professional role for the pharmacist does a disservice to new graduates when they enter the real world of retail pharmacy. In the real world, newly minted PharmDs are in for a rude awakening as they quickly discover that they're being paid to use their hands and feet, not their brains. They quickly discover what veteran pharmacists have known for decades: the chains have always been antagonistic to the concept of clinical pharmacy.

I don't like the phrase "pharmacy practice" because I feel that it is pompous and pretentious. A "practice" is something that professionals engage in. If a pharmacist doesn't have time for bathroom breaks or meal breaks, I do not consider him to be a professional. I consider him to be a wage laborer. Who are we kidding in calling ourselves professionals if we don't even have rights that most other employees take for granted? Until we recognize the cold and hard facts about our working conditions, we will be easy prey for the corporate bosses who play hard ball with us, while we consider it beneath us to stand up to these playground bullies.

We need to realize that retail pharmacy is a distributive enterprise, not a cognitive enterprise. Until pharmacists realize that our employers are playing hard ball with us, we will be unable to take the actions required to ameliorate our pathetic working conditions. The big employers treat us arrogantly as wage laborers while we view ourselves as professionals who are above unions.

If our professors had accurately described us as wage laborers, pharmacy students would realize that our best ally is aggressive labor leaders, not ivory tower academicians who fill our heads with subjects like chemistry that we never use in the real world.

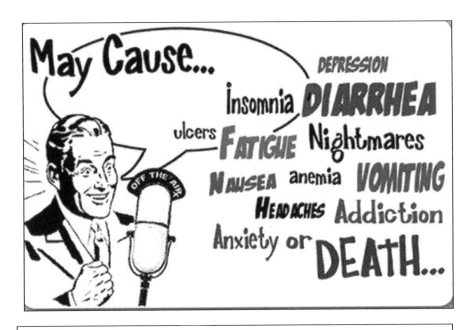

PART XII

HOW TO AVOID BECOMING A PHARMACY STATISTIC

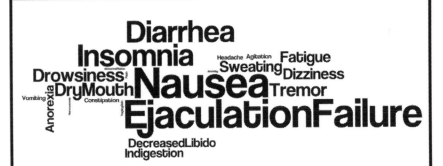

62

"Why do my pills look different this time?"

In general, when customers question the color or shape of the pills they receive at the pharmacy, the most common answer they're given by pharmacists and techs is that the medication is a generic equivalent or that it is made by a different company. This explanation is usually correct, but there are cases in which pharmacy clerks have given this answer even though they are clearly not qualified to do so.

When your medication looks different from what you were expecting, verify the contents with the pharmacist. Some pharmacy clerks have heard the "generic equivalent" or "different company" explanation so often that the clerks use it themselves reflexively when questioned by a customer. You need to know that newly hired pharmacy clerks may not clearly understand the ramifications of giving this explanation all the time. Many pharmacy clerks clearly do not have the experience or authority to make the determination whether your medication is a generic equivalent, whether it is made by a different company, or whether it is indeed an instance of the pharmacy dispensing the wrong drug. In most cases, the "generic equivalent" or "different company" explanation is correct. However, in some cases the drug the customer has received looks different because it is indeed the wrong medication.

The "generic equivalent" explanation often comes in very handy when there has indeed been a pharmacy error and the pharmacy staff tries to obfuscate this fact. I think it would be fair to say that a large number of pharmacists have used this explanation to cover up what is indeed a mistake. I've used this explanation myself to get out of a fix on more than one occasion. Here's the scenario: A customer brings her container back to me and asks why the pills look different from what she expected. My heart rate immediately goes into the danger zone as I experience another instance that pharmacists have nightmares about: *Another pharmacy error!!*

I have, on occasion, lied to such customers and said that the pills are "a generic." I've seen a few other pharmacists use the same lie. It gets us out of a very touchy situation. Most customers obviously don't know that we're lying to them. They trust us and accept our explanation.

Many pharmacists (myself included) feel that if the corporation provided us with adequate staffing, errors would be a rarity. Therefore, why should we, as pharmacists, offer our head on a platter by admitting an error and thus possibly prompting a lawsuit? It's so much easier to lie to the customer by telling him or her that it's a generic equivalent. Few pharmacists are eager to open a huge can of worms by admitting negligence. Of course, if we perceive that the customer may be at some risk as a result of the wrong medication, we are much less likely to engage in a cover-up. Most pharmacists tell the customer something like "I'll be happy to give you the brand you had before." This is an easy way for us to correct the error without the customer realizing that an error has indeed occurred. Let me emphasize that we do indeed correct the error when it is pointed out to us and, in the most serious instances, we notify the patient's doctor.

Certainly, lying to customers about the occurrence of an error is strictly against corporate policy. Corporate policy states that we should admit our error to the customer, apologize, give the customer a refund for the prescription, and give the customer the proper medication at no charge. Since many pharmacists blame the corporation for the environment in the drugstore that makes errors inevitable, many pharmacists question why should we have to endure the wrath of an angry customer ourselves and why should we make ourselves an easy target for a lawsuit.

I once worked with a pharmacist who was an absolute stickler for rules. He seemed to be one of those people who loved to follow rules to the *nth* degree. But one day I found out that he was actually selective about which rules he enforced. One day I observed him as he spoke with a customer who asked him why her pills looked different this time. He told her that they were a generic equivalent. He said, "They're a generic made by a different company but I'll give you the ones you've had before if you like." She answered "yes." So he gave her the proper pills. After she walked away, this pharmacist passed by me and said something like "Jim [a substitute pharmacist] gave her the wrong pills yesterday but I didn't want to get tangled in a big mess so I just told her that it was a generic." He wasn't necessarily proud of himself for lying but his attitude seemed to reflect the impossible position we pharmacists are placed in.

The point is that it is handy to use the "It's a generic" explanation in instances in which that is indeed the case, and also in instances in which a real error has occurred. William Winsley, executive director of the Ohio State Board of Pharmacy, comments on this tendency to freely use the "It must be a generic" explanation ("Are All Drug Errors System Errors?" *Drug Topics*, April 15, 2002, pp. 18, 20). He says that several cases of severe patient harm have resulted from using this explanation too freely:

> When a patient calls the pharmacy and asks if the medication he just received is correct since it has a different color or shape than what he was expecting, the prudent pharmacist reviews the prescription, the patient record, and asks for the color, shape, and identifying marks on the dosage form received by the patient. In several cases this board [the Ohio State Board of Pharmacy] has dealt with, the pharmacist did none of these steps. Instead, he told the patient that the dosage form must have been a generic equivalent and should be safe to take. Several cases of severe patient harm have resulted, followed by board hearings, due primarily to the pharmacist's carelessness.

Here is an actual example of an error that occurred as a result of a pharmacy customer not questioning a change in medication appearance. In this case, methotrexate, an extremely powerful drug used for various conditions (rheumatoid arthritis, some forms of cancer, severe psoriasis), was mistakenly dispensed by a pharmacy instead of the blood pressure drug minoxidil. (Institute for Safe Medication Practices, "Medication Errors," *U.S. Pharmacist*, October 2006, p. 144)

As the number of generic products continues to increase, it seems that both patients and practitioners have become desensitized to changes in medication appearance. Patients may not even question a change, or if they do, practitioners may just reassure them that it was due to a change in manufacturer, without actively investigating the reason. It is not uncommon for ISMP [Institute for Safe Medication Practices] to receive reports from practitioners and consumers that a change in medication appearance was not fully investigated and subsequently contributed to an error.

In one case, a man shared an account of what his 86-year-old father experienced over the course of nine days after his prescription for minoxidil was mistakenly refilled with another medication. He had been taking minoxidil 2.5 mg for years, at a dose of 5 mg (two tablets) twice daily. Due to his failing vision, he did not realize that his minoxidil tablets looked different. His daughter noticed the change but was unconcerned, because the tablets had changed in appearance before. Within a few days, he began to experience a diminished appetite, complained of a sore throat, and felt like he was coming down with a cold. Soon after, he developed a rash on his face, had trouble maintaining his balance, and wished to remain in bed. When a family friend (a nurse) came to see him, she noticed a red, raised rash on his abdomen that looked like a medication rash. She was told that he was not taking any new medications, but that the minoxidil tablets looked different than before. The pharmacy was contacted about the change, and a staff member explained that it was a different generic for minoxidil and that the pills could be exchanged for those that the man usually received. There was no mention of a mistake being made when the medication was exchanged. He was taken to the hospital the next day, when he could barely walk. After the incident was explained to hospital staff, they contacted the pharmacy. It was revealed that the man had been given methotrexate by mistake, because the bottles were stored next to each other. By this time, he had taken 36 methotrexate 2.5 mg tablets, and he was in critical condition. We later learned that he died during the hospital visit.

How could this pharmacy mix-up have occurred? The pharmacy customer was taking minoxidil in the 2.5 mg strength. Sitting on the pharmacy shelf next to the minoxidil 2.5 mg tablets were methotrexate 2.5 mg tablets. Whenever two drug names are somewhat similar, and whenever those two drugs are available in the same strength (in this case 2.5 mg), and whenever those drugs are sitting on the pharmacy shelf next to each other (probably due to these drugs being shelved in alphabetical order), the opportunity for error increases significantly.

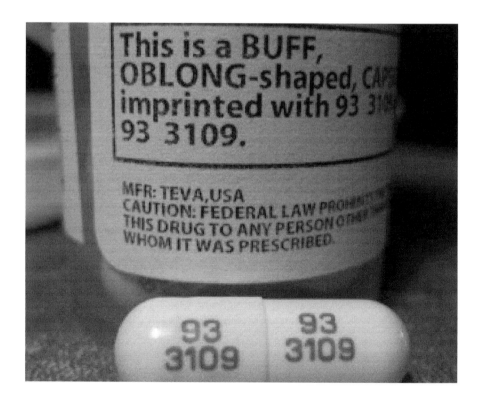

63

Identifying generic drugs is not as difficult as it used to be

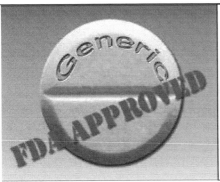 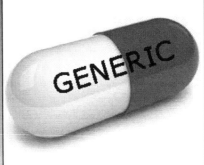

Identifying generic drugs used to be much more difficult (for pharmacists and consumers) than identifying brand name drugs. Generic drugs are very often garden variety white tablets, i.e., they have few, if any, unique distinguishing characteristics that make them readily identifiable except for the product number which may be too small to read easily. The manufacturers of brand name products seem to take more pride in the appearance of their tablets and in making sure that the tablets don't crumble too easily. Brand name products are intentionally made with a unique appearance to gain patient loyalty and expectation. Customers ask the pharmacist, "I've been on this light blue blood pressure pill for two years. Why did you refill my prescription with red pills? Did the pharmacy make a mistake?" Sometimes the highly embarrassing answer is *yes*.

If all the tablets in the pharmacy were round and white like many generics, errors would probably be more frequent. The endless variation in shapes, sizes, and colors helps pharmacists and techs cut down on pharmacy errors. Customers often ask the pharmacist to identify a tablet. Tablets that are easy to identify are more likely to have a unique appearance. It is obviously helpful to have the name of the manufacturer on the pill. Most pills are imprinted with a product number. Some pills are imprinted with the brand name of the product, a practice which I wish all companies would adopt. In general—but certainly not always—generic names are longer than brand names. This makes it more difficult to stamp long generic names like hydrochlorothiazide, methocarbamol, amitriptyline, or cyclobenzaprine on small tablets. Thus, it is often easier to identify brand name pills than generics. Generic tablets are much more likely to be unremarkable in appearance. Many generic pills are, however, quite distinct in their appearance.

In the last few years, websites have become available that greatly simplify the process of identifying tablets and capsules, whether they are brand name drugs or generics. Search Google for *pill identifier* and you will find several websites. For example: 1) drugs.com, 2) webmd.com, 3) healthline.com, and 4) health-tools.aarp.org, and 5) rxlist.com

Usually all that you have to do to identify your tablets and capsules is enter the numbers, letters, or words on those pills. Even though my mother died over ten years ago, I have kept all the pills that she was prescribed during her treatment for colon cancer that spread to her liver. I grabbed ten of those pill bottles containing mostly generic drugs and entered the numbers, letters, and words into the appropriate fields on the drugs.com website. I was quickly given the precisely correct identity of each pill. Below you will see the info I entered and the results:

1.	54 543	Correctly identified as Roxicet
2.	Mylan 155	Correctly identified as generic Darvocet
3.	SP 4220	Correctly identified as Niferex-150
4.	Endo 602	Correctly identified as Endocet
5.	INV 276 10	Correctly identified as prochlorperazine 10 mg
6.	M 15	Correctly identified as generic Lomotil
7.	Watson 349	Correctly identified as generic Vicodin
8.	KU 108	Correctly identified as generic Levbid
9.	MP 85	Correctly identified as generic Septra DS
10.	OC 20	Correctly identified as Oxycontin 20 mg

It is not rare that adults ask pharmacists to identify some tablet or capsule found at home. In my career, sometimes I had the impression that this was a parent who had discovered that pill in his or her child's room or in the child's clothing while emptying pockets before doing laundry. I was somewhat uncomfortable under these circumstances because I suspected that if the pill I identified were a controlled substance, the son or daughter would soon be in for a world of hurt, i.e., confronted by a very angry parent.

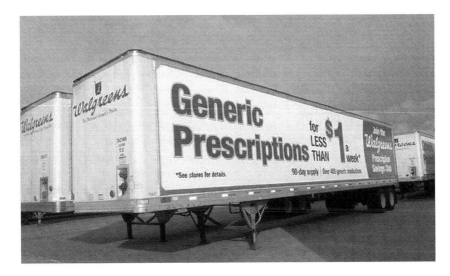

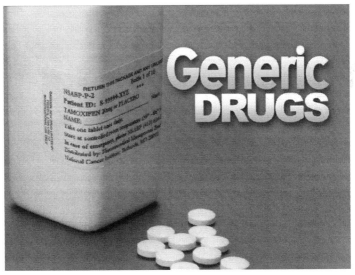

64

Your confusion with brand and generic names can have disastrous consequences

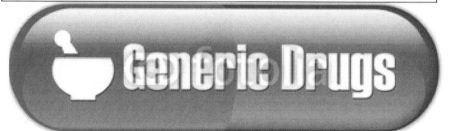

Another issue regarding confusion with generic drugs involves what is known as "therapeutic duplication." It is extremely important that consumers learn both the brand and generic names of all their drugs so that they don't end up taking the exact same drug under two different names. For example, if you were taking the generic thyroid hormone levothyroxine and your doctor wrote you a prescription for Levothroid, Levoxyl, Euthyrox, or Synthroid, would you know that all of these are simply brand names for levothyroxine? If you were taking generic theophylline for asthma, and your doctor wrote you a prescription for Slo-Phyllin, Slo-bid, Theo-Dur, Theo-24, or Uniphyl, would you know that these are simply brand names for theophylline? If you were taking generic lithium carbonate for manic depression and your doctor wrote you a prescription for Cibalith, Eskalith, Lithobid, Lithotabs, or Lithonate, would you know that these are simply brand names for lithium carbonate? If you were taking Lanoxin for your heart and your doctor wrote you a prescription for digoxin, would you know that these are the same drug? If you were taking the blood thinner Coumadin and your pharmacy filled a new prescription for warfarin, would you know that these are the same drug?

Reports of concurrent use of digoxin and Lanoxin have been reported in the past, sometimes with unfortunate outcomes. Such situations tend to occur when the same medication is prescribed by brand name by one physician and by generic name by another physician, or when the medications are dispensed from different pharmacies. This problem is becoming more common as healthcare becomes increasingly fragmented. Dupont, manufacturer of the blood thinner Coumadin, says that several cases of therapeutic duplication have been reported to the company. In one case, a 69-year old female inadvertently taking both warfarin and Coumadin was admitted to the hospital with massive rectal and nasal bleeding and an international normalized ratio (INR) of 30.9. During her hospitalization, she suffered a myocardial infarction that was attributed to her blood loss. In another case, a patient received prescriptions for Coumadin from one physician and generic warfarin from another. She ended up hospitalized as a result of "bleeding from her ears and eyes." Fortunately, treatment with vitamin K resolved the patient's symptoms and she was subsequently discharged. (Susan Proulx, "Medication Errors," *U.S. Pharmacist*, June 1998, p. 95)

Whenever you receive a prescription for a drug that you're not familiar with, you should never assume that your doctor has put you on an entirely different medication. It could be the same drug under a different name. Pharmacists see many instances in which customers are not aware that indapamide is the same as Lozol, alprozolam is the same as Xanax, lorazepam is the same as Ativan, atenolol is the same as Tenormin, furosemide is the same as Lasix, gemfibrozil is the same as Lopid, piroxicam is the same as Feldene, methocarbamol is the same as Robaxin, etc.

Trying to decide whether you have a generic drug by comparing it to the brand name is usually a bad idea. Sometimes the generic name does resemble the brand name in some ways. For example, digoxin sounds somewhat like Lanoxin. Naproxen sounds a lot like Naprosyn. Cefaclor sounds like Ceclor. Clonazepam sounds a little like Klonopin. Roxicet and Percocet share "cet" (denoting aCETaminophen). Amoxicillin, Trimox, and Amoxil all share "mox." But in most cases, the generic name does not look anything like the brand name. For example, ranitidine shows absolutely no resemblance to Zantac. Guanfacine shows absolutely no resemblance to Tenex. Glyburide shows no resemblance to Diabeta or Micronase. Ketoprofen shows no resemblance to Orudis. Nortriptyline shows no resemblance to Pamelor.

Here's an actual case illustrating the confusion that can be caused by generic names. Attorney Dan Frith from the Frith Law Firm in Roanoke, Virginia, writes: ("Pharmacy Mistakes Kill," Feb. 13, 2008. Accessed Feb. 28, 2008.
http://roanoke.injuryboard.com/medical-malpractice/pharmacy-mistakes-kill.php?googleid=14934]

My law firm is getting ready to try a case against a local pharmacy which filled and dispensed a doctor's prescription for medication to which our client was allergic. You may ask, "Why did the client take a medication to which she knew she was allergic"? The answer is that she was given the generic form of the drug—the pills did not look the same and the generic name was nowhere close to the name of the medication to which she was allergic. The prescribing doctor has accepted his responsibility and paid money damages to our client but the pharmacy has not.

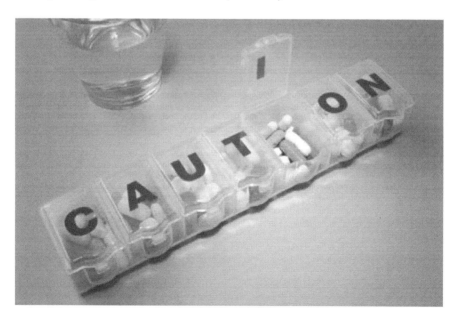

65

Pharmacy customers routinely fail to understand the medications they consume

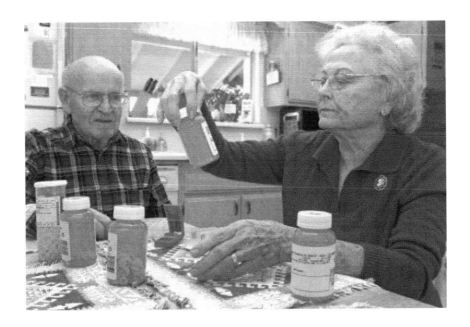

Both of my parents were simply overwhelmed with the volume of medications their doctors prescribed during the last few months of their lives. When my mother was released from the hospital following colon cancer surgery, she was given a long list of drugs, most of which were simply for relief of symptoms. My mother was one of the most organized people in the world, but the sheer volume of pills she was supposed to take at home was very unsettling to her. She had difficulty understanding what each pill was used for and which ones were strictly for relief of symptoms. At one point as I watched her, she gagged as she was preparing to take more pills. She then told me she was no longer going to take any more of those pills unless they were absolutely critical.

My mother took very few prescription drugs until the few months of her life following her colon cancer diagnosis. Her colon cancer was not diagnosed until it was at an advanced stage and had spread to her liver. Even though many pharmacy customers are very knowledgeable about drug names and drug uses, my mother had little need during most of her life to gain such knowledge. So she was at a disadvantage after her cancer diagnosis when the number of prescribed drugs she was given increased dramatically.

At different points during the last six months of her life, she was prescribed four pain pills—Darvocet, Vicodin, Percocet, and Oxycontin—the first three of which were filled generically, increasing her confusion. The generic Darvocet was labeled PROPO-N/APAP 100-650. The generic Vicodin was labeled HYDROCO/APAP 5-500. The generic Percocet was labeled OXYCODONE/APAP. She did not know that Darvocet was the mildest of the pain pills. She did not know that Vicodin was intermediate. And she did not know that Percocet and Oxycontin were the strongest. She received the generic for Bactrim DS (labeled SMZ/TMP DS 800-160MG) but the label did not tell her that this drug was being used for her urinary tract infection. She received the generic for Levbid (HYOSCYAMINE 0.375 CR) with no indication on the label that these pills were for her stomach spasm and gastrointestinal cramps. She received Actigall with no indication on the label that these pills were being used to decrease her liver enzyme levels. She received the generic for Lomotil (DIPHEN/ATROP 2.5 MG) with no indication on the label that these pills were for diarrhea. She received Cipro with no indication on the label that these pills were for her urinary tract infection. She received Prilosec with no indication on the label that these pills were for stomach acid. She received the generic for Zyloprim with no indication on the label that these pills were being used to counter some of the effects of her chemotherapy.

My mother decided to write the intended use of each medication directly on each bottle. It would, of course, have been so much easier if the pharmacist or tech had typed the intended use on the label. But I do not blame the pharmacists or techs for not indicating on the label the precise use of each medication. If doctors don't specify the precise reason they are prescribing each drug, the pharmacist cannot simply take an educated guess as to why the doctor has prescribed the drug. So the pharmacist cannot add the intended use to the label unless the doctor indicates that on the prescription. For example, Actigall is usually used to dissolve gallstones, rather than to decrease liver enzymes. If the pharmacist had taken an educated guess and labeled the Actigall as being used to help dissolve gallstones, he would have been wrong in my mother's case.

Including the intended use on the label of each medication is not always desired by our pharmacy customers since family members, friends, and neighbors may notice these bottles lying around your house in your kitchen, bathroom, or elsewhere. When the medication is used to treat a sexually transmitted disease, clearly most people would prefer that this detail not appear on the label. I assume that some users of antidepressants don't want the phrase "for depression" on the label. Throughout my entire career, I don't recall ever including any of the following "indications" (intended uses) on customers' labels: "for psychosis," "for shyness," "for attention deficit/hyperactivity," "for excessive handwashing or other obsessive-compulsive behavior," "for AIDS," "for bedwetting," "for lice," "for erectile dysfunction," or "for cancer." Doctors usually specify the more formal "for loose stools" rather than "for diarrhea" and "for nasal congestion" rather than "for runny nose."

Our medical system functions best when patients are highly sophisticated and informed. This system essentially throws potent pills at people and expects everyone to understand their proper use. Yet every pharmacist knows that too many customers take medications incorrectly. For example, pharmacists routinely see customers return for a refill on their medications after, say, fifteen days when these customers were given a thirty day supply with instructions to take one tablet per day.

One Sunday a female customer in perhaps her thirties came to the pharmacy and told me that she was having severe pain in her abdomen. She told me that she had taken a very large number of the non-prescription analgesic Aleve over the previous few days in an attempt to relieve her stomach pain. She told me that she had been released from Duke Hospital in Durham, North Carolina a few days or weeks prior. I think she said she was at Duke for some type of abdominal problem, but I can't recall precisely. It appeared to me that it was possible that her severe abdominal pain could have been caused or exacerbated by her gross overuse of Aleve. Non-steroidal anti-inflammatory drugs like Aleve and many others are well-known for their potential to cause stomach irritation with ulceration and/or gastrointestinal bleeding in more serious cases. Even though it was a Sunday afternoon, I asked her if it was okay for me to try to reach her doctor at Duke. She said that was okay and luckily her doctor happened to be at Duke when I called. When the switchboard operator connected me with her doctor, I briefly informed her doctor about this young lady's severe abdominal pain, then I handed the phone to this young lady. Her doctor proceeded to tell warn her about the risks of taking too many drugs like Aleve. My feeling was that this young lady needed to head straight for the emergency room. Unfortunately, I don't know how this story turned out but I think it illustrates how poorly so many pharmacy customers understand how easy it is to get into trouble with pharmaceuticals when they're not used properly.

I suspect that many pharmacists have reached the conclusion that it is unrealistic to expect all of our customers to be able to follow the manufacturer's directions on non-prescription labels. Clearly many pharmacy customers have difficulty understanding the directions that pharmacists and techs type on prescription labels. Regardless how much verbal counseling pharmacists provide, and regardless how much written information we provide, some of our customers simply do not seem to be able to manage their medications properly. In the real world, millions of users of prescription drugs have extreme difficulty managing their medications because they have diminished eyesight and mental acuity, because they are marginally literate or illiterate, because English is not their native language, etc.

Pharmaceuticals are potent substances that require competent prescribers and competent patients who are capable of understanding and following directions on labels. We have a sophisticated medical system in this country based on complexity. It appears to me that millions of people in this country fall through the cracks in our complex system every day.

Here's an example from the Institute for Safe Medication Practices of the kind of confusion that pharmacists see all the time, especially among elderly patients. In this example, an elderly patient died after chewing a medication that was not supposed to be chewed. ("To Chew, Or Not To Chew? Patient Dies After Chewing Medication," Institute for Safe Medication Practices, Accessed March 7, 2008.
http://www.ismp.org/Newsletters/consumer/alerts/chewable.asp)
With the McDonald's model of pharmacy, incidents like this are inevitable.

Some medications should never be chewed, cut, crushed, or diluted. The only way to know is to read label instructions carefully and/or ask your pharmacist or physician how each drug should be taken. Unfortunately, not all patients read the directions or receive and follow this kind of advice from health providers. The following case illustrates the dangers when patients are not given appropriate instructions or do not question how to take medication.

An 83-year-old patient was given Cardizem CD (sustained release diltiazem capsules) for blood pressure control. Because the capsule was too large to swallow, the patient chewed the medication. As a result, her pulse twice slowed to low levels and the family contacted the pharmacist for advice. Upon learning that she was chewing the medication, the pharmacist suggested that the physician substitute immediate release diltiazem tablets, which are easier to swallow. The prescription was changed and the patient did well for several months

Months later the patient returned to her physician for a check up. She was again put on Cardizem CD because the physician apparently did not review the patient's previous medication use and neither the patient nor her caregiver reminded the doctor about the prescription change. Since the patient had either forgotten or never been warned about the danger of chewing Cardizem CD, she again began chewing the larger capsules. She became progressively weaker and died three weeks later. According to her family, the patient had been alert and intelligent but had too much faith in her health providers to question their instructions.

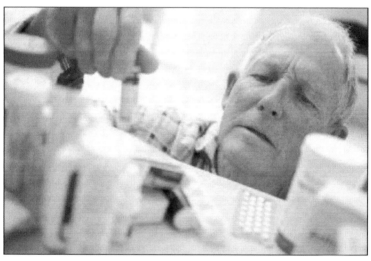

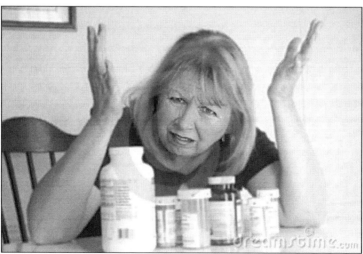

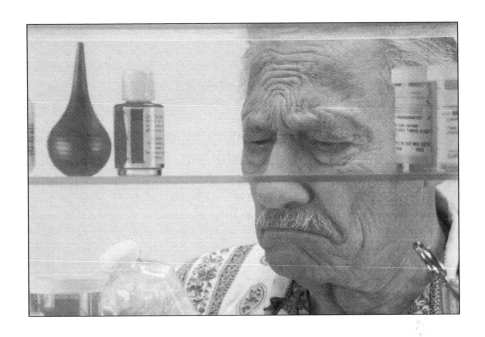

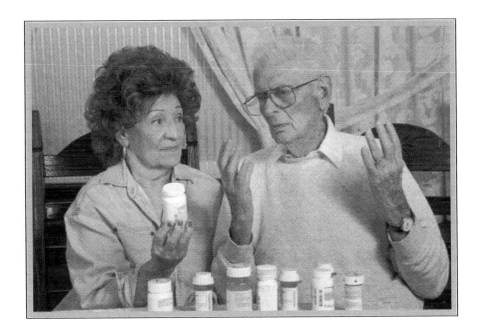

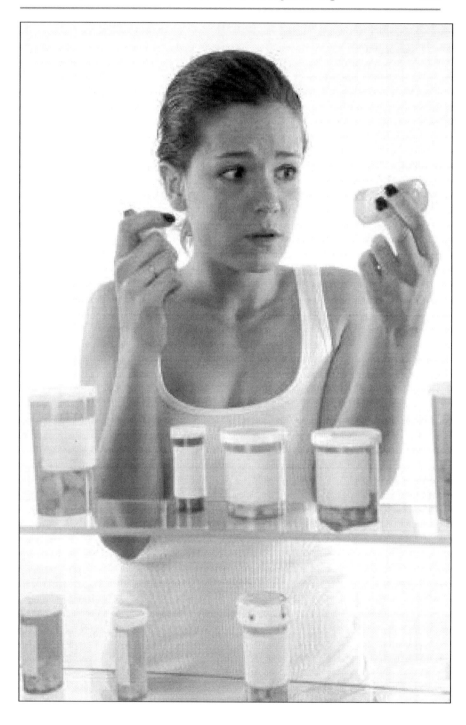

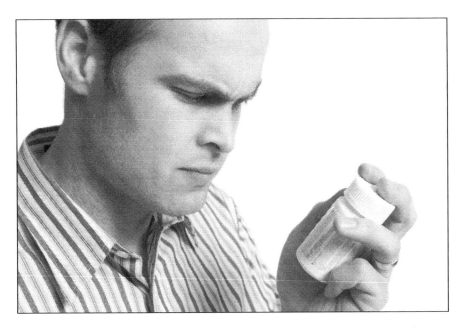

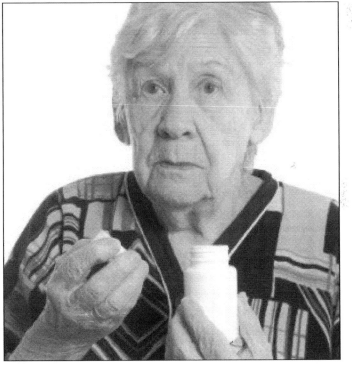

66

"Take as directed"
—What does that mean?

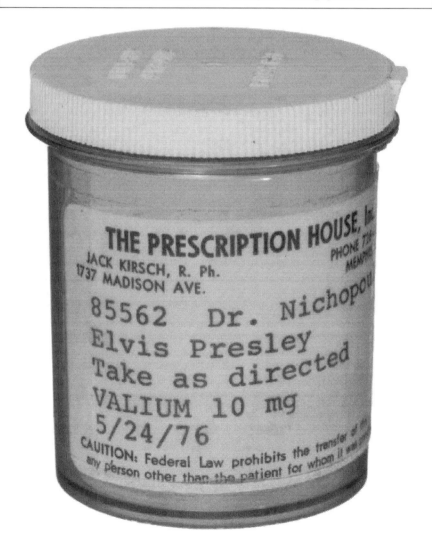

THE PRESCRIPTION HOUSE, Inc.
JACK KIRSCH, R. Ph.   PHONE 73
1737 MADISON AVE.   MEMPHIS

85562   Dr. Nichopou
Elvis Presley
Take as directed
VALIUM 10 mg
5/24/76
CAUTION: Federal Law prohibits the transfer of this
any person other than the patient for whom it was

Have you ever obtained a prescription medication from your pharmacy with the following directions printed on the label that is attached to the vial or bottle: "Take as directed"? These three simple words appear on your prescription label for one of two reasons. The most common reason is because that is precisely what your doctor specified. Supposedly the doctor told you how to use the medication during your office visit, or you've been on the medication for some period and you're familiar with how to take it. But there is also an interesting second reason why the three words "Take as directed" appear on your prescription label. If the pharmacist can't read your doctor's handwriting, and the pharmacist doesn't have the time or desire to contact your doctor's office for clarification, the pharmacist may simply punt and type "Take as directed" on your prescription label.

The nice thing about this, from the pharmacist's perspective, is that it is (or has been—see below) basically legal in addition to being extremely convenient. In other words, "Take as directed" is (or has been) a legally accurate statement in which the pharmacist (if he can't read the doctor's prescription) is telling you *Just take the damn medication like your doctor told you!* I've read a few commentaries written by pharmacists or pharmacy professors stating that use of the "Take as directed" shortcut is not good pharmacy practice and that the pharmacist should make every effort to contact the physician before resorting to the "Take as directed" cop-out.

Of course, when the pharmacist can't read the doctor's directions but goes ahead and types "Take as directed" on your prescription label, the pharmacist is doing you no favor. The pharmacist is attempting to place the ball in your court, hoping that you will call the doctor's office yourself for clarification if you forgot how the doctor told you to take the drug.

When there is grossly inadequate staffing in the pharmacy, the pharmacist's use of "Take as directed" is understandable but, in the eyes of many pharmacists, regrettable. I would predict that nearly every community pharmacist in America has had at least a few instances wherein he or she was so slammed with prescriptions that he or she simply punted and typed "Take as directed" on the prescription label. I've done it myself more times than I am proud to admit—at least once a month, I would guess.

Some pharmacists are uncomfortable punting the ball like this, while other pharmacists seem to be totally fine with it. The latter group rationalizes the situation as follows: *If the doctor doesn't take the time to write clearly and if my employer doesn't provide enough staffing for clearing up problems like this, why should I care?* With adequate staffing in pharmacies, shortcuts like this would be less necessary.

So if you receive a prescription medication from your pharmacy with the directions "Take as directed" on the label and you are confused about this, consider the two major possibilities: 1) Your doctor told you how to take this medication during your office visit and you simply forgot what he said, or 2) Your pharmacy couldn't read your doctor's handwriting and your pharmacist didn't have the time or desire to contact your doctor for clarification.

It appears that the "Take as directed" or "Use as directed" shortcut may indeed get the pharmacist into trouble in the event of a lawsuit stemming from a customer's confusion about how to take or use the prescribed medication. Jesse Vivian, a professor at the Wayne State University Collge of Pharmacy with degrees in pharmacy and law, wrote three full pages on this subject in the February 2012 issue of *U. S. Pharmacist*. Vivian describes a lawsuit against a pharmacist involving the "Use as directed" directions and a customer's confusion and harm after a change in warfarin dosage. Vivian suggests that the courts may be heading toward holding pharmacists partly liable for parroting the doctor's directions and typing on the label, "Take as directed" or "Use as directed." Vivian says the pharmacist should always clarify the directions with the prescriber. He states, "It's time to finally end the confusing practice of putting 'Use as directed' on prescriptions." (page 60). And he concludes by saying "It is way past time for this nonsense to end." (page 67). (See also, David B. Brushwood, "As directed prescription exposes pharmacy to liability," *Pharmacy Today*, 2011; 17(7): 24)

67

Request a print-out when your doctor transmits your prescription to your pharmacy

Whenever you are at your doctor's office and he tells you that he will transmit your prescription to your pharmacy, you should request a print-out of that prescription so you'll know what to expect when you pick up that medication at the pharmacy. Here is a possible real world scenario from *Pharmacy Times* (Michael J. Gaunt, Pharm.D., "Electronic Prescribing: Potential Areas of Weakness," *Pharmacy Times*, published online Oct. 15, 2009 http://pharmacytimes.com-/issue/pharmacy/2009/october2009/MedicationSafety-1009)

A girl was recently taken to a doctor by her parents for evaluation of a skin rash. The doctor prescribed a topical corticosteroid, using a handheld device to place the order electronically. He had asked the couple which pharmacy they'd like to use, which seemed very efficient, except for one issue: the doctor never told the family exactly which drug he was prescribing. He just instructed the parents to pick up the medication at their community pharmacy.

This raises an important question when prescriptions are sent electronically to a pharmacy: How will the patient know what they are supposed to receive, if they are not told the prescribed medication, strength, and directions for use, and given a written copy of the information to compare with the dispensed medication?

In this situation, electronic prescribing (e-prescribing) may lead to an unintended weakness in the system if the patient does not know what to expect when he or she picks up prescriptions at the pharmacy. Ideally, with e-prescribing, patients should receive verbal instructions from the prescriber, be given an opportunity to ask questions, and also be provided with a corresponding voucher listing the prescribed medication, dose, and directions for use. This way, the patient can use the information to check the prescription in the pharmacy by matching the voucher to what he or she actually receives to assure it is correct.

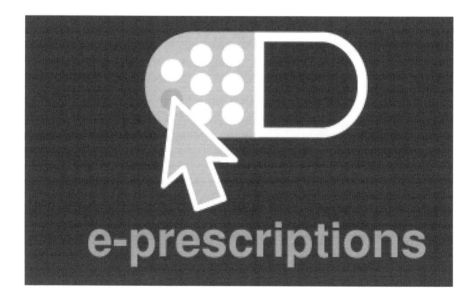

68

Confusing label directions can be deadly

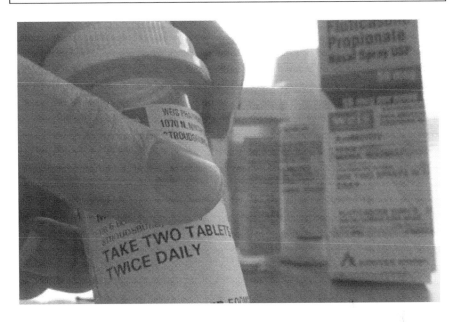

In my 25-year career as a pharmacist, I saw a huge number of instances in which pharmacists and techs typed unclear or confusing label directions. I blame two factors: 1) Some pharmacists and techs are simply careless and don't really care whether the label directions are easy to follow. These pharmacists and techs see their job as one of quantity rather than quality. 2) The big pharmacy chains and indeed our entire health care system find increased profits in understaffing. This understaffing makes it much more difficult for pharmacists and techs to do our jobs with a degree of professionalism that the public assumes and expects.

Auburn University School of Pharmacy is one of the leading centers in America for the study of pharmacy errors. In 2007 several professors at this pharmacy school cooperated with ABC News' 20/20 in an undercover investigation of pharmacy mistakes. A total of 100 pharmacies in Atlanta, Tampa-St. Petersburg-Clearwater, and New York City-Newark were randomly selected for the study. Trained patient actors presented a new prescription for one of several study drugs to each pharmacy. (E. Flynn, K. Barker, et. al., "Dispensing Errors and Counseling Quality in 100 Pharmacies— Study Summary," Auburn University School of Pharmacy, March 30,   2007 abcnews.go.com/images/WNT/ross_auburn_final_summary.pdf) With an estimated 3.8 billion prescriptions filled in America each year, the hundred prescriptions filled during this undercover investigation represent an infinitesimally small percentage. Nevertheless, potentially serious errors were discovered in this tiny investigation. For example, out of this sample of a hundred prescriptions, the study found two prescriptions that were filled with directions that were quite unclear and potentially dangerous.

One significant error involved the blood-thinner Coumadin. Coumadin is potentially the most dangerous drug in the drugstore. This drug a) must be dosed precisely by doctors, b) must be filled precisely by pharmacy staff, and c) must be taken by patients precisely according to directions. If the dose of Coumadin is too high, the patient can hemorrhage or bleed to death. If the dose is too low, clotting could occur which could have devastating consequences. The Auburn study noted the following with regard to the unclear directions on the label for Coumadin: "...the instructions on a Coumadin prescription read 'Take 1 tablet by mouth daily as needed' instead of 'Take 1 tablet by mouth every day and as directed.'"

Taking Coumadin "as needed" is absurd and potentially deadly. This is like handing a loaded gun to a patient. Blood thinners like Coumadin are absolutely unlike drugs that can indeed be taken "as needed" such as some pain pills.

Another significant error discovered in this study involved the incomplete or truncated directions that the pharmacy staff typed on the label for the insulin product Novolog:

[Another] significant error was on a label for Novolog Mix 70/30 insulin where the instructions were cut off. The label read "Inject 15 units subcutaneously 15 minutes before breakfast, and 15 units 15 minutes", leaving off "before dinner." The incomplete instructions may result in the patient injecting the second dose at an inappropriate time, leading to high or low blood sugars.

Why were parts of the directions cut off? The most likely explanation is that the directions exceeded the maximum number of characters the computer allows in the "directions" field. Computers are great for many things but they can introduce an entirely new set of potential errors that did not occur twenty or thirty years ago when pharmacists used typewriters to type directions on labels. When pharmacists using typewriters ran out of room on labels, this would be immediately obvious to the pharmacist. However, computers facilitate the filling of prescriptions at lightning speed without notifying pharmacists/techs that the maximum number of characters in the directions has been exceeded. In my experience, the computer merrily proceeds to print the label without informing the pharmacist or tech that part of the directions were cut off. Bells and whistles don't sound when things like this occur.

Here's one example from my career that stands out in my mind. One day a customer returned to the pharmacy for a refill on triamcinolone cream. Triamcinolone is a cortisone-type drug used for a variety of skin conditions. I happened to look at the directions that were typed on the label by another pharmacist who was filling in at our store. It is possible that the directions had been typed by a pharmacy technician and the pharmacist on duty failed to check the directions. (Pharmacists are responsible for all the work done by technicians.) The pharmacist on duty may have failed to insist that a tech make the directions clearer to the patient. The pharmacy label directions for this triamcinolone cream read *exactly* as follows: "Apply thin film twice daily *times two (2) weeks*, then *as reduce* as tolerated. Avoid mucous **memb** and genitals." I have added bold italic type to indicate the parts that I consider to be unclear or confusing.

Here is how this label should have been typed to be clearer to the customer: "Apply a thin film twice a day for 2 weeks, then reduce as tolerated. Avoid mucous membranes and genitals."

The errors that I find in the original label are as follows: 1) I looked at the doctor's original handwritten prescription. The doctor wrote "X 2 weeks." The pharmacist or tech should have transcribed this as "for two weeks" rather than "times two weeks." It is simply easier to understand "for" rather than "times." 2) The pharmacist or tech has a grammatical error (or typographical error) when he or she typed "then as reduce as tolerated." The first "as" should not have been there. 3) The pharmacist or tech should have typed out the word "membrane" rather than use the shorthand "memb." Not everyone knows what a "mucous membrane" is but even fewer people know what a "mucous memb" is.

What reaction does the customer have when reading this label? Does she know what "times two weeks" means? Does she see the poor grammar? Does she know what "mucous memb" means?

Here are two examples from the *North Carolina Board of Pharmacy Newsletter* in which a pharmacist or tech typed unclear directions. The consequences in these two examples are far more serious than one would expect from confusion in the above example involving triamcinolone cream. A patient died, at least in part as a result of not understanding the directions. The drug involved in this patient's death was methotrexate, a potentially risky drug even when taken properly. (*North Carolina Board of Pharmacy Newsletter,* Item 846—Critical Doses, October 1995, p.4)

A patient received a prescription to treat psoriasis, which was written for methotrexate 2.5 mg with the directions stating, "Two tablets every 12 hours for three doses each week." The patient who was marginally literate had her husband pick up the prescription. He customarily asked store clerks to make out his checks for him, which is one of the cardinal signs of a marginally literate or illiterate patient. …The patient consumed two tablets every 12 hours for six consecutive days until she was hospitalized. She eventually expired.

The patient obviously understood the directions as two tablets every 12 hours each day in contrast to what the physician had intended. The prescriber meant for her to take two tablets one day in the morning, two tablets 12 hours later in the evening, and two tablets the next morning. The directions were obviously unclear and subject to several different interpretations. The patient's death was due, at least in part, to methotrexate toxicity.

The same issue of the *North Carolina Board of Pharmacy Newsletter* describes another incident in which the label directions were incorrectly understood and resulted in another patient's death. This incident involved another powerful drug, melphalan. Melphalan is used to treat multiple myeloma and ovarian cancer. (*North Carolina Board of Pharmacy Newsletter*, Item 846—Critical Doses, October 1995, p. 4)

...a prescription for melphalan whose directions were for the patient to consume six tablets for four days each month was incorrectly understood by the patient. The decedent took two consecutive courses for a total of 48 doses, and expired due to the melphalan overdose.

When you pick up your prescription medications from the drugstore and you look at the directions typed on your label(s) by pharmacists/techs, don't assume that you must be dumb for not clearly understanding how your doctor intends for you to take those medications. Due to the assembly-line nature of pharmacy today, pharmacists and techs too often don't have the time to make sure that the directions are easily understandable. Call the pharmacist and ask him or her to clarify the directions. You're not stupid. Unclear or confusing label directions are much more common than you know. The chains' focus on quantity rather than quality means that too many drugstores in America are an accident waiting to happen.

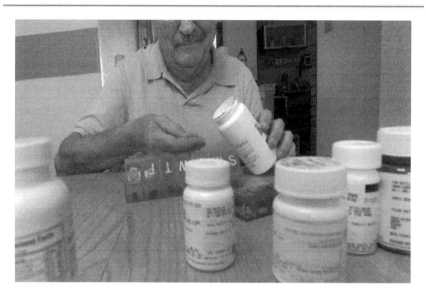

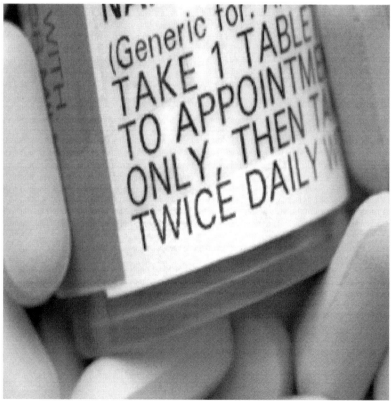

69

Spanish-speaking customers beware: Computer translations of prescription directions can cause dangerous confusion

Here's a common scenario: Say a doctor's prescription for a Hispanic patient has a standard abbreviation that doctors use for all of their patients. Say the doctor indicates on the prescription pad, "1 tab tid." This means "1 tablet three times a day." Most pharmacy computers are programmed to recognize Latin abbreviations like "tid." So, for example, in this case, the pharmacist might enter the following into the computer: "T 1 T TID." The computer will translate this to "Take 1 tablet three times a day" when it prints on the customer's label.

Many pharmacists routinely instruct the computer to translate the directions to Spanish for our Hispanic customers, thinking we're helping those customers. But, according to an article on HealthDay.com, this translation can be unclear, resulting in a hazardous situation. For simple directions like "Take one tablet three times a day," the pharmacy computer probably does a pretty good job in translating this to Spanish. But, in a very large number of cases, the doctor's directions are not so simple and straightforward, resulting in confusing translations.

I was never a big fan of the computer's translation skills when translating from Latin or English to Spanish. I never felt comfort-

able dispensing a prescription for which I had no idea whether the directions on the label were clear to our customers, or worse, inaccurate. So I think I never translated a doctor's directions from Latin or English to Spanish, even for the simplest directions like "Take one tablet 3 times a day." My hope was that these Hispanic customers would show the label to a bilingual person who could read English directions and translate those directions to Spanish. From the HealthDay News article (D. Thompson, "Prescriptions Translated to Spanish Could Be Hazardous to Health: Computer Translation Programs Give Confusing, Incomplete Instructions, Study Finds," HealthDay.com, April 8, 2010
  http://consumer.healthday.com/Article.asp?AID=637694):

Many Spanish-speaking people in the United States receive prescription instructions from the pharmacy so poorly translated that the medications are potentially hazardous to their health, a new study shows.

The errors occur largely because of deficiencies in computer programs that most pharmacies rely on to translate medication information from English to Spanish, said lead researcher Dr. Iman Sharif, chief of the division of general pediatrics at the Nemours/Alfred I. duPont Hospital for Children in Wilmington, Del.

"The technologies that are currently available to produce instructions in the patient's language are inadequate," Sharif said.

Half of the Spanish-language prescription labels reviewed for the study contained errors, and some of those errors could result in life-threatening situations if misinterpreted by the patient, Sharif said.

The study is published in the May [2010] issue of *Pediatrics*.

Of the New York City pharmacies surveyed that provide Spanish-language labels, more than four of every five used a computer program to translate their labels from English to Spanish. Nearly all the pharmacies said they had someone double-check the labels for errors, but researchers found dozens of examples of poorly translated instructions.

A common problem was "Spanglish," Sharif said. The programs produced a mix of English and Spanish on the labels, creating confusing and difficult-to-read instructions.

The use of "Spanglish" also created some potentially dangerous situations. For example, the word "once" means "eleven" in Spanish. "You mean to say 'once,' as in 'take once a day,' and a Spanish-speaking person could interpret that to mean 'eleven,'" Sharif said. Such a mistake could result in an overdose.

Other phrases that weren't accurately translated include "dropperfuls," "apply topically," "for seven days," "for 30 days," "apply to affected areas," "with juice" and "take with food."

Misspellings also created errors. Incorrect use of the word "poca" for the word "boca" meant patients were told "by the little" instead of "by the mouth." One set of instructions included "dos besos," which means "two kisses"; the intended instructions likely were "dos veces," which means "two times."

Poor translations specifically cited in the study included:
• "Take 1.2 aldia give dropperfuls with juice eleven to day."
• "Taking 0.6 mL 2 times to the day by the little with juice."
• "Apply to affected area twice to the indicated day like."

Dr. David Flockhart, director of the division of clinical pharmacology at the Indiana University School of Medicine in Indianapolis, said it's not surprising that these computer-generated errors are occurring.

"Word-for-word, you probably could get it right, but you can't get the entire sense of what's being communicated through a computer program," Flockhart said.

Translated Drug Labels Are Often Wrong

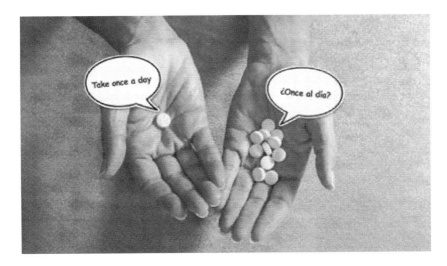

The directions on your pill bottle could put your health at risk. Here's how to protect yourself.
by Claudia Forestieri, <u>AARP VIVA</u>, Spring 2011

http://www.aarp.org/health/drugs-supplements/info-03-2011/drug-wrong-translation.html

If your pharmacist uses translation software and isn't bilingual, the directions on your pill bottle could be dead wrong.

Fifty percent of all prescription labels translated from English to Spanish are wrong or incomplete, according to a recent study, with potentially hazardous results.

For instance, the word "once," as in "take once a day,"means "one time" in English, but "11" in Spanish.

"Orally," *por la boca*, was confused with *por la poca*, "by the little."

Phrases such as "take with food" and "for 7 days" were dropped entirely.

Protect Yourself From Translation Errors

1. Ask your doctor about the medicine before filling the prescription.

2. At the pharmacy, ask for a Spanish speaker to explain the instructions to you verbally and to double-check what's said against the printed instructions.

3. Repeat the instructions back to the person to ensure that you understood them correctly.

4. Finally, never worry about sounding stupid.

In a recent interview, Walkiris Fernandez Raineri, RPh, a Chicago-area bilingual pharmacist with 24 years' experience, spoke about translation errors and offered tips for consumers.

Q: How does your pharmacy handle the translation of prescriptions?
A: Our pharmacy has a computer software program that translates the directions, but it has the information printed in Spanish and in English so that the pharmacist knows what's prescribed. That's one of the safeguards. Mistakes can occur when it's dispensed at the drive-thru window if the pharmacist doesn't go through the instructions with the patient. I

have an advantage because I speak Spanish, so I know what I'm dispensing.

Q: Did you ever find any mistakes or misinterpretations in the translations?

A: I can't think of anything specifically, but these programs translate literally — they don't translate exactly the way the prescription should be worded in Spanish for someone to understand. If the patient doesn't speak English, and the professional doesn't speak Spanish, and you're translating it through this computer program, it's tough. There's still that human error there that you really can't correct if you don't speak the language.

Q: If a person's English is not up to par and he or she needs to have a prescription translated, what precautions should be taken?

A: Before you get to the pharmacy, ask your doctor about the medicine prescribed. Most of the time, when patients come to the pharmacy they have no idea what's been prescribed to them. The doctor just hands them the prescription and says, "Get this filled." Patients should make sure they understand what they're being given and why. If you get your medicine from a pharmacist who doesn't speak Spanish, ask for one who does. Patients can also call the pharmacy anytime and ask questions if they have any doubts.

70

Chain drugstores too often have inadequate staffing to answer your questions and give advice

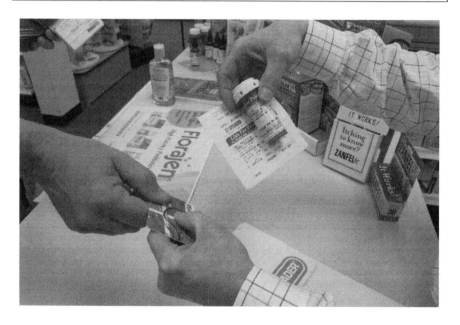

Try explaining the pharmacy counseling law to a non-pharmacist. Good luck.

A federal law passed in 1990 called the Omnibus Budget Reconciliation Act (OBRA '90) contains a provision stating that pharmacists must offer to counsel our customers on new prescriptions. Here are some questions I commonly get when I try to explain this counseling regulation to family members and non-pharmacist friends.

What does it mean that pharmacists must offer to counsel customers?

We must offer to discuss their medications.

That seems awfully vague. What specifically do you have to discuss?

Here's what a pharmacist-lawyer at the University of Florida College of Pharmacy says (David B. Brushwood, R.Ph., J.D, "The pharmacist's legal duty to counsel patients," *Drug Topics*, April 17, 2006, p. 56):

> According to the OBRA '90 standard, pharmacists must offer to discuss prescribed medications with patients or family caregivers. The subject of the discussion is up to the individual pharmacist. The flexible requirement is that the discussion between the pharmacist and the patient must pertain to matters deemed significant by the pharmacist. These matters may include common side effects, techniques for self-monitoring, and action to be taken in the event of a missed dose, if the pharmacist deems them significant. Patients or their family caregivers may refuse consultation if they wish.

If customers accept the offer to be counseled, we can tell them such things as the purpose of the drug, the most common side effects, how to take the drug (like the number of times per day), whether or not to take it with food, what foods to avoid while on the medication, how to store the medication, what to do if they miss a dose, and things like the necessity to refrigerate, shake well, avoid sunlight, etc.

Sometimes I've concluded that no verbal communication is best. I've always felt that written information is better because most people don't remember what we tell them or they are confused by what we tell them or they mistakenly do precisely opposite what we tell them. For example, some antibiotics are not supposed to be taken with milk. I have felt that some of our customers are so easily confused that, once at home, they'll remember only that I mentioned milk so they'll take it *with* milk. So I've felt sometimes that the best verbal instructions I can give are no verbal instructions. If pharmacists have the right to decide what we deem relevant, it seems to me that we ought to be able to decide when it is best to leave well enough alone. For example, in this case, we usually put a "Do not take with milk" sticker on the prescription vial. The right to tell customers what we feel is best for them should also include the right to *not* counsel customers whom we feel will be confused.

In my opinion, written information in the quiet of the customer's home is the simplest and clearest communication. I've always found written information to be much more helpful than trusting my recollection of what someone tells me. After I speak with a dentist or mechanic, I always write down their recommendations for what work needs to be done. Whenever I call my car insurance agent or bank, I always take notes. I don't recall a customer ever taking notes when I counsel them.

You've told me that you don't have time to eat lunch or go to the bathroom. Do you have time for a discussion with each of your customers?
Absolutely not. And many customers aren't interested anyway. Many customers just want to get their drugs and go home or go to the supermarket or go to work. Most pharmacists just have time to say something like "Be careful. This medication may make you drowsy."

How could the federal government pass a law that's so vague?
Most pharmacists don't realize that the idea for the OBRA counseling regulation originated in the pharmacy community with the National Community Pharmacists Association (NCPA), the trade group that represents independent pharmacists. (The National Association of Chain Drugstores represents the chains.) Contrary to the belief of many pharmacists, the impetus for this regulation did not originate with the federal government. Certain leaders at NCPA approached members of Congress and requested that the offer to counsel become law. Prior to that, the federal government showed no interest in whether pharmacists counseled. NCPA felt that the counseling requirement would give the profession more respect and would help to convince certain payers that pharmacists do much more than transfer pills from big bottles to little bottles.

Pharmacists are trying to convince insurance companies and the general public that we should be paid for our counseling, just like you pay a doctor or lawyer for a consultation.

What reaction do customers have when they're asked if they want to be counseled by the pharmacist?

Most customers don't really understand what they're being asked. Often a technician or clerk will simply ask the customer, "Do you have any questions for the pharmacist?" And customers don't understand why we're requiring them to sign a counseling log. They think they need to sign the log to indicate that they've received their prescriptions. Most customers don't know the log has anything to do with accepting or declining the offer to be counseled by the pharmacist.

What if the prescriptions are picked up at the drive thru window?

We have to fight the noise from the car engine, from the car radio, and from the children screaming or crying. Unless we have a secure drive thru with pneumatic tubes like at a bank drive-thru, we end up inhaling a good dose of fumes from the auto exhaust.

What if a 16-year-old son or daughter picks up the prescriptions? How do you counsel them?

We don't. Some pharmacists throw a few words at them like "Tell your mother to take this antibiotic until it's all gone." I don't know whether there are any statistics on this but I bet that around half the time the person picking up the prescription is not the actual person for whom the prescription was filled. It is often the spouse or teenage son or daughter. Counseling a family member is usually very problematic because that person may have less interest in what I have to say.

Some state boards of pharmacy enforce the counseling law more aggressively than other state boards. Some state boards send undercover inspectors around to pharmacies to see whether we offer to counsel customers. Pharmacists who don't offer to counsel can be cited by the state board and fined. A pharmacist in Wisconsin sent me an e-mail saying he had just received a citation for failure to counsel. He told me that he was hit with a fine of $250.00 and $400.00 in court costs. He wrote:

> When the inspector introduced herself after this so-called violation, I felt like I was caught in an ambush. I was FURIOUS. And like a cornered cat, the hair on my back stood up. I had to calm myself down before calling the prosecuting attorney, so that I would be polite when I informed her that the terms of the citation were not acceptable and I would be seeking legal counsel to fight these charges.

Later this pharmacist e-mailed me:

> I did seek the advice of legal counsel. I faxed the info to him and he looked it over. He agreed that it was nitpicking, but he looked up the statute and stated that "They got you, and while it is a picky little matter, it is their way of showing you that they are in charge." The lawyer also stated that the $400.00 court fee is "made up" and that, if I have a hearing, the court fee will be $1200.00 whether I win or lose!!!

With the slight possibility that an undercover board of pharmacy inspector is watching me, I usually throw a few words at whatever family member happens to pick up the prescription. That is, unless I'm really stressed out, or really exhausted, or mad at the world, or the person picking up the prescription appears highly unlikely to remember a single word I say. I don't really know what the OBRA counseling regulation has to say with regard to what is required of pharmacists when a family member or friend or neighbor picks up the prescription. That is a vague part of a very vague law.

I wonder whether there are lots of other laws that Congress passes that are as vague as the law that requires pharmacists to offer to counsel customers on new prescriptions. Laws like this breed cynicism among pharmacists because we don't have enough staffing to allow us to tell our customers nearly as much as we would like. This is the first law I've ever heard of that requires someone to do what he feels is right, i.e., to tell customers whatever the pharmacist thinks is important. This is like a law for highway safety that states "You are not allowed to exceed the speed limit but you are allowed to determine what the speed limit should be."

Lawyers are having a field day with this law, increasingly accusing pharmacists of negligence for anything negative that occurs as a result of drug therapy. Once we initiate the act of counseling a customer, lawyers say we have a duty to be complete in our answer. For example, if we tell a customer that the medication can cause drowsiness, lawyers will accuse us of negligence for not telling that customer every other possible adverse effect.

Mail order pharmacists are exempt from the requirement to verbally offer to counsel customers—as long as these mail order pharmacists provide their customers with a toll-free number. Many pharmacists wonder why the exemption allowing mail order pharmacists to have a toll-free number doesn't apply to all pharmacists. The law seems to be picking on community pharmacists and giving special leniency to mail order pharmacists. Whatever happened to the "equal protection" clause in the U.S. Constitution which states that all citizens shall be treated equally? Many community pharmacists are angry that mail order pharmacists have this exemption from the counseling regulation. Mail order pharmacists are given this exemption because they obviously can't provide face-to-face communication with someone who lives hundreds or thousands of miles away. I suspect that many pharmacists working for the big chain drugstores feel we deserve an exemption because we're not given enough staffing to allow us time for counseling.

The fact that the trade group representing independent pharmacists pushed for a counseling regulation is a sign of the weakness and vulnerability of community pharmacists. Pharmacists see that mail order pharmacy is growing rapidly. We see that the big pharmaceutical companies and the big drugstore chains would like to decrease the role of pharmacists. We see that the market views pharmaceuticals like widgets. Bruce Roberts, executive VP-CEO of the National Community Pharmacists Association, describes the threat to the future of retail pharmacists (Carol Ukens, "R.Ph.s must act to protect profession," *Drug Topics*, March 20, 2006):

Outside forces, including politicians, the government, and pharmacy benefit managers are trying to turn medications into just another commodity and to disenfranchise retail pharmacy, said Roberts. "It's painfully obvious what's up with regard to pharmacy. I don't think we'll be able to continue down this path and have a sustainable model for the long term. Mail order is growing like crazy. People believe that all we're selling is widgets, nothing that inherently needs the guidance of a pharmacist. If we're just a business model competing head-to-head with mail order, it doesn't bode well for the future."

When an industry or profession finds itself at risk, it often seeks government protection, as NCPA did with OBRA. The community drugstore model is endangered by mail order pharmacies, so NCPA sought to shore up the status of the independent pharmacy by requiring that pharmacists voluntarily offer to counsel our customers. However, many of the state boards of pharmacy were not happy with such an amorphous regulation. Some state boards wanted a regulation with more teeth. Even though NCPA wanted a voluntary regulation requiring the offer to counsel customers, many state boards have aggressively gone after pharmacists who do not offer to counsel customers. Many pharmacists view this as a power play by the state boards to increase their visibility and influence. (Similarly, many pharmacists view the requirement that all graduating pharmacists now have a doctorate as a power grab by the schools of pharmacy.)

The big pharmaceutical manufacturers ("Big Pharma") feel that pharmacists are unnecessary middlemen between the doctor and the patient. Big Pharma prefers the model of mail order pharmacy where prescription drug orders are filled the same way that Amazon.com fills orders for books. To Big Pharma, a pharmacist's advice or guidance are unnecessary. Big Pharma promotes the idea that pharmaceuticals are no different from any other consumer product: no more complicated, no less safe. Big Pharma does not believe that consumers of pharmaceuticals need pharmacists' counseling or drug information leaflets explaining proper use, side effects, etc. Big Pharma thinks that all the customer needs to know is, for example, "Take one tablet three times a day." Possible side effects? Drugs don't cause side effects!!

Many pharmacists feel that the writing is on the wall, that the future of the community pharmacist is in jeopardy, that market forces will continue to minimize the role of the pharmacist, and that we'll end up working as a drone at some huge mail order facility. Even though the big chains are opening up shiny new drugstores on every corner, corporate management at those chains would like to staff the stores with the smallest possible number of pharmacists, preferring less expensive techs and robotics instead. The big chains certainly don't want their pharmacists spending time advising customers. The big chains feel that counseling is a major drag on productivity. The big chain drugstores never embraced the OBRA counseling regulation. The big chains have never felt that they have a duty to educate our customers. When the Wisconsin pharmacist who was cited for failure to counsel wrote to me, he said that when he informed his supervisor of the citation, the supervisor said, "Bullshit."

Counseling in the real world

Let me make it perfectly clear that, if I had adequate staffing, I would be 100% in favor of counseling. All the arguments in favor of counseling are absolutely correct. Counseling saves lives. Lots of errors are caught during counseling. I agree that many customers are in a complete fog about their medications and counseling can clear this up. Pharmacists: How many times have you had a customer ask you, "What's this drug used for?" How many times have you wondered how someone could leave his doctor's office without really understanding the purpose of the medication his doctor has prescribed?

My techs tell me that I spend too much time talking to customers. To be honest, I'd much rather counsel customers than fill prescriptions. Running the computer and counting pills can be boring while counseling can be fulfilling. I'd much rather interact with customers all day than stare at a computer. Unless a pharmacist suffers from what Big Pharma terms "social anxiety disorder" (a.k.a., shyness), counseling is the easiest job in the pharmacy. With each of our customers' patient leaflets in front of us, counseling should be a breeze. I am totally exhausted at the end of most days when I fill two hundred prescriptions, but I bet if I did nothing but counsel all day, I'd feel like I had the day off.

Most pharmacists would desperately love to thoroughly counsel every customer. The boards of pharmacy seem incapable of understanding that basic reality. They seem to be incapable of understanding that the reason we don't counsel is not because we don't want to counsel. It is because, too often, there is simply inadequate time and staffing for counseling. Since counseling is the easiest and most fulfilling job in the pharmacy, it should tell the boards of pharmacy something when they discover instances of "failure to counsel."

Do the boards of pharmacy think we are simply being recalcitrant? Do the boards of pharmacy think we're willfully and wantonly trying to flaunt their counseling regulations? Do the boards of pharmacy think we're akin to misbehaving kids who need to be spanked? Most pharmacists I know would love to do nothing but counsel all day long. When are the boards of pharmacy going to see the real world for what it is? The boards of pharmacy have the luxury of passing regulations while sitting in comfy chairs. At the same time, pharmacists are filling prescriptions as fast as they are physically capable.

The boards of pharmacy are good at passing regulations that don't take into consideration real world working conditions. Boards of pharmacy have shown themselves to be too timid to pass regulations that require safe levels of staffing in pharmacies. I wish the boards of pharmacy would pass a regulation that mandates that pharmacists have enough staffing so that counseling is possible.

We fear the pharmacy boards because of their power to discipline us for failing to counsel. Yet, at the same time, the boards are doing nothing substantial to address our dangerous working conditions. Pharmacy boards say that they can only pass regulations that protect the public safety. But surely unsafe working conditions endanger the public safety.

Many pharmacists are contemptuous of the pharmacy boards for threatening disciplinary action for failure to counsel. The boards readily tell us that our job entails counseling. Yet, when we say the boards should perform their job (protect the public safety by addressing pharmacists' working conditions), we're met with arrogant indifference.

The counseling regulation is unquestionably well intended. In my opinion, pharmacists should counsel because it is the right thing to do, not because it is a regulation passed by the board of pharmacy. In the end, regulations that don't acknowledge the real world breed cynicism.

Our professors in pharmacy school do a brilliant job of preparing us to counsel our customers—in a sterile environment. Don't these professors realize what the real world is like? Professors and boards of pharmacy need to instruct us how to counsel customers in a hyper-stressful environment in which we're running an or hour or two behind, customers are yelling at us, people at the drive-thru window are honking their horns, all four phone lines are for the sole pharmacist on duty, and we haven't had a meal or bathroom break all day. On top of that, customers are telling the clerk at the register, *I've waited long enough! Tell the pharmacist I want my prescriptions back so I can go somewhere else to get them filled!*

Proper counseling technique involves such things as asking open-ended questions. Don't tell the customer what the drug is used for. Instead, ask him if he knows what it's used for. Open the pill container and show the customer the pills. That way we can catch errors. Indeed, most pharmacists would love to practice this type of pharmacy. When we protest that there's simply no time, the boards and professors and legal experts tell us "Well you'd better find the time! It only takes a few seconds." The legal experts tell us "You'd better find the time to counsel because a jury won't believe you when you say you didn't have enough time to tell Mr. Jones that his anxiety medication could make him too drowsy to drive."

It is a sad commentary on the current state of affairs that pharmacists feel we need to minimize customer contact because it slows down production. When we start talking to customers, some of them do indeed have lots of questions. Some of them want to tell us their complete medical history. Some of them want to tell us about their grandchildren. Customers look at the pills we're showing them and say "They're so big they must be horse pills." Or they see us take the lid off the vial and say "I don't want those safety caps! I have to get the kids to take them off for me!" All the questions, comments, and jokes from customers put us even further behind. Unfortunately, we can't catch up by counseling customers. The boards need to acknowledge that there is simply an incredibly powerful conflict between the need to counsel and the need to produce.

In the real world, almost any words spoken to customers seem to pass for counseling. "Call me if you have any questions" probably passes for counseling in some states. "This may cause drowsiness" probably passes and, indeed, this is a very important warning. "Take this until it's all gone" probably passes for antibiotic counseling.

What legally constitutes adequate counseling? If we need to tell the customer the most common uses of the drug, the most common side effects, warnings, and contraindications, the best time to take the drug, and what to do if you forget to take a dose, then the vast majority of pharmacists in America are breaking the law. How many possible side effects do we need to mention? The top two, top five, top ten?

The big chains and managed care are pushing pharmacists in one direction (speedily herding customers) while lawyers are pushing us in the opposite direction (giving more warnings to our customers).

Some chains advertise that their pharmacists are eager to counsel customers about medications. The truth is that the chains don't value pharmacists who spend too much time counseling customers. The chains can tolerate counseling only as long as it doesn't slow our processing of customers. Chains give lip service to counseling, but most pharmacists learn quickly that our No. 1 job (by far) is filling prescriptions as fast as we can (i.e., faster than we should).

When I shop at Home Depot or Office Depot, I am amazed that, most of the time, the salespeople have plenty of time to answer my questions. Pharmacists would love to have as much time to discuss medications with our customers. The difference is that the big pharmacy chains have adopted the fast food model.

Our pharmacy leaders say that pharmacists need to assume more liability through counseling if we want to be recognized by payers (insurance companies, state Medicaid programs, Medicare Part D, etc.) as independent professionals who should be compensated for our cognitive services rather than just for the products we dispense. This means acceptance of a duty to warn customers about potential dangers associated with drug therapy. With an increased counseling role and a duty to warn come increased liability and lawsuits. Even though I am absolutely 100% in favor of counseling, somehow I bet that the people advocating all this increased liability for pharmacists aren't themselves actually filling prescriptions all day long. Educators and boards of pharmacy are good at promoting regulations that affect others, not themselves.

Did our pharmacy leaders understand the extent to which the OBRA counseling provision would increase pharmacists' legal liability? Thanks to aggressive lawyers, in the not-too-distant future, pharmacists may have recurrent nightmares as a result of these three words: "failure to warn."

It used to be that, if the pharmacist dispensed the right drug, the right dose, the right directions, and gave it to the right customer, we were free of liability. Things have become a lot more complicated lately. Our profession has succeeded in tremendously increasing the liability on front line pharmacists. I propose that our educators and associations institute a moratorium on finding new ways to increase pharmacists' liability, unless these advocates of expanded pharmacist liability first figure out some way to fix the horrendous problem of understaffing that endangers the safety of our customers. I think the boards of pharmacy need to acknowledge the real world when they find instances of "failure to counsel." I think that the enormous problem of understaffing needs to be fixed before pharmacists are disciplined.

Some pharmacy leaders believe there's no future in "dispensing" alone, because of mail order mills, robotics, and the tremendous power of insurance companies (also known as pharmacy benefit managers or PBMs). Therefore pharmacists must embrace cognitive roles, i.e., advising customers about the proper use of their medications. Pharmacy associations, pharmacy school faculty, and boards of pharmacy have embraced the expanded cognitive role for pharmacists, but have they fully recognized the legal jeopardy to pharmacists who actually do the dispensing? These groups seem to be completely oblivious to the harsh reality of filling prescriptions at incredible speeds with woefully inadequate staffing.

Most pharmacists have time for, at best, a very few sentences such as "Be careful. This may make you drowsy." Or "Be sure to take this antibiotic till it's all gone." A few words of advice to the customer are usually better than nothing, but I think it needs to be pointed out that this level of communication is nowhere near being adequate in the eyes of aggressive lawyers. Lawyers see pharmacists as tasty targets because our employer has deep pockets. Lawyers often sue everyone they can, including the doctor, the pharmacist, the drugstore, and the drug manufacturer. Lawyers hope something sticks. Pharmacists have made lawyers' jobs easier since we have proclaimed that we want more responsibility in drug therapy management. Lawyers are happy to oblige pharmacists' desire for expanded responsibility. Lawyers will increasingly sue pharmacists when anything goes wrong as a consequence of a patient's drug therapy.

Lawyers envision pharmacists' responsibilities as going far beyond our simple warning to a customer that a medication may cause drowsiness or an antibiotic needs to be taken till it's all gone. Many pharmacists feel if we say something to customers—*anything*—then we've satisfied the OBRA counseling requirement. Lawyers don't look at the situation in such simplistic terms. Even though understaffing forces pharmacists to adopt a minimalist approach to counseling, lawyers will, in court cases, contend that we must have a maximalist approach. Lawyers will claim that our customers deserve no less, i.e., our customers deserve to know every possible adverse consequence of every drug that is being prescribed.

Pharmacists have effectively placed a bullseye on our forehead and it seems clear that lawyers will increasingly take aim at us. Lawyers are ecstatic to see pharmacists embracing a greater role in drug therapy. Doctors, on the other hand, are often leery of pharmacists' expanded roles in drug therapy because doctors often view pharmacists as encroaching on the doctors' turf.

Even though I am one hundred percent in favor of counseling customers about medications, I am also one hundred percent in favor of having adequate staffing so that counseling is possible. I sometimes read "letters to the editor" from pharmacists proudly stating that they counsel every customer. I assume these pharmacists are working in slow stores.

I wonder whether there are other professionals in our society who have so willingly and eagerly exposed themselves to increased liability. It is as if we're saying to lawyers, "Come and get us!" Did the people in pharmacy who eagerly advocated OBRA '90 fully appreciate the extent to which pharmacists would be vulnerable to aggressive lawyers? The desire to move ourselves away from the product has opened a Pandora's box of expanded liability. Did our brilliant leaders fully appreciate the incredible liability this places on the shoulders of pharmacists on the front lines?

While pharmacists on the front lines suffer under the burden of expanded liability, certain groups in pharmacy seem to be quite contented: pharmacy professors, boards of pharmacy, and that small subset of pharmacists who have both R.Ph. and J.D. after their names (i.e., registered pharmacist and attorney). All these groups seem to view the expanded liability very differently from those pharmacists who actually dispense drugs. The professors, the boards, and the pharmacist-lawyers seem to view pharmacists' expanded liability as, perhaps, "deliciously terrible." The expanded liability is terrible for those pharmacists on the front lines but it increases the relevance, visibility, and importance of professors, board members, and R.Ph.-J.D.'s.

Whenever legal experts comment on pharmacy errors, I often wonder what planet they're living on. When, for example, a legal expert asks how it is possible that we placed Coumadin in a bottle labeled Cardura, I often wonder how long it has been since they dispensed drugs themselves, assuming these legal experts were actually pharmacists at some point. Errors often occur while we're running one or two hours behind, while people at the drive-thru window are honking their horns, and while the non-pharmacist store manager is on the store intercom rudely telling us (sometimes almost yelling) that all four phone lines are for the pharmacist. This environment is worlds apart from examining an error in hindsight, after the fact, like during a court case. Of course, in hindsight, we know it's an error. We didn't make the error because we didn't know the difference between Coumadin and Cardura. We made the error because the pharmacy was in chaos from being dangerously understaffed, forcing us to fill prescriptions at lightning speed.

Here are some scenarios that aren't too difficult to imagine in which we will be sued at some point in the not-too-distant future. Pharmacists would love to be able to spend the time with each customer that would allow us to prevent every possible adverse consequence. Unfortunately, the chains don't see things the same way that we do.

The following questions are directed at pharmacists:

1. Can you see yourself being sued for failure to warn a customer and call his or her doctor and emphasize that using albuterol asthma inhaler too often means asthma is out of control? If such a customer were to end up in emergency room, can you see yourself being sued for not notifying the doctor and/or not adequately stressing to the customer the significance of overuse of this inhaler.

2. Can you see yourself being sued for failure to notify all the doctors who prescribe pain medications that their patient is becoming addicted? Every pharmacist has many customers who appear to be addicted to pain pills. Will some lawyer say that you have a duty to discuss each of these customers in detail with all the doctors who prescribe these pain pills, even when the patient utilizes many doctors to get access to these drugs?

3. Can you see yourself being sued for filling prescriptions with potentially interacting drugs even though you call the prescribing doctor and he says to go ahead and fill them? Here's an instance a neighbor told me about. A doctor prescribed Zocor 80 mg daily, gemfibrozil 600 mg daily, niacin 1000 mg daily, and Zetia 10 mg daily. The *Physicians' Desk Reference* says to use no more than 10 mg of Zocor daily in patients receiving gemfibrozil. It also says that niacin doses of 1000 mg or more increase the risk of muscle damage and that Zetia is not recommended with gemfibrozil. When I showed my neighbor these warnings in the *PDR*, he asked his doctor if there's anything to be concerned about. I was told that the doctor replied, "You've had two heart attacks. We're treating you aggressively." If this patient were your customer and he developed rhabdomyolysis (a serious muscle disorder), would he sue you for continuing to fill these prescriptions?

4. Can you see yourself being sued for filling prednisone prescriptions in the following scenario: A customer with rheumatoid arthritis develops osteoporosis and needs a hip replacement as a result of long term use of prednisone. Will some aggressive lawyer say you should have refused to fill these prescriptions and/or called the doctor to express your concern?

5. Can you see yourself being sued for failure to ask every customer every time for an update on all the over-the-counter medications they're taking so that you can enter that information into your computer in order to screen for possible interactions (like serotonin syndrome from the combination of Robitussin DM and Paxil)?

6. Can you see yourself being sued by a customer with rheumatoid arthritis who develops lymphoma from long-term use of methotrexate? Will some lawyer say you were negligent for continuing to fill methotrexate prescriptions long term, in view of the fact that the link to lymphoma is part of the black box warnings in the labeling?

When we call a doctor about a drug interaction and he tells us to go ahead and fill the prescription, do we need to second-guess the doctor and refuse to fill the prescription? If the customer suffers adverse consequences from the drug interaction, lawyers will say that we as pharmacists should indeed have second guessed the doctor and refused to fill the prescription. In any large statistical sample, some people will experience adverse consequences from a drug interaction, others will not. In my opinion, it should be the doctor's responsibility to make the final decision regarding potential drug interactions, not the pharmacist's.

Legal experts tell us that we need to give our customers what seems like an ever-increasing volume of information. We are told that our medication leaflets need to be the most detailed ones available anywhere. With an oversupply of lawyers in America, pharmacists can count on being sued more often for failure to list less common or rare side effects in our leaflets or for failure to verbally warn customers about these side effects. When customers experience uncommon adverse consequences, pharmacists are being sued for providing lists containing only the most common side effects.

Two separate lawsuits against pharmacists are based on the failure to warn about the risk of priapism (an abnormally persistent erection) from two different drugs: Desyrel and Caverject. In the first case, the patient (who had an erection lasting over four hours after taking the anti-depressant Desyrel), sued the pharmacy, claiming that the pharmacist should have told him about this risk. He literally claimed that the pharmacist had a legal duty to tell patients of risks foreseeable to health care practitioners when ordinary people would not know enough about a drug to know which questions to ask. In this case, the Court of Appeals held that the pharmacist could not be held liable under the circumstances.

In the case involving the erectile dysfunction drug Caverject, the patient injected the medication into his penis as directed, and suffered a severely painful erection that lasted almost 72 hours. On June 3, 2002, the patient underwent surgery to reduce the erection. As a result of the incident, the patient was diagnosed with priapism, resulting in permanent and non-reversible impotence. The patient argued that the law should impose a duty on pharmacists to warn of foreseeable risks known to be associated with the use of particular drugs, and that the failure to do so renders the prescription as not properly dispensed. The court decided that, if the legislature wanted to require pharmacists to warn customers of the side effects associated with prescription drugs, it would have done so by statute.

In commenting on these two cases, pharmacist-lawyer Jesse Vivian, B.S. Pharm., J.D., a professor in the Dept. of Pharmacy Practice at Wayne State University, says that we should "not take this as a free and clear message that pharmacists are legally immune from civil liability for failing to warn about known adverse effects associated with the use of a particular drug. ...there are, in fact, several courts that have come to the opposite conclusion of the judges involved in this case. ...While both of these cases were correctly decided under prevailing laws—especially considering the lack of any discernible legislative intent to the contrary—it is not hard to imagine that sometime in the near future, the courts are going to take judicial notice that the practice of pharmacy is moving away from a strict dispensing of a product model and into an information management model. In this context, courts may well impose new and greater expectations in the context of liability when things happen that could have been easily avoided with just a bit of counseling." (Jesse Vivian, "Legislative Intent, *U.S. Pharmacist*, Nov. 2005, pp. 92-97)

A Texas lawsuit involved a pharmacist's failure to warn about a very uncommon adverse reaction in the death of a 14-year old Austin boy. The lawsuit charged that the pharmacist failed to warn about potential adverse reactions from desipramine. After taking the antidepressant for two years, he developed a chronic allergic reaction to the medication. The suit contended that the pharmacist failed to warn the boy's mother. An expert witness for the dead child's family testified that the pharmacist had a duty to tell the mother more than just that the drug could cause dry mouth or constipation. On appeal, the court ruled for the pharmacist after finding that the adverse reaction was a rare side effect of the medication. (*Drug Topics*, April 19, 1999, p. 43 and *Drug Topics*, Sept. 18, 2000, p. 38)

Nothing makes me angrier than pharmacy "experts" (often a hired-gun pharmacy professor) who testify in lawsuits that pharmacists have a duty to warn the customer about an ever-increasing list of possible adverse consequences. These "experts" are not living in the real world. They are being paid 200 or 300 dollars per hour to testify that pharmacists have a duty to warn. I doubt seriously that these professors would provide more counseling than average when faced with the overwhelming workload that is typical of many drugstores across this country. I'd like to put my pharmacy professors and heads of boards of pharmacy in a high volume store and see how well they counsel customers. I'd like to see them thoroughly counsel every customer without having a dozen misfills and lines all the way to the parking lot. I'd like to see how well these "experts" tell every customer about every conceivable consequence of every medication. I'd like to see how long chain management tolerates that.

I bet that most pharmacists are more exhausted after a day's work than heads of boards of pharmacy or pharmacy professors. One pharmacist told me that she goes home each day after her shift and sits in a dark room just to decompress. I wonder how many board members and professors do likewise. I wonder how many heads of boards and professors don't have time to eat or go to the bathroom.

If we are forced to defend ourselves in a court case in which a customer is harmed as a result of some drug therapy, we would, of course, like to make the critical point that we'd absolutely love to have the time to tell customers everything they could possibly need to know about the drugs their doctor has prescribed. But lawyers will ask us, "Why have you agreed to work for an employer that does not allow you time to counsel customers? Are you being forced to work for that employer? If you feel that conditions with that employer are dangerous, you have a duty to quit and to report your employer to the board of pharmacy." We reply "But working conditions with all the big chains are becoming absurd everywhere. If we report our chain to the board of pharmacy, we fear that our bosses will make life so miserable for us that we will end up quitting. The board of pharmacy will send an inspector to investigate our store only."

Pharmacy school professors seem to think the environment in the drugstore is as relaxed as that at pharmacy school, and that pharmacists have the time to sit down with each customer for a leisurely conversation, sharing several cups of coffee, maybe a Danish. The professors seem to think we've got an hour to discuss with each customer their entire medical history and every possible adverse drug effect. The reality is that pharmacists too often have time for only one or two short sentences with customers.

Pharmacy school professors don't seem to realize that most customers simply want to get their prescriptions filled as quickly as possible so they can get out of the drugstore and go home or go to work or to the supermarket. Pharmacy school professors don't seem to realize that many customers don't want a lot of information about their drugs. We know that many customers throw away the drug leaflets we give them without reading a single word. Some customers tell us that they don't want to learn about the drug their doctor has prescribed because they wouldn't want to take the medication after reading all the possible side effects. I have found that nearly 100% of people who look up their drug in the *Physicians' Desk Reference* (at a library or bookstore) become less enthusiastic about taking that drug after they see the list of potential side effects. The list in the *PDR* is usually far more comprehensive than the list we provide our customers in our leaflets.

Our pharmacy professors say they are not expecting us to practice medicine, but that is exactly what they are expecting us to do. When we are responsible for second-guessing every prescription the doctor writes, we are indeed practicing medicine. The individual pharmacist is being forced to play a role that should be played by state medical licensing boards and physician continuing education. Pharmacists don't have the time to second-guess every prescription decision made by every doctor. It seems that, because of OBRA, lawyers are, in fact, expecting us to practice medicine.

I am continually amazed by the huge disconnect between pharmacy school professors and the real world. It is as if the pharmacy school professors have no clue what it's like in the real world, or else they have a tremendous disincentive to acknowledge the real world. Many pharmacists say that pharmacy school professors embraced the counseling requirement to increase the visibility and importance of professors and to justify the requirement that all graduating pharmacists now have a doctorate, known as a

Pharm.D. degree. Many pharmacists feel the requirement for a doctorate as the entry level degree was a power grab by the schools of pharmacy.

Do professors realize the absurdity of pharmacy schools producing drug experts in an environment in which the big chains don't want drug experts? The big chains want pharmacists who can dispense at lightning speed. The big chains are dripping with disdain for pharmacists who spend too much time counseling customers. The pharmacy professors are loath to acknowledge the fact that the real world is the opposite of pharmacy school.

The state boards of pharmacy are the governmental regulatory entities that have the responsibility to protect the public safety. So why don't the boards step in and require working conditions that are conducive to the safe filling of prescriptions? In my opinion, the boards of pharmacy have as much backbone as a banana. The state boards of pharmacy appear to be strongly intimidated by the legal and political clout of the big chains. Consequently, the state boards take the wimpish approach of targeting individual stores and individual pharmacists as a result of complaints from the public, rather than targeting the chain drugstore industry as a whole for operating stores in a manner that makes errors inevitable.

I once spoke with the head of one state board of pharmacy. I asked him why the board of pharmacy doesn't do something about pharmacists' working conditions. He told me that if I knew a specific store that had dangerous working conditions, the board would investigate that store. I told him that this misses the point. It is not fair to investigate individual stores because pharmacists' employers (i.e., chain management) would be extremely unhappy if they found out we had reported them to the board of pharmacy. I told him that the board of pharmacy needs to investigate the big chains as a whole. This head of the state board of pharmacy told me that his worst days are when he has to fight the corporate lawyers from the big chains.

Here are two e-mails I received from pharmacists as a result of my editorial in *Drug Topics* titled "Counseling in the real world." (December 8, 2003, pp. 24, 26)

Subj: Counseling in the real world
Date: 1/31/04
From: [Pharmacist M. K.]
To: dmiller1952@aol.com

I just finished reading your "Counseling in the real world" article and I'm really glad someone is finally speaking out. I'm a third year pharmacy student at USC and I'm already feeling very frustrated. This is definitely a catch 22 situation and pharmacists really need to get some support from our employers and the pharmacy boards. I work at Kaiser Permanente and it is an extremely busy place w/the long lines, phones ringing off the hook, etc. Already as an intern I feel I'm being pulled 10 different ways. So I am dreading getting my license and having to worry about the liability.

In school they teach us counseling and, as you said, the professors preach on about the amount of stuff that we must convey to the patient, not realizing that there is just no time. The pharmacy resident who facilitates my discussion group told us that when we counsel patients on their hypertension meds, we must discuss lifestyle changes as well. That discussion should include a detailed exercise regimen like how often they should get on a treadmill, for how long, and at what speed. Isn't that insane? Not only is there not time for that in the outpatient, retail setting, but we do not get trained here at USC on things like physical fitness. I don't even know how long I should be on the treadmill. We also don't get the opportunity to review the patient's chart in an outpatient setting so there's no way we could even comment on that aspect of things (at a hypertension clinic, yes; at the 24 hour outpatient pharmacy, no).

It's so funny that you are comparing pharmacy to fast food. Maybe I'm a little out of the loop here, and maybe this comparison has been made by others but I haven't heard it yet. I thought I was the only one who saw such a similarity between the two. Last week, I went inside the local In & Out (do you have that in Florida?). It was the first time I had been in a fast food joint in a long time. While I was waiting for my order, I watched the workers do their thing and I started to get a bit of anxiety, as it seemed all too familiar, despite the fact that I had never ever worked fast-food before. And then of course it hit me. It reminds me of work at the pharmacy. The fast pace, the long lines, the hierarchy, the audience watching and waiting for their order, the drive through!!! I went home and told my mom that I'm nothing but a glorified fast food clerk. Sometimes I'm even the cook. We do compounding at our pharmacy and the standards we use really suck, just like at a fast food place.

You are so right about the fast food model and I'm so glad someone with your experience and background sees it that way too. I thought I was going nuts. I feel better now. Thank you so much for sharing your insight with the rest of us.

My point is that I completely agree w/everything you said. Professors preach and employers are all about the bottom line. We are getting the short end of the stick here and something has to be done about it. Once again, thank you for speaking up. You said it perfectly. I'm going to send a couple of my profs the link in case they haven't already seen it yet.

Sincerely,
[Pharmacist M. K.]

Subj: Re: Counseling in the real world
Date: 12/31/03
From: [Pharmacist S. T.]
To: Dmiller1952

Thank you for your editorial in *Drug Topics*. You are so right about everything! I just don't understand why pharmacists don't come together and do something about it. In my state, pharmacists are not required to counsel every single patient. However, I still try to counsel patients because it's my duty to counsel as a pharmacist. Unfortunately, after we moved to a new pharmacy, with a drive through, and after the budget cut, I hardly have any time to counsel anymore. Instead, I write down all the important information on the labels and have my tech inform the patients. That's wrong and I know it! But, that's the only way for me to convey my messages to the patients because I am the only pharmacist on duty with only 2 hours of overlap every day. Sometimes things get so hectic that I just want to walk out and quit. I didn't go to school to learn how to fill and verify as fast as I can. Anyway, I do make sure I counsel patients, personally, if they just get out of surgery, or ER, or if they have more than 4-5 prescriptions. I do take the time to make sure they know what they are taking. But you are right, some of the patients don't even want to listen to us. All they want is to get their medications and get out of the pharmacy as quickly as possible! They think we are McDonald's or Burger Kings. Patients need to be educated!

It's very frustrating to be a pharmacist anymore. No lunch, no breaks, and not enough tech help. All we ever hear from our supervisors is the KPI's (don't even know what it stands for anymore). We get graded for things we do such as how fast the scripts go from one station to another station. If we get a D or and F, we get lectured. We always get yelled at about the phone hold time. Don't they see that there is a problem with the pharmacy if we consistently get D's and F's? KPI's should be used as a tool to tell them whether we need more help or not. Well, first of all, there are only 2 people in the pharmacy and there is only so much we can do. We have to fill scripts, ring customers up in the out-window and the drive through. We have to answer questions from customers, we have to get doctor's calls, and we have to check voice mails, etc.! I think it's absurd to grade us on how fast we can fill a script because that's not the only thing I do. I am probably telling you things that you already know. I guess I am just venting. I cried twice last week because of the workload and not enough tech help. Every day I come home, I am so exhausted that I don't even want to do anything else. Most of the time, I just doze off on the couch after work.

I'm sorry for bothering you, but thanks for letting me vent my frustration. My job is eating me alive!

Thank you.
[Pharmacist S. T.]
P.S. I hope I didn't get myself into trouble by whining too much. :)
Thanks for reading.

71

Some of my favorite pharmacy pictures demonstrating the meticulous work done by pharmacists and technicians

The next few pages consist of some of my favorite pharmacy pictures which don't seem to fit well in other parts of the book. These pictures, gathered from the Internet, show pharmacists and technicians in mostly real-life situations. I hope these pictures give a sense of what it looks like in the real world behind the pharmacy counter. I do not know any of these people and I don't know anything about them. As I stated in the front of this book, the pictures in this book are for demonstration purposes only. My inclusion of these images in an exposé of chain drugstores should NOT in any way suggest or imply that the people depicted do anything less than exemplary work. In this book I am trying to describe how meticulous and exacting the work done by pharmacists and technicians is. I like these pictures because they show pharmacists and technicians who seem to have a focused look on their faces. Pharmacists and technicians are expected to be one hundred percent accurate. Even though that is an impossibility, it is my hope that these pictures give an idea of the extremely serious work that pharmacists and technicians do, and the potentially disastrous consequences when customers rush the pharmacy staff.

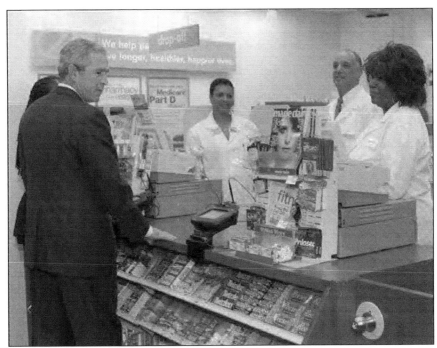

President Bush at CVS

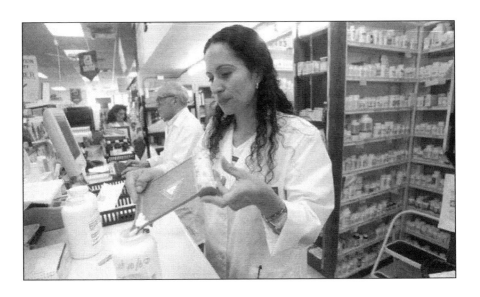

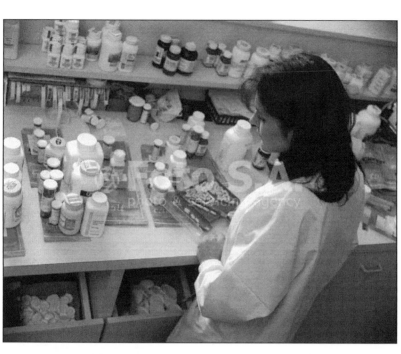

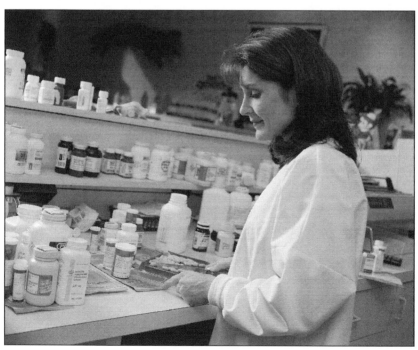

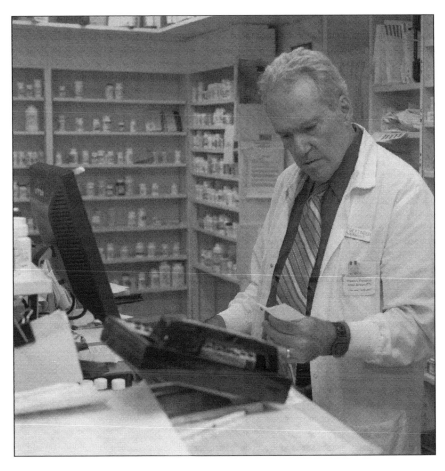

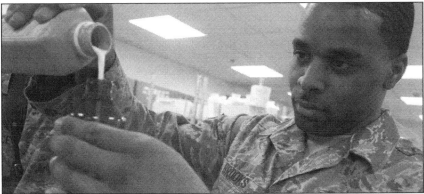

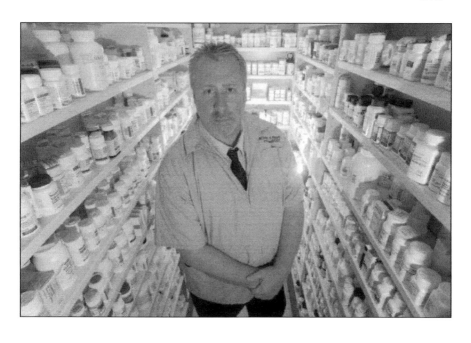

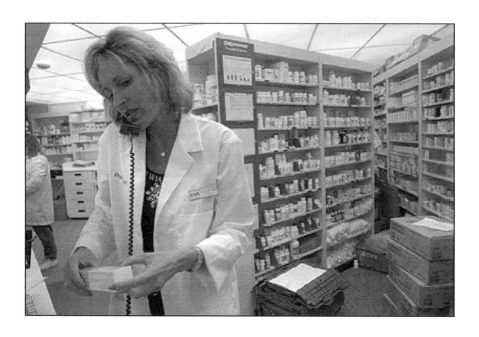

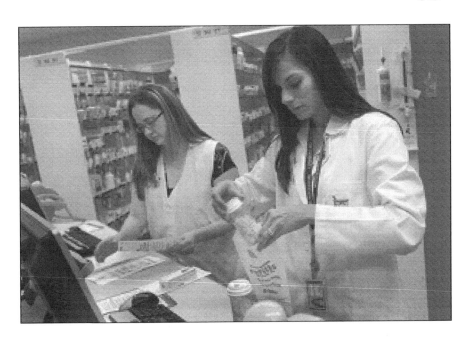

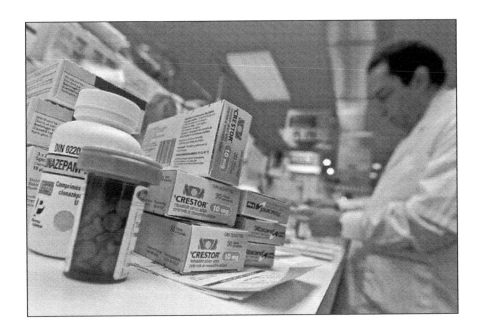

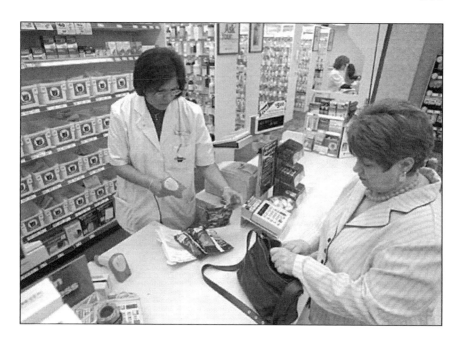

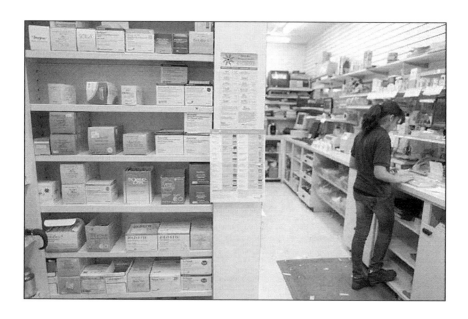

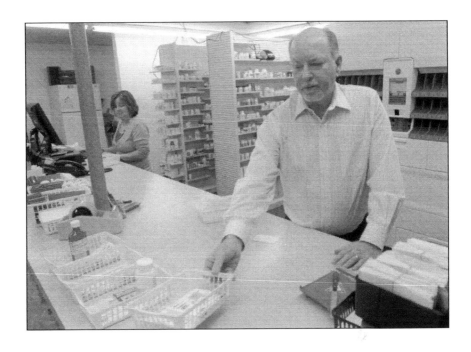

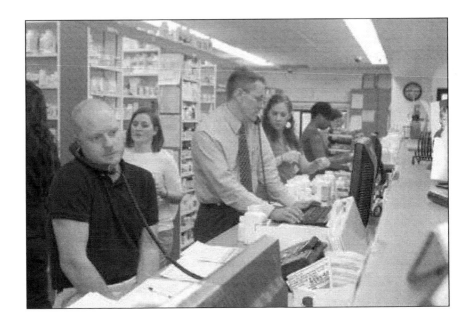

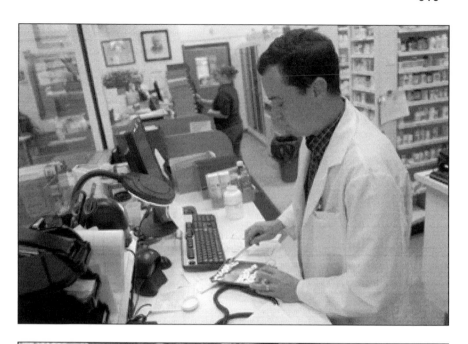

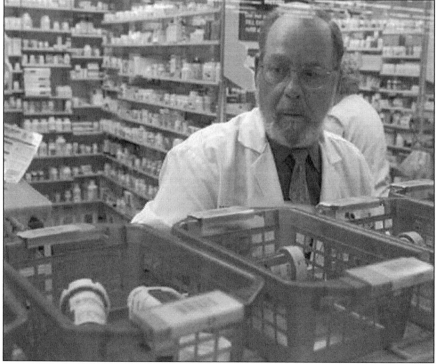

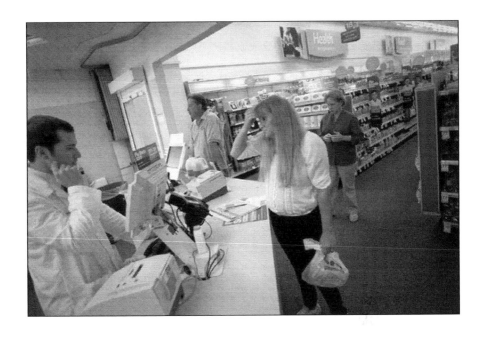

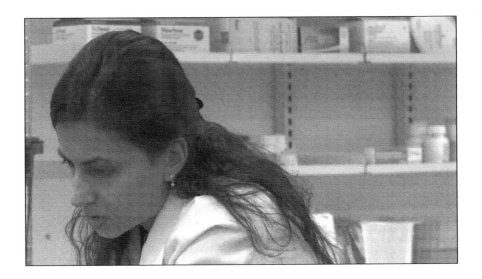

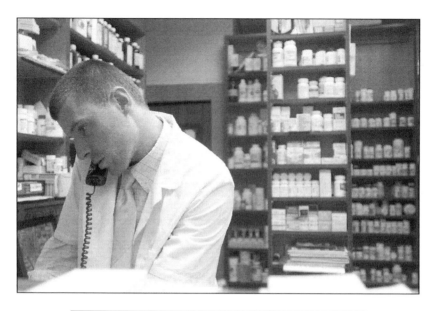

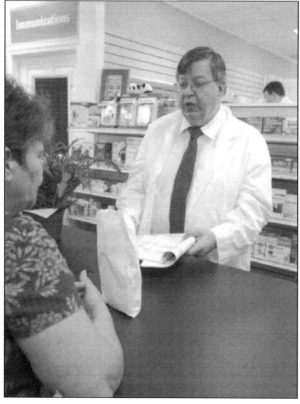

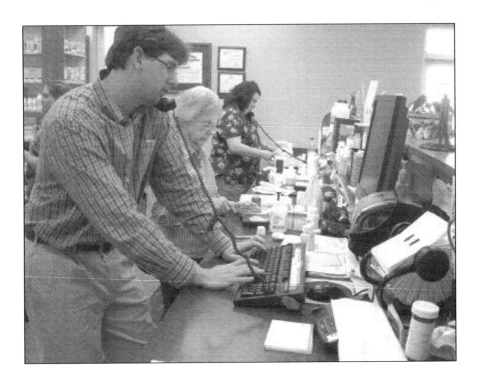

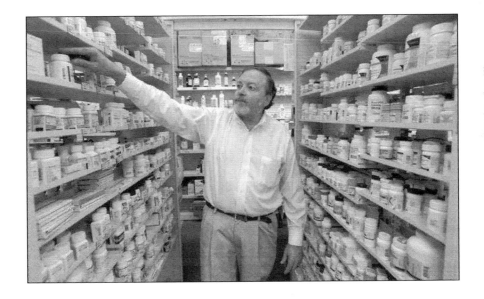

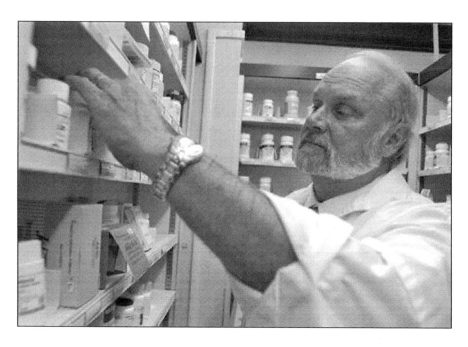

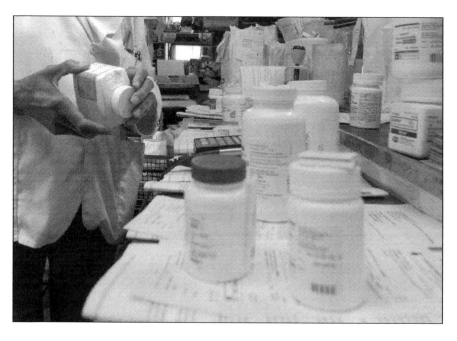

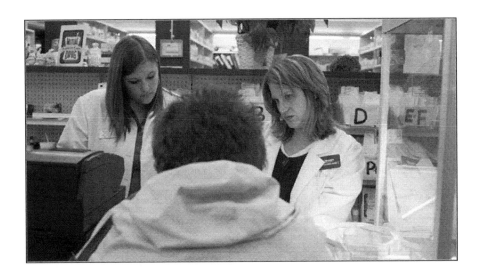

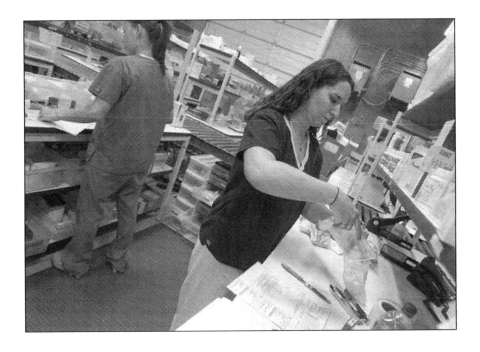

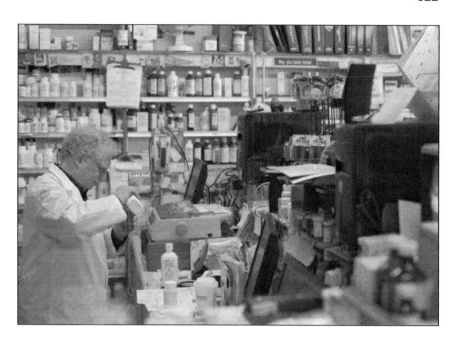

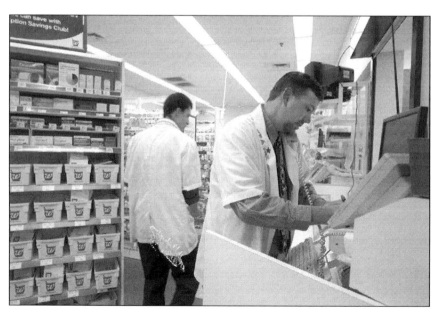

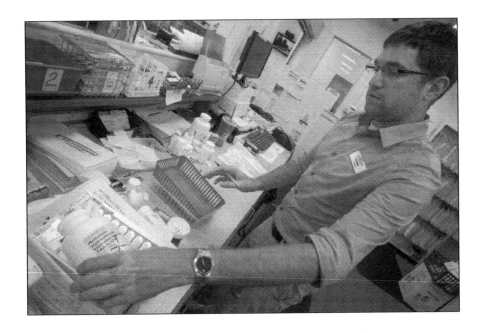

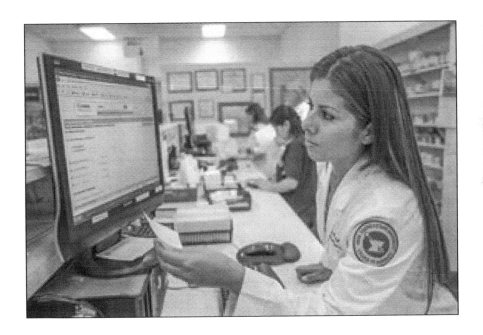

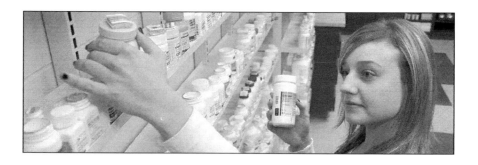

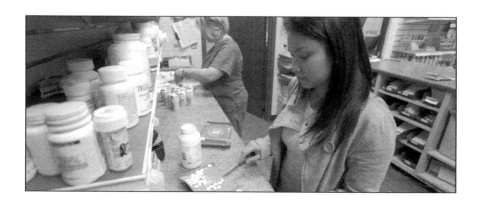

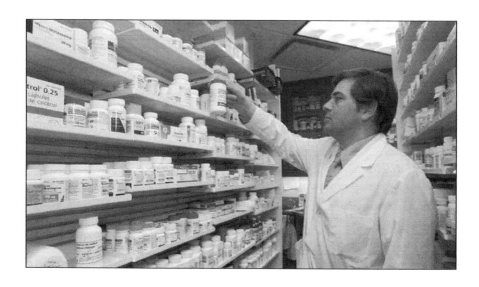

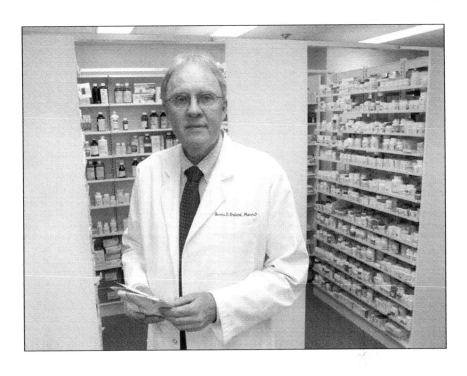

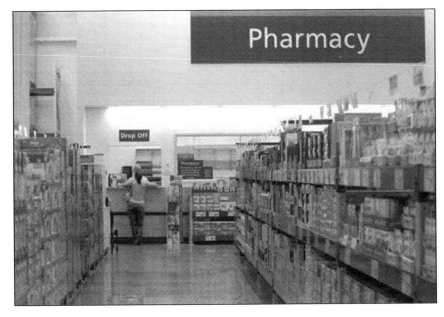

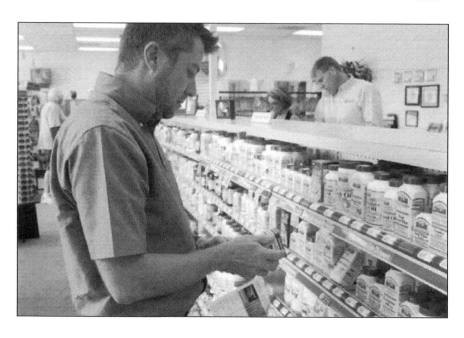

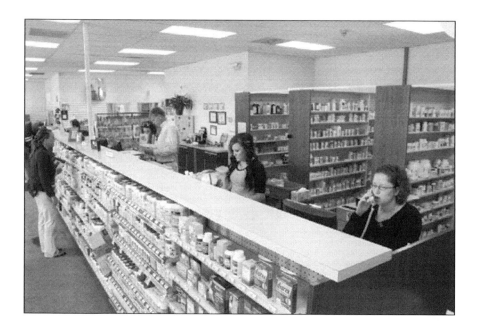

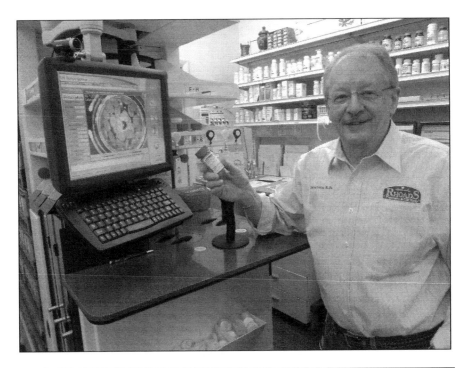

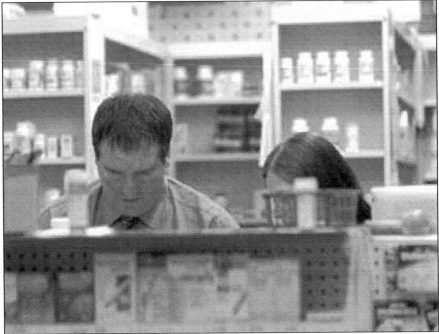

ABOUT THE AUTHOR

The author graduated from West Virginia University School of Pharmacy in 1975. Over the next twenty-five years, he worked for three of the largest drugstore chains in America. He worked as a pharmacist in West Virginia (primarily in Charleston, Huntington, and Summersville) and in North Carolina (primarily in Raleigh, Durham, Chapel Hill, Burlington, Oxford, and Henderson). He has worked as a staff pharmacist and as pharmacist-in-charge. He was the manager of the entire store several years ago in Burlington, North Carolina when the Revco chain had pharmacist store managers.

The author has spent the last several years researching and writing this book and writing articles/editorials for major national pharmacy magazines. He has written a total of eighteen editorials for *Drug Topics*. He has also written two articles for *American Druggist* which were subsequently reprinted in the physicians' newsmagazine *Medical Tribune*. He wrote a 25-page chapter on pharmacy errors for a book published in 2005 for lawyers and judges (*Drug Injury: Liability, Analysis, and Prevention*, Phoenix, Arizona: Lawyers and Judges Publishing Company). He was a major source for an article on pharmacy errors in the June 2005 issue of *Good Housekeeping*. Several of the author's editorials are available on the *Drug Topics* website (drugtopics.com) by entering "Dennis Miller" in the search field.

The author welcomes comments, suggestions, and corrections at dmiller1952@aol.com.

The author is not related to another pharmacist named Dennis Miller who wrote a book on manic depression.

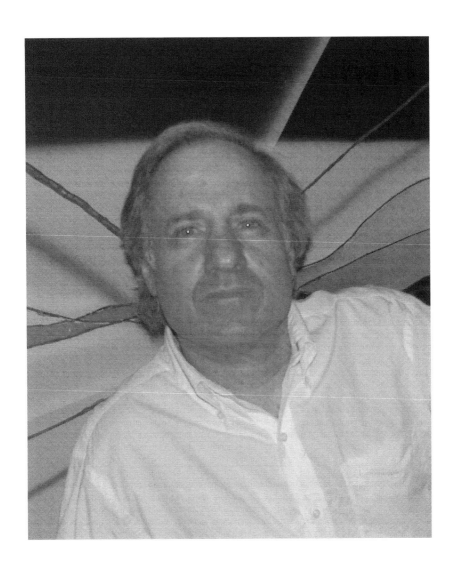

Made in the USA
Lexington, KY
22 May 2014